Difficult Clinical Problems in Psychiatry

Difficult Clinical Problems in Psychiatry

Edited by

Malcolm Lader OBE, DSc, PhD, MD, FRCPsych.
Head, Section of Clinical Psychopharmacology (MRC)
Professor of Clinical Psychopharmacology
Institute of Psychiatry
De Crespigny Park
London SE5 8AF, and
The Maudsley
London SE5 8AZ, UK

Dieter Naber MD, DSC
Professor of Psychiatry
Director, Department of Psychiatry
University Hospital Hamburg
Universitäts-Krankenhaus Eppendorf
D-20246 Hamburg
Germany

Martin Dunitz

© Martin Dunitz Ltd 1999

First published in the United Kingdom in 1999 by
Martin Dunitz Ltd
The Livery House
7–9 Pratt Street
London NW1 0AE
Tel   +44 (0)20 7482 2202
Fax   +44 (0)20 7567 0159
Email   info.dunitz@tandf.co.uk
Website   http://www.dunitz.co.uk

Reprinted 2001

Distributed in the United States by:
Blackwell Science Inc.
Commerce Place, 350 Main Street
Malden, MA 02148, USA
Tel: 1-800-215-1000

Distributed in Canada by:
Login Brothers Book Company
324 Salteaux Crescent
Winnipeg, Manitoba, R3J 3T2
Canada
Tel: 1-204-224-4068

Distributed in Brazil by:
Ernesto Reichmann Distribuidora de Livros, Ltda
Rua Coronel Marques 335, Tatuape 03440-000
Sao Paulo
Brazil

A CIP catalogue record for this book is available from the British Library.

ISBN 1–85317–550–1

Composition by Wearset, Boldon, Tyne and Wear
Printed and bound in Great Britain by Biddles Ltd,
Guildford & King's Lynn

Contents

Contributors   vii

Introduction – Difficult clinical problems   1

1   Refractory schizophrenia   3
Dieter Naber, Michael Krausz, Martin Lambert and Stefan Bender

2   Treatment of tardive dyskinesia   23
Stephen R Marder

3   Unstable manic-depressives   37
Michael Bauer

4   Treatment-resistant unipolar depression   57
Graham D Burrows and Trevor R Norman

5   Treatment of the difficult panic patient   77
Antoine Pélissolo and Jean-Pierre Lépine

6   Treatment of the difficult obsessive–compulsive disorder patient   97
Dan J Stein and Robin A Emsley

7   Anorexia nervosa   109
Janet Treasure

8   Treatment of chronic fatigue syndrome   135
Trudie Chalder, Alicia Deale and Simon Wessely

9   The psychopharmacological treatment of substance abuse (including alcoholism)   155
Michael Soyka

10   Behavioural disturbances in old age   181
Franz Müller-Spahn and Christoph Hock

11   The violent patient in the community   199
Siegfried Kasper

12   The hyperactive child   213
Peter Hill

13   Ways of improving compliance   229
Martina Hummer and W Wolfgang Fleischhacker

Index   239

Contributors

Michael Bauer
Neuropsychiatric Institute and
Hospital, Department of Psychiatry
and Biobehavioral Sciences, UCLA
Medical School, Los Angeles,
CA 90095, USA

Stefan Bender
Department of Psychiatry, University
Hospital, Essen, Germany

Graham D Burrows
Professor, Department of Psychiatry,
University of Melbourne, Austin and
Repatriation Medical Centre,
Heidelberg 3084, Victoria, Australia

Trudie Chalder
Academic Department of Psychological
Medicine, Guy's, King's and St Thomas'
School of Medicine and the Institute of
Psychiatry, London SE5 8AZ, UK

Alicia Deale
Academic Department of Psychological
Medicine, Guy's, King's and St Thomas'
School of Medicine and the Institute of
Psychiatry, London SE5 8AZ, UK

Robin A Emsley
Professor and Chairman, Department
of Psychiatry, University of
Stellenbosch, P.O. Box 19063,
Tygerberg 7505, South Africa

W Wolfgang Fleischhacker
Professor, Department of Biological
Psychiatry, University of Innsbruck,
A-6020 Innsbruck, Austria

Peter Hill
Professor, Great Ormond Street
Hospital for Children, London
WC1N 3JH, UK

Christoph Hock
Consultant Psychiatrist, Department of
Psychiatry, University of Basel, CH-4025
Basel, Switzerland

Martina Hummer
Department of Biological Psychiatry,
University of Innsbruck, A-6020
Innsbruck, Austria

Siegfried Kasper
Professor and Chairman, Department
of General Psychiatry, University of
Vienna, A-1090 Vienna, Austria

Michael Krausz
Professor, Department of Psychiatry,
University Hospital, Hamburg,
Germany

Martin Lambert
Department of Psychiatry, University
Hospital, Hamburg, Germany

Jean-Pierre Lépine
Professor of Psychiatry, Department of
Psychiatry, Hôpital Lariboisière
Fernand Widal, Assistance Publique
Hôpitaux de Paris, F-75475 Paris
Cedex, France

Stephen R Marder
Psychiatry Department, West Los
Angeles Veterans' Affairs Medical
Center, and Professor, Department of
Psychiatry and Biobehavioral
Sciences, UCLA School of Medicine,
Los Angeles, California, USA

Franz Müller-Spahn
Professor, Department of Psychiatry,
University of Basel, CH-4025 Basel,
Switzerland

Dieter Naber
Professor of Psychiatry, Director,
Department of Psychiatry, University
Hospital Hamburg, Universitäts-
Krankenhaus Eppendorf, D-20246
Hamburg, Germany

Trevor R Norman
Associate Professor, Department of
Psychiatry, University of Melbourne,
Austin and Repatriation Medical
Centre, Heidelberg 3084, Victoria,
Australia

Antoine Pélissolo
Department of Psychiatry, Hôpital
Lariboisière Fernand Widal,
Assistance Publique Hôpitaux de
Paris, F-75475 Paris Cedex, France

Michael Soyka
Senior Psychiatrist, Psychiatric
Hospital, University of Munich,
D-80333 Munich, Germany

Dan J Stein
Director, MRC Research Unit on
Anxiety Disorders, Department of
Psychiatry, University of Stellenbosch,
P.O. Box 19063, Tygerberg 7505,
South Africa

Janet Treasure
Consultant Psychiatrist, Eating
Disorders Outpatient Unit, The
Maudsley, London SE5 8AZ, and
Senior Lecturer, Institute of Psychiatry,
London SE5 8AZ, UK

Simon Wessely
Academic Department of Psychological
Medicine, Guy's, King's and St Thomas'
School of Medicine and the Institute of
Psychiatry, London SE5 8AZ, UK

Introduction – Difficult clinical problems

Although it appears that the classification and description of psychiatric conditions have made major strides in the last few decades as witnessed by the DSM and ICD systems, these categories may not be helpful in actual day-to-day practice. Indeed, there has been a proliferation of diagnostic categories; for example, the DSM system has multiplied enormously in over 30 years. Are these really all separate conditions, are we making false distinctions, or are they just symptom clusters that are too closely related to be separated out clearly? That we are not sure about this is reflected in the dispute over hierarchical models versus coexisting pathology models. In other words, the complex conditions we see may contain symptom patterns within an overall disorder but they may represent the common co-occurrence of various disorders. Indeed, some people have suggested that a dimensional approach is more profitable but no one agrees as to which should be the major dimensions. The therapeutic relevance of some psychiatric diagnoses is limited – psychopharmacological treatment is particularly syndrome orientated and not yet specified according to disorders or diagnostic entities.

Another problem is comorbidity, which may reflect the inchoate nature of our classificatory schemes, but increasingly it is a result of genuine multiple diagnoses. The most notorious example is perhaps the increasing complication of alcohol and substance abuse in our patients, particularly younger patients. This complicates the diagnosis but even more so the treatment and prognosis. In the move to evidence-based medicine, we are all often hard put to justify our treatments in a single disorder, let alone in multiple disorders, where very few studies have actually been carried out.

The change in emphasis of treatment has often suggested an unreal high degree of specificity, for example, benzodiazepines for anxiety, tricyclic antidepressants for depression and antipsychotic drugs for schizophrenia. The advent of new drugs which are more selective has still not resulted in any more specific treatments. Indeed, if anything, some of these drugs used in depression, such as the specific serotonin reuptake inhibitors, are used in other conditions such as panic disorder, obsessive–compulsive disorder and social phobia. Mood regulators including lithium are also being supplemented by anticonvulsants such as carbamazepine and valproate. Clozapine is effective in a useful pro-portion of schizophrenic patients who are otherwise treatment resistant, but also seems effective in mania and other psychotic depression indications.

What seems immutable about treatment problems is the constant proportion of patients who respond. In condition after condition and treatment after treatment around 70% of patients show a worthwhile response to the first treatment. They therefore do not present management difficulties. However, the substantial minority, namely 30% or so, who are left are problematic to treat and this is particularly the province of the psychiatrist. There are also nonspecific features, such as lack of insight leading to poor compliance for unwanted effects, giving the same end result.

Because of all these factors we thought it opportune to gather together a series of clinically relevant topics which, we believe, often present problems to the practising psychiatrist, and to ask international experts in each of these areas to provide us with their solutions. We are well aware that sometimes these opinions have to be based on uncontrolled clinical impressions, but nevertheless some treatment paradigms can provide a useful guideline for the generalist psychiatrist. We are delighted that so many people answered our invitation to provide chapters and we believe that these contributors have produced a book of uniformly high quality. The topics selected cover a wide field and we are well aware that there may be other topics that could well have been included but for reasons of space had to be excluded.

We are particularly grateful to Ruth and Martin Dunitz, our publishers, for supporting this venture and for their constant encouragement and help during the planning and execution of this project. We are also grateful to the numerous contributors who gave their time to provide us with these expert chapters. We hope our readers will find this book of continuing help in their clinical practices.

1
Refractory schizophrenia

Dieter Naber, Michael Krausz, Martin Lambert and Stefan
Bender

Definition

The benefit of neuroleptic drugs in the treatment of schizophrenic
patients is beyond doubt: numerous double-blind studies have documented their efficacy in acute or chronic psychotic patients and in the
prophylaxis of relapse. Despite these advances in the treatment of
schizophrenia, all studies since the introduction of the first neuroleptic
drugs have identified a subgroup of patients who are either partially or
totally unresponsive to therapy. Studies into therapy resistance or refractory schizophrenia face two major problems: first, the difficulties of definition, and secondly, differentiation from chronicity. For many years,
refractory schizophrenia was often defined according to chronicity or the
frequency of hospitalization.[1–3] However, there is no doubt that the
chronicity of schizophrenic illness is not restricted to severe psychopathology.[4] Therapy resistance is, in the main, defined by a minimal
severity of psychopathology and, particularly, by continuous positive
symptoms.[5] Since the chronicity of schizophrenia is influenced by many
nonpharmacological variables (such as inadequate psychosocial treatment or aggressive behaviour[6]), it might be concluded that chronicity *per
se* is not a valid predictor for neuroleptic nonresponse.[7] The problem
when considering chronicity as a major condition of refractory schizophrenia is exemplified by studies on risperidone. In an investigation by
Marder and Meibach, risperidone was found to be superior to haloperidol
in reducing positive symptoms in patients hospitalized for more than 6
months.[8] The authors concluded that risperidone might have a special
effect in therapy-resistant patients. However, other authors do not support this assumption.[9–11] Altman, cited by Buckley et al.,[12] found that 40%
of patients who did not improve with risperidone showed a marked
reduction of psychopathology with a subsequent treatment with clozapine. However, only 15% of clozapine nonresponders improved under
risperidone treatment. Similar data were found by Pajonk et al., who also
concluded that risperidone is less effective than clozapine in the treatment of therapy-resistant patients.[13]

Various definitions of the criteria for treatment-resistant schizophrenia have been proposed. An international study group[6] pursued three objectives: clarify the concept; suggest criteria for defining or rating the degree of treatment refractoriness; and explore the role of psychosocial and drug therapies in increasing the responsiveness of the treatment-refractory patient. They recommended a multidimensional definition since the construct of treatment refractoriness is complicated, and various areas, such as psychopathology (continuing positive and/or negative symptoms), substantial functional disability and behavioural deviance, have to be considered. It is not a categorical but a dimensional approach that is suggested by their rating scale. Similar (but using six different levels instead of seven) are the 'degrees of therapy resistance' (see Table 1.1) proposed by May et al.[14]

The parameters necessary for trials of different neuroleptic drugs, dosage and duration of treatment have often been discussed during the last years and decades. Most of the criteria in the definition of therapy resistance were developed by Kane and co-workers:[15]

1) Persistence of positive psychotic symptoms in at least two out of four items of the Brief Psychiatric Rating Scale (BPRS) positive scale with a score of $\geqslant 4$;

2) A BPRS total score of $\geqslant 45$ and a Clinical Global Impression (CGI) score of $\geqslant 4$;

3) Persistence of the illness without any period of good social or vocational functioning during the last 5 years; and

4) At least three unsuccessful trials with conventional neuroleptics conducted during the last 5 years.

The neuroleptic drugs should represent two different chemical groups, each with a dosage $\geqslant 1000$ mg chlorpromazine equivalence, administered for 6 weeks without a reduction of at least 20% of the BPRS total score. At least one trial with haloperidol (10–60 mg/day for at least 6 weeks) should have been tried, and discontinued because of inefficiency or intolerability. These criteria used in the definition of therapy resistance include the severity and persistence of positive symptoms despite an adequate neuroleptic treatment, and they were used to find that clozapine is effective in these patients.[15]

The fourth criterion for treatment resistance (three drug trials) has since been modified because several studies have shown that only 3–7% of schizophrenic patients benefit from a third trial with conventional neuroleptics.[16] Therefore, failing two drug trials is now generally accepted as a criterion for treatment resistance,[17] and most authors recommend a switch to an atypical neuroleptic after only one unsuccessful trial with a typical one. The dosages and the treatment duration to define an

Table 1.1   Degrees of resistance proposed by May et al.[14]

Level 1	Excellent responders	Total remission within 1 week, whatever treatment is given
Level 2	Very good responders	Good response within 1 month when antipsychotic medication is given in standard dosages
		'Clinical remission': patients can return to the same social situation as before the illness with little, if any, residual scarring
Level 3	Good responders	Major reduction of symptoms within 1 month but definite signs of residual schizophrenic disorder, e.g. autistic thinking or behaviour, disturbed ego identity
		'Social remission': patients can return to their earlier social situation but show some (although not great) reduced ability to study or to work
Level 4	Fair responders	Slow and incomplete recovery; structured rehabilitation programme needed in addition to antipsychotic medication, because of a long or fairly long hospital stay
		No clinical remission and only partial social remission: patients can leave hospital but continued support and rehabilitation are needed
Level 5	Poor responders	Insufficient remission of psychotic symptoms or disturbed behaviour to permit entry into ordinary group rehabilitation programmes, despite standard-dose antipsychotic medication for $\geqslant 6$ months and standard rehabilitation and nondrug programmes at a defined support level *or* withdrawal from treatment because of toxicity or other unwanted effects
		No social or clinical remission: patients will remain in hospital for a long period or in some alternative form of caring milieu, such as a hostel or family care
Level 6	Severe treatment resistance	Failure to respond to any useful extent after 6 months of hospital treatment, including antipsychotic drugs given with measured and presumably adequate plasma levels and accompanied by an intensive level of psychosocial intervention.
		Patients remain in hospital or equivalent care

adequate drug trial have also undergone revisions. There is now at least some agreement that a duration of 4–6 weeks is sufficient to evaluate antipsychotic response.[18] Regarding the dosage of conventional neuroleptics, a minimal dosage of 1000 mg chlorpromazine equivalence was suggested. However, in vitro receptor-binding studies showed that dosages of only 400 mg chlorpromazine equivalence result in blockade of 80–90% of dopamine-D2 receptors.[19] Accordingly, an elevated dosage of classical neuroleptics does not induce better antipsychotic efficacy, but increases the rate of extrapyramidal side-effect(s) (EPS).[20,21] Therefore, 400–600 mg of chlorpromazine equivalence is mostly recommended as a standard dosage.[17,22] These criteria were also used for the guidelines of the American Psychiatric Association.[23]

A major problem with the old definition of therapy resistance in schizophrenia was the concentration mostly or exclusively on positive symptoms. There is now wide agreement that negative symptoms (of major importance regarding long-term prognosis) need to be considered further. Recent investigations, therefore, have focused on the problem of persisting negative symptoms.[24–26] Clozapine and other atypical neuroleptics, such as risperidone, olanzapine and sertindole, have shown better efficacy on negative symptoms in comparison with haloperidol in several double-blind controlled studies.[8,27,28] However, there is an ongoing controversy whether these atypical neuroleptics influence the negative symptoms directly or through a reduction of depressive symptoms or through less-frequent EPS.[29,30]

Prevalence

The prevalence of therapy resistance in schizophrenic patients depends on the definition used. Most studies agree that between 20 and 30% of all patients with schizophrenia do not respond adequately or do so only partially to drug treatment. This percentage of drug-resistant schizophrenic patients seems to be consistent over time.[4,14] The survey of Davis et al.[31] summarized changes in psychopathology during acute treatment: a good or excellent response in 70%, a moderate response in 22%, no response in 5% and a worsening in 3%. A recent investigation by Juarez-Reyes et al. in a group of 293 patients found therapy resistance in 43%.[32] The criteria used were two unsuccessful neuroleptic trials for at least 4 weeks with a dosage of at least 600 mg chlorpromazine equivalence or tardive dyskinesia or a score of global assessment of functioning of less than 61. The prevalence was lowered to 13% when the criteria of Kane et al.[15] were used. These data agree somewhat with those of May et al., who found 20% to be nonresponders.[14] McMillan et al. found that in a group of patients with first-episode schizophrenia 7% did not respond to neuroleptic treatment.[33] Essock et al.[34] examined therapy-resistant hospitalized patients and used the following criteria: at least two unsuccessful neuro-leptic trials for a minimum of 6 weeks with a minimum of 1000 mg chlor-promazine equivalence; hospitalization for at least 4 months; and a total hospitalization during the last 5 years for at least 24 months. They found that 40% of all hospitalized schizophrenic patients fulfilled these criteria of therapy resistance.

Factors associated with treatment resistance

A variety of clinical, neurobiological, brain morphological and pharmaco-logical factors have been found to be associated with treatment resis-tance. Male gender, early age of onset, negative symptomatology, more severe illness, poor premorbid social and work adjustment, poor initial outcome and neurological soft signs are the clinical factors that are found to be significantly correlated with insufficient response.[34-40] However, the clinical relevance of these factors is very limited. The same is true for neurobiological or brain morphological factors, which help little in pre-dicting individual response to neuroleptic drugs. Neurotransmitter studies showed a reduced catecholamine level in the cerebrospinal fluid (CSF) of therapy-resistant schizophrenics,[41] but a low level of homovanillic acid in the CSF of clozapine responders.[42] Computed tomography (CT) and magnetic resonance imaging abnormalities were also associated with insufficient neuroleptic response,[37,43-46] particularly in patients who had mostly negative symptoms.[47] Moreover, an insufficient response to the first neuroleptic medication seems to be associated with a later non-response.[44,45,48]

A major factor in insufficient treatment response is noncompliance. A majority of patients with poor outcome could be undertreated. More than 30% of inpatients and 40–65% of outpatients are at least episodically noncompliant with their regular treatment. The reasons for noncompli-ance include adverse effects as well as psychological, familial and social factors.[6,14,18]

Pharmacological treatment

Typical neuroleptics

First, psychiatrists should distinguish apparent nonresponse from authen-tic treatment resistance by either measuring neuroleptic plasma concen-tration or switching to a depot preparation. If noncompliance can be excluded, the dosage of the typical neuroleptic may be increased. There are several reports indicating that at least some schizophrenic patients may respond to a marked increase in the usually recommended dosage.[49-51] However, with the availability of clozapine and other atypical neuroleptics, high-dosage strategies remain controversial and should be used only if atypical neuroleptics do not improve psychopathology. In the majority of patients there is evidence of a ceiling effect. The increase does not lead to better improvement but to a higher prevalence of adverse effects. Of 6 randomized, double-blind trials comparing parallel standard and high doses of neuroleptics in refractory patients, 4 did not find any difference between high and standard dosages, and one found greater improvement for the low dosage. Only one study supports the use of the high dosage.[20,21] Thus, high doses of typical neuroleptics are not associated with an obvious advantage for the vast majority of treatment-refractory patients, except in those where rapid metabolism or poor absorption might lead to low neuroleptic plasma concentrations. High doses of typical neuroleptics are a last resort for use in well-selected and supervised patients.

Most treatment guidelines recommend that if therapy with one typical neuroleptic does not result in marked improvement another typical neuro-leptic of a different chemical class should be used.[52] The efficacy of this common procedure is not supported by published studies. In more than 100 investigations where two or more conventional neuroleptics were compared, only a few found a significant difference.[53,54] The conclusion of these studies is that conventional or typical neuroleptics do not differ in their antipsychotic efficacy in schizophrenic patients. Regarding the sub-group of therapy-resistant patients, differences between typical neurolep-tics cannot be excluded but are, rather, unlikely. Most controlled trials show that fewer than 5% of patients improve after being switched from one typical neuroleptic to another.[15,55] Kinon and co-workers also showed that neither a change of fluphenazine to haloperidol or a threefold increase of the fluphenazine dosage resulted in marked improvement of psychopathology; only 9% of patients subsequently responded.[38]

The choice of the 'right' conventional neuroleptic is often difficult or even not possible. If previous neuroleptic treatment is known, and good efficacy as well as good tolerability under one drug are documented, this should be used first. If after treatment for 6–8 weeks with at least 300–600 mg chlorpromazine equivalence no improvement of psy-chopathology is found, compliance should be examined and possible EPS treated by reducing the dosage or by using anticholinergic drugs.

Atypical neuroleptics

There are several sequential advantages of atypical neuroleptics, which are strong arguments for the broad use of these drugs – and not only in therapy-resistant or otherwise negatively selected patients. Because of the lack of relevant motor or affective side-effects with atypical neurolep-tics, compliance is relatively high and patients are less often rehospitalized. Therefore, these patients are better able to participate in long-term psychosocial rehabilitative treatment that might finally lead to an improvement of negative symptoms, in subjective well-being and of quality of life. Moreover, several studies indicate that early[56] and continuous neuroleptic treatment[57] is of major importance for long-term prognosis. Therefore, it might be possible that the broad use of effective, tolerable and socially accepted atypical neuroleptics also results in a markedly better long-term prognosis. In general, typical neuroleptics should no longer be used, and it is certainly in the patient's interest to use an atypical neuroleptic at the beginning of antipsychotic treatment (at least after the first unsuccessful trial with a typical neuroleptic) and not to conduct a second or a third trial with another conventional neuroleptic. Efficacy in therapy-resistant patients is best-documented for clozapine, the oldest atypical neuroleptic.[58-62] However, there is the well-known but low risk of agranulocytosis, which needs to be considered in evaluating the benefit/risk ratio. For the other new atypical neuroleptics, an elevated risk of agranulocytosis is not known. The efficacy regarding therapy-resistant schizophrenic patients has been investigated in double-blind controlled trials of risperidone, olanzapine and zotepine. Regarding other atypicals (e.g. sertindole, quetiapine, ziprasidone and amisulpride), only case reports or open trials have been published, and studies comparing sertindole and quetiapine with risperidone or chlorpromazine are ongoing.

Clozapine
Since the well-known study of Kane et al.,[15] clozapine is indicated in patients with no adequate response to typical neuroleptics. For many years it was the only drug recommended for this negatively selected group of patients.[7,17,63,64] To increase tolerability or to reduce side-effects induced by clozapine's anticholinergic properties, the dosage of clozapine should be increased only gradually. Generally, clozapine therapy is begun while patients are still being treated with the previous neuroleptic. While the clozapine dosage is increased, the typical neuroleptic is reduced, and usually discontinued within 7–14 days of starting clozapine treatment. The clozapine dosage should be increased in the following way: 12.5 mg on day 1, 25–50 mg on days 2–4, 50–100 mg on days 5–7, 100–200 mg on days 8–14, 200–400 mg on days 15–21 and 400–600 mg on days 22–28.[58] If severe side-effects (such as sedation, hypotension or delirious states) occur, an even more gradual increase will lead to better tolerability. Most clozapine studies show discontinuation as a result of side-effects for only 6–8% of patients, and its temporary combination with sympathomimetics to counter hypotension or with pirenzepine or other peripherally acting anticholinergics to treat hypersalivation is advisable.

Aside from the study by Kane et al.,[15] there are several other double-blind controlled studies that showed clozapine to be more effective than chlorpromazine or haloperidol in patients who did not respond to conventional neuroleptics.[55,65] Moreover, there are numerous open long-term investigations documenting a marked reduction of psychopathology in 30–60% of chronic patients and/or therapy-resistant patients.[58–62,66] This improvement is more or less similar in first-episode and other patients, and occurs mostly within 6–12 weeks of treatment. The necessary duration of clozapine treatment to evaluate its efficacy 'finally' is controversial. Conley et al.[67] found that therapy-resistant patients improved in the main during the first 8 weeks of clozapine treatment; others found a shorter or longer duration of treatment.[30,59] The tolerability of clozapine, its efficacy and the tolerability of previous neuroleptics (including other atypicals), possible alternatives (other atypicals?) and patients' subjective experiences need to be considered when deciding if and when clozapine should be discontinued. The underutilization of clozapine in many countries probably reflects the costs and complexities of therapy with this old atypical neuroleptic. In addition to the need for the long-term haematological monitoring for agranulocytosis, the most relevant side-effects are weight gain, sedation and hypersalivation. However, beside the particular efficacy of clozapine in therapy-resistant patients, there are other arguments in favour of administering this neuroleptic: a reduction of aggressive behaviour,[55,68] a reduction of the symptoms of tardive dyskinesia[58–62,66,69] and a reduction of suicidal behaviour.[70]

Risperidone

Several investigations have demonstrated the efficacy of risperidone in the treatment of positive and negative schizophrenic symptoms. In these investigations, a risperidone dosage of less than 6 mg/d did not induce EPS more frequently than did placebo. Regarding the efficacy of risperidone in chronic or severely ill schizophrenic patients, the US multicentre trial indicates that risperidone has greater efficacy than haloperidol.[8] To date there is no evidence of superior efficacy in rigorously defined treatment-resistant patients, but some open-label or retrospective studies have described patients with poorly responsive schizophrenia who showed some improvement under risperidone.[71–74] The first data on the use of risperidone in therapy-resistant patients were presented by Lindenmayer et al.:[75] of 82 patients, 27% were found to show marked, and 37% minimal, improvement. Daniel and Whitcomb have recently reviewed 10 risperidone trials and they concluded that the data are far from being complete but that they provide 'an overall sense of optimism for risperidone's role in treatment-resistant/intolerant patients'.[76] In view of the numerous comparisons between clozapine and risperidone, this conclusion might be premature or too optimistic (see below).

Olanzapine

Olanzapine has a receptor-binding profile similar to clozapine, in vivo as well as in vitro. Better tolerability and similar or better efficacy in the treatment of schizophrenic patients were found in 6-week trials where the drug was compared with haloperidol.[77] These data were confirmed by clinical experience with 150 schizophrenic inpatients: the only EPS was akathisia, which occurred in 4 patients, all treated with doses above 20 mg/d. Weight gain seems to be the only side-effect of major relevance (Lambert et al., in preparation). First trials on therapy-resistant patients yielded somewhat conflicting results regarding the usefulness of olanzapine in this special population. A recent double-blind controlled comparison over 8 weeks between 25 mg/d of olanzapine and 1200 mg/d of chlorpromazine plus 4 mg/d of benztropine mesylate in 84 treatment-resistant patients (similar to those in the study by Kane et al.[15]) showed better tolerability for olanzapine but no significant difference regarding efficacy:[25] 7% of the olanzapine patients responded with a 20% reduction in total BPRS; however, no chlorpromazine patients responded. Since in most clozapine studies on comparable populations, 30–70% fulfilled the response criteria, the data might indicate that olanzapine is less effective than clozapine. However, the data might also be explained by a more negatively selected patient population. A Spanish 6-week prospective open-label study on 25 schizophrenic patients with documented lack of response to two conventional antipsychotic drugs showed a considerable treatment response (≥35% decrease in BPRS) in 36% of patients.[78]

Zotepine

The few studies on the efficacy of zotepine in therapy-resistant patients were not conducted in populations defined according to the criteria by Kane et al.[15] Harada et al. examined efficacy in 22 patients treated with 50–500 mg zotepine for 12 months.[79] According to the CGI, 10 patients showed marked, 7 moderate and 5 slight improvement. Another study, again by Harada and co-workers, showed significant improvement of BPRS (at least 20%) in 85% of 45 patients.[80]

Which atypical neuroleptic is the best?

There have not yet been many double-blind controlled studies in which the different atypical neuroleptics have been compared regarding their efficacy in patients not responding to conventional neuroleptics. Therefore, the scientific basis in deciding which atypical is best is still very limited. Moreover, the data from the few clinical trials that have been conducted are of marginal relevance for the individual patient. Vulnerability and tolerability regarding certain side-effects are rather different and impossible to predict. For example, sedation is not always an adverse effect, and hypersalivation (induced by clozapine) is a severe burden for one patient but only a minor annoyance for another. For such a patient – perhaps a musician – it might be of vital importance not to have even the slightest EPS.

Most trials comparing two atypicals have involved clozapine and risperidone. Klieser et al. reported a similar efficacy for both drugs in chronic schizophrenic patients.[81] However, subjects were not categorized as treatment resistant and the number of patients was too low to test adequately for a differential effect between the drugs. The other double-blind study, comparing 6.4 mg risperidone with 291 mg clozapine in 86 chronic schizophrenic patients who were resistant to or intolerant of conventional neuroleptics, did not reveal a significant difference either: 67% of the risperidone group and 65% of the clozapine group had a reduction of 20% or more in total using the Positive and Negative Symptom Scale (PANSS).[25] In contrast, there are numerous open crossover studies showing that risperidone is effective in only 0–15% of clozapine nonresponders,[12,13,82,83] but that clozapine improved 40–80% of risperidone nonresponders.[12,13,84] Although one crossover study by Daniel et al.[85] on 20 therapy-resistant patients did not find a significant difference between both atypicals, both open comparisons with a higher number of subjects indicated that clozapine had better efficacy than risperidone.[86,87]

The only double-blind controlled comparison between clozapine and zotepine (150–450 mg/d each) in 50 therapy-resistant patients did not reveal any significant difference: both drugs induced 'a relevant improvement' in 52% of patients.[88]

The efficacy of olanzapine in therapy-resistant patients or in those who did not tolerate or did not respond to other atypicals was investigated in several open trials and in one double-blind study, not yet published: 23 of 34 (68%) risperidone nonresponders improved under olanzapine for at least 20% of the BPRS total score.[89] Regarding clozapine nonresponders, 18 of 45 (40%) or 6 of 16 (38%) responded with at least a 20% reduction in PANSS total score.[90,91] However, there are also patients who do not respond to olanzapine but improve under clozapine. This was the case for 11 or 21 patients (52%) in the study by Conley et al.[25] The double-blind study compared 15–25 mg olanzapine and 200–600 mg clozapine over 18 weeks in 180 patients (Beuzen et al., in press). Some 107 patients completed the study (olanzapine 60%, clozapine 59%), and the rates of discontinuation due to adverse events were lower for olanzapine than for clozapine (4.4% vs. 15.6%, $p = 0.013$). There was no significant difference regarding efficacy: 60% of olanzapine and 54% of clozapine patients improved by at least 20% in PANSS total score.

Other pharmacological possibilities

If atypical neuroleptics do not lead to a major improvement of psychopathology, other psychopharmacological drugs might be used. No controlled trials have been conducted in populations based on the criteria by Kane et al.,[15] but three studies reported a significant benefit from additional treatment with lithium (particularly in excitement) in 30–50% of patients.[2,92,93] Four-week treatment seems to be sufficient to evaluate the success of lithium treatment, and patients with depressive symptoms seem to improve the most.[2] Christison et al. also reported that lithium particularly influences hostility and aggressive behaviour in therapy-resistant schizophrenic patients.[7] However, there is also one single-blind study which did not find any symptomatic improvement in 44 patients receiving either placebo or lithium in addition to neuroleptic medication.[93] Moreover, it must be borne in mind that this treatment is associated with an elevated risk of severe side-effects, such as delirious states, encephalopathy or neurotoxicity.[17]

Other drugs recommended as additives to neuroleptics in therapy-resistant schizophrenic patients are anticonvulsants, carbamazepine and valproic acid, as well as benzodiazepines.[3,17,23,63,64] Many open trials and case studies – some of them rather impressive – indicate that these drugs are at least worth trying. However, despite the large volume of literature, small sample sizes and other methodological flaws do not allow any conclusions to be drawn as to which of these drugs should be used first and in which patients.[94]

To date, there have been no controlled investigations on electroconvulsive treatment (ECT) in treatment-resistant schizophrenic patients. One open trial indicated that the combined use of typical neuroleptics and ECT might be beneficial for some patients in this population.[95] There have been two other open studies of additional ECT in patients with no or only partial response to clozapine, both of which showed some improvement after ECT.[96,97]

Treatment recommendations

Table 1.2 gives an example of one of the generally accepted guidelines for the treatment of an inadequate response to conventional antipsychotic drug therapy.[23] It reflects most or all of the well-documented studies. Certain issues (e.g. when atypical neuroleptics should be given) are, however, controversial.

With the development of several new atypical neuroleptics, already or soon to be on the market, it is likely that the guidelines will change as new data become available. The neuroleptic-resistant patient requires a systematic and comprehensive plan, including pharmacological and nonpharmacological treatment. The patient and his or her relatives or partners should be informed as thoroughly as possible about the expected benefits, the potential adverse effects and the reasons for choosing and changing treatment. Frequent mistakes in the pharmacological treatment of the difficult, severely ill or therapy-resistant schizophrenic patient may reflect insufficient patience on the part of psychiatrists. It is well known that sedating and most other adverse

Table 1.2   Strategy for the treatment of an inadequate response to conventional antipsychotic drug therapy

1) Optimize trial of antipsychotic medication:

   a. Use 300–600 mg chlorpromazine equivalents for 6–8 weeks
   b. Consider a trial of depot neuroleptic, if not yet done
   c. Treat any underlying EPS

      i. Consider dose reduction if EPS is present
      ii. Add adjunct anticholinergic medication, if needed

2) If no response to above, switch medication to novel antipsychotic. Cross-taper off conventional antipsychotics for 2–4 weeks. Continue anticholinergic medication until conventional antipsychotics have been discontinued for at least 2 weeks. Choices include the following:

   a. Risperidone, 2–6 mg/d for 6–8 weeks
   b. Olanzapine, 15–25 mg/d for 6–8 weeks
   c. Sertindole, 20–24 mg/d for 6–8 weeks
   d. Quetiapine, 300–450 mg/d for 6–8 weeks

3) If no response to above, switch to clozapine

   a. Increase gradually to 200–400 mg for 4–6 weeks
   b. If no response, increase gradually to 500–600 mg for 6 weeks
   c. If no response, increase gradually to 700–900 mg for 6 weeks

      i. Carefully monitor for side-effects
      ii. Do not increase dose if myoclonus is present.

4) If no response to clozapine, discontinue

   a. Reinstitute best prior drug therapy
   b. Consider adjunct medication

      i.   Lithium
      ii. Anticonvulsants

         (a) Valproic acid
         (b) Carbamazepine

      iii. Benzodiazepines
      iv. Propanolol
      v.   Antidepressants
      vi. Higher doses of conventional antipsychotics

5) If no response to best prior drug therapy or adjunct medications, consider ECT

Source:
Adapted from Frances et al.[23]

effects occur within hours of administrating neuroleptic drugs, but that antipsychotic efficacy is often not obvious until 3 or 5 days later, in some patients even longer. Good pharmacological concepts are often not realized because medication, substance and dosage (as well as comedication) are changed too fast and too often. In particular, if adjunctive treatment is used in combination with a neuroleptic, these combinations must be assessed carefully to allow for clear conclusions regarding potential benefits or risks (e.g. no more than one drug should be changed at a time).

Resistance to neuroleptic treatment, at least in part, is rather common and occurs in 70–80% of schizophrenic patients. Although in the most often used definition (that by Kane et al.[15]), 'treatment resistance' is defined operationally as a categorical diagnosis, response to treatment is along a continuum from the poor to the full remission of symptoms. That means that a carefully planned scheme should determine the treatment of neuroleptic-resistant patients and also should be applied to all schizophrenic patients. First, the diagnosis should be reassessed and potential factors contributing to treatment resistance examined: the presence of mood disorder, substance abuse or personality disorder; neurological or internal diseases; and nonpsychopharmacological medication. Secondly, noncompliance as the reason for nonimprovement should be excluded, either by a trial with a depot neuroleptic or with measurements of plasma concentrations. Thirdly, the appropriateness of the kind and dosage of the antipsychotic should be assessed. Although most guidelines for the treatment of schizophrenia recommend a trial with typical neuroleptics, there are strong arguments to suggest using an atypical neuroleptic as the drug of first choice.[98]

Some psychiatrists are sceptical about the efficacy of atypical neuroleptics and assume that acutely psychotic patients do not benefit sufficiently from atypical compounds. However, this belief is not supported by scientific data. Multiple comparisons between an atypical and a typical neuroleptic exist only for clozapine, which was compared in 20 control trials mainly to chlorpromazine or haloperidol.[99] Clozapine was found to be more effective than chlorpromazine in 6 out of 13 studies. Four out of a further 6 studies also found clozapine to be superior to haloperidol. Only one study found clozapine to be less effective than other neuroleptics, but the clozapine dosage was of much lower equivalence than that of the typical neuroleptic.

Not only the famous study by Kane et al.[15] (revealing the superiority of clozapine over chlorpromazine in therapy-resistant patients) but also all studies in which an atypical neuroleptic was compared to a typical or classical drug showed either no difference or an advantage of the atypical compound. No study shows that a typical neuroleptic has more antipsychotic efficacy than an atypical one. There are also no data indicating a delayed efficacy of atypical neuroleptics. One exception might be clozapine, where a slow and gradual increase in dosage is required to improve tolerability by preventing the side-effects that are induced by its anticholinergic properties.

At the moment there are only three major reasons to prescribe typical neuroleptics:

1) *Longer experience of these drugs.* This argument is certainly not valid for most of the atypical neuroleptics. Clozapine has been on the market (at least in Europe) for more than 20 years. Risperidone and olanzapine have each been prescribed to more than one million patients worldwide, and it is not very realistic to expect any unknown, late-occurring, clinically relevant side-effect. The same is true for amisulpride, which has been available in France and other European countries for 10–15 years.

2) *No depot formulation available.* Depot injections are valuable in those patients who are noncompliant regarding oral medication due to, for example, cognitive deficits. This subgroup of mostly chronic schizophrenic patients might indeed benefit more from a depot injection with a typical neuroleptic than from oral atypicals.

3) *Price.* Atypical neuroleptics are 5–10 times more expensive than typical ones. The relevance of this argument differs from country to country depending upon different medicoeconomic systems. Pharmacoeconomic studies have shown for clozapine,[100,101] as well as for risperidone,[102,103] that the cost of outpatient treatment does increase. However, this is more than compensated for by the reduced cost of inpatient treatment as a result of the need for less rehospitalization.

Summary

Therapy-resistance, occurring in 10–40% of schizophrenic patients, requires systematic and comprehensive planning for its management. Patients should, first, be assessed to verify that they are indeed resistant to neuroleptic drugs as opposed to being noncompliant or undertreated. If possible, the dosage of the existing antipsychotic should be increased, and extrapyramidal or other side-effects treated. Treatment with typical neuroleptics is still most often recommended, but there are already strong arguments to use atypicals as drugs of first choice. Most data on the usefulness of atypical neuroleptics in patients not responding to conventional drugs are known for clozapine, but olanzapine, risperidone, zotepine and others might be valuable alternatives. In patients failing to respond to any single antipsychotic, the combination with lithium, carbamazepine, valproic acid and benzodiazepines should be tried.

References

1. Holden J. Thioridazine and chlordiazepoxide, alone and combined, in the treatment of chronic schizophrenia. *Compr Psychiatry* (1968) **9:** 933–43.

2. Carman J, Bigelow L, Wyatt R. Lithium combined with neuroleptics in chronic schizophrenic and schizoaffective patients. *J Clin Psychiatry* (1981) **42:** 124–8.

3. Wolkowitz O, Pickar D, Doran A, Breier A, Tarell J, Paul S. Combination alprazolam-neuroleptic treatment of the positive and negative symptoms of schizophrenia. *Am J Psychiatry* (1986) **143:** 85–7.

4. McGlashan T. A selective review of recent North American long-term followup studies of schizophrenia. *Schizophrenia Bull* (1988) **14:** 515–42.

5. Meltzer H. Commentary: defining treatment refractoriness in schizophrenia. *Schizophrenia Bull* (1990) **16:** 563–5.

6. Brenner H, Dencker S, Goldstein M et al. Defining treatment refractoriness in schizophrenia. *Schizophrenia Bull* (1990) **16:** 551–61.

7. Christison G, Kirch D, Wyatt R. When symptoms persist: choosing among alternative somatic treatments for schizophrenia. *Schizophrenia Bull* (1991) **17:** 217–45.

8. Marder S, Meibach R. Risperidone in the treatment of schizophrenia. *Am J Psychiatry* (1994) **151:** 825–35.

9. Cohen S, Underwood M. The use of clozapine in a mentally retarded and aggressive population. *J Clin Psychiatry* (1994) **55:** 440–4.

10. Cardoni A. Risperidone: review and assessment of its role in the treatment of schizophrenia. *Ann Pharmacother* (1995) **29:** 610–18.

11. Shore D. Clinical implications of clozapine discontinuation: report of an NIMH workshop. *Schizophrenia Bull* (1995) **21:** 333–8.

12. Buckley P, Buchanan R, Schulz S, Tamminga C. Catching up on schizophrenia. The Fifth International Congress on Schizophrenia Research, Warm Springs, VA, April 8–12, 1995. *Arch Gen Psychiatry* (1996) **53:** 456–62.

13. Pajonk F, Naber D, Hippius H. Alternativen zum Clozapin? Klinische Erfahrungen mit Risperidon. In Naber D, Müller-Spahn F (eds) *Clozapin. Pharmakologie und Klinik eines atypischen Neuroleptikums* (Heidelberg: Springer, 1997): 89–104.

14. May PR, Dencker SJ, Hubbard JW. A systematic approach to treatment resistance in schizophrenic disorders. In Dencker SJ (ed) *Treatment Resistance in Schizophrenia* (Braunschweig: Vieweg, 1988): 22–33.

15. Kane J, Honigfeld G, Singer J, Meltzer H, the Clorazil Collaborative Study Group. Clozapine for the treatment-resistant schizophrenic. A double-blind comparison with chlorpromazine. *Arch Gen Psychiatry* (1988) **45:** 789–96.

16. Kinon B, Kane J, Perovich R, Ismi M, Koreen A. Influence of neuroleptic dose and class in treatment-resistant schizophrenia relapse. Paper presented at the 32nd Annual Meeting of the New Clinical Drug Evaluation Unit, Key Biscayne, FL, May 1992.

17. Barnes T, McEvedy CJB. Pharmacological treatment strategies

in the nonresponsive schizophrenic patient. *Int Clin Psychopharmacol* (1996) **11:** 67–71.

18. Kane J, Marder S. Psychopharmacologic treatment of schizophrenia. *Schizophrenia Bull*
(1993) **19:** 287–302.

19. Farde L, Nordström A, Wiesel
F-A, Pauli S, Halldin C, Sedvall
G. PET analysis of central D1-
and D2-dopamine receptor
occupancy in patients treated
with classical neuroleptics and
clozapine: relation to extrapyramidal side effects. *Arch Gen
Psychiatry* (1992) **49:** 538–44.

20. Kane J. The use of higher-dose
antipsychotic medication. Comment on the Royal College of
Psychiatrists' consensus statement. *Br J Psychiatry* (1994)
164: 431–2.

21. Möller H. Treatment of schizophrenia: state of the art. *Eur Arch
Psychiatry Clin Neurosci* (1996)
246: 229–34.

22. Dixon L, Lehman A, Levine J.
Conventional antipsychotic medications for schizophrenia. *Schizophrenia Bull* (1995) **21:** 567–77.

23. Frances A, Docherty J, Kahn
D. The expert consensus guidelines series: treatment of schizophrenia. *J Clin Psychiatry* (1996)
57: 11–50.

24. Kane J, Mayerhoff D. Do negative symptoms respond to pharmacological treatment? *Br J
Psychiatry* (1989) **155(Suppl 7):**
115–18.

25. Conley R, Tamminga C, Bartko J
et al. Olanzapine compared with
chlorpromazine in treatment-
resistant schizophrenia. *Am J
Psychiatry* (1998) **155:** 914–20.

26. Bondolfi G, Dufour H, Patris
M et al., the Risperidone
Study Group. Risperidone versus
clozapine in treatment-resistant
chronic schizophrenia: a randomized double-blind study.
Am J Psychiatry (1998) **155:**
499–504.

27. Beasley C, Tollefson G, Tran P,
Satterlee W, Sanger T, Hamilton
S. Olanzapine versus placebo
versus haloperidol. Acute phase
results of the North American
double-blind olanzapine trial.
Neuropsychopharmacology
(1996) **14:** 111–23.

28. Zimbroff D, Kane J, Tamminga J
et al., the Sertindole Study
Group. Controlled dose-response
study of sertindole and haloperidol in the treatment of schizophrenia. *Am J Psychiatry* (1997)
154: 782–91.

29. Meltzer H. An overview of the
mechanism of action of clozapine. *J Clin Psychiatry* (1994) **55:**
47–52.

30. Carpenter W, Conley R,
Buchanan R, Breier A, Tamminga C. Another view of clozapine treatment of schizophrenia.
Am J Psychiatry (1995) **152:**
827–32.

31. Davis J, Schaffer C, Killian G,
Kinard C, Chan C. Important
issues in the drug treatment of
schizophrenia. *Schizophrenia
Bull* (1980) **6:** 70–87.

32. Juarez-Reyes M, Shumway M,
Battle C, Baccetti P, Hansen M,
Hargreaves W. Effects of stringent criteria on eligibility for
clozapine among public mental
health clients. *Psychiat Serv*
(1995) **46:** 801–6.

33. MacMillan J, Crow T, Johnson A,
Johnstone E. Short-term outcome in trial entrants and trial eli-
gible patients. *Br J Psychiatry*
(1986) **148:** 128–33.

34. Essock S, Hargreaves W, Dohm
F et al. Clozapine eligibility
among state hospital patients.
Schizophrenia Bull (1996) **22:**
15–25.

35. Kolakowska A, Williams T, Arden
M. Schizophrenia with good and

poor outcome. I. Early clinical features, response to neuroleptics and signs of organic dysfunction. *Br J Psychiatry* (1985) **146:** 229–46.

36. Kolakowska T, Williams AO, Jambor K, Ardern M. Schizophrenia with good and poor outcome. II. Neurological soft signs, cognitive impairment and their clinical significance. *Br J Psychiatry* (1985) **146:** 348–57.

37. Kccfc R, Mohs R, Davidson M et al. Kraepelinian schizophrenia: a subgroup of schizophrenia? *Psychopharmacol Bull* (1988) **24:** 56–61.

38. Kinon B, Kane J, Johns C et al. Treatment of neuroleptic-resistant schizophrenic relapse. *Psychopharmacol Bull* (1993) **29:** 309–14.

39. Bareggi S, Mauri M, Cavallaro R. Factors affecting the clinical response to haloperidol therapy in schizophrenia. *Clin Neuropharmacol* (1990) **13(Suppl 1):** 29–34.

40. Prudo R, Munroe Blum H. Five-year outcome and prognosis in schizophrenia: a report from the London Field Research Centre of the international pilot study of schizophrenia. *Br J Psychiatry* (1987) **150:** 345–54.

41. van Kammen D, Schooler N. Are biochemical markers for treatment-resistant schizophrenia state dependent or traits? *Clin Neuropharmacol* (1990) **13:** 516–28.

42. Pickar D, Breier A, Kelsoe J. Plasma homovanillic acid as an index of central dopaminergic activity: studies in schizophrenia patients. *Ann N Y Acad Sci* (1988) **537:** 339–46.

43. Friedmann L, Knutson L, Shurell M, Meltzer H. Prefrontal sulcal prominence is inversely related to response to clozapine in schizophrenia. *Biol Psychiatry* (1991) **29:** 865–77.

44. Lieberman J, Jody D, Alvir J et al. Brain morphologic features, dopamine, eye-tracking abnormalities in first episode schizophrenia: prevalence and clinical correlates. *Arch Gen Psychiatry* (1993) **50:** 357–68.

45. Stern R, Kahn R, Davidson M. Predictors of response to neuroleptic treatment in schizophrenia. *Psychiatr Clin N Am* (1993) **16:** 313–38.

46. Bilder R, Wu H, Chakos M et al. Cerebral morphometry and clozapine treatment in schizophrenia. *J Clin Psychiatry* (1994) **55(Suppl B):** 53–6.

47. Ota P, Maeshiro H, Ishido H et al. Treatment-resistant chronic psychopathology and CT scans in schizophrenia. *Acta Psychiatr Scand* (1987) **75:** 415–27.

48. Kinon B, Kane J, Chakos M, Munne R. Possible predictors of neuroleptic-resistant schizophrenic relapse: influence of negative symptoms and acute extrapyramidal side effects. *Psychopharmacol Bull* (1993a) **29:** 365–9.

49. Prien R, Cole J. High-dose chlorpromazine therapy in chronic schizophrenia. *Arch Gen Psychiatry* (1986) **18:** 482–95.

50. Rifkin A, Quitkin F, Carrillo C, Klein D, Oaks G. Very high dosage fluphenazine for nonchronic treatment-refractory patients. *Arch Gen Psychiatry* (1971) **25:** 398–403.

51. Ereshefsky L, Saklad S, Mings T. Management of chronic refractory schizophrenic patients with high-dose loxapine. *Psychopharmacol Bull* (1983) **19:** 600–3.

52. Kane J. New developments in the pharmacological treatment of schizophrenia. *Bull Menninger Clin* (1992) **56:** 62–75.

53. Klein D, Davis J. *Diagnosis and Drug Treatment of Psychiatric Disorders* (Baltimore, MD: Williams & Wilkins, 1969).

54. Janicak P, Davis J, Preskorn S, Ayd F. *Principles and Practice of Psychopharmacotherapy* (Baltimore, MD: Williams & Wilkins, 1993).

55. Breier A, Buchanan R, Kirkpatrick B et al. Effects of clozapine on positive and negative symptoms in outpatients with schizophrenia. *Am J Psychiatry* (1994) **151:** 20–6.

56. Wyatt R, Damiani L, Henter I. First-episode schizophrenia. Early intervention and medication discontinuation in the context of course and treatment. *Br J Psychiatry* (1998) **172(Suppl 33):** 77–83.

57. Szymanski D, Cannon T, Gallacher F, Erwin R, Gur R. Course of treatment response in first-episode and chronic schizophrenia. *Am J Psychiatry* (1996) **153:** 519–25.

58. Naber D, Holzbach R, Perro C, Hippius H. Clinical management of clozapine patients in relation to efficacy and side-effects. *Br J Psychiatry* (1992a) **160(Suppl 17):** 54–9.

59. Meltzer H. Multiple-outcome criteria in schizophrenia: an overview of outcome with clozapine. *Eur Psychiatry* (1995) **10(Suppl 1):** 19–25.

60. Lindenmayer J-P, Grochowski S, Mabugat L. Clozapine effects on positive and negative symptoms: a six-month trial in treatment-refractory schizophrenics. *J Clin Psychopharmacol* (1994) **14:** 200–4.

61. Alvarez E, Barón J, Puigdemont José Soriano D, Masip C, Perez-Solá V. Ten years' experience with clozapine in treatment-resistant schizophrenic patients: factors indicating the therapeutic response. *Eur Psychiatry* (1997) **12(Suppl 5):** 343–6.

62. Lindström L-H. The effect of long-term treatment with clozapine in schizophrenia: a retrospective study in 96 patients treated with clozapine for up to 13 years. *Acta Psychiatr Scand* (1988) **77:** 524–9.

63. Conley R, Buchanan R. Evaluation of treatment-resistant schizophrenia. *Schizophrenia Bull* (1997) **23:** 663–74.

64. Jalenques I. Drug-resistant schizophrenia. Treatment options. *CNS Drugs* (1996) **5:** 8–23.

65. Claghorn J, Honigfeld G, Abuzzahab FS et al. The risks and benefits of clozapine versus chlorpromazine. *J Clin Psychopharmacol* (1987) **7:** 377–84.

66. Small J, Milstein V, Marhenke J, Hall D, Kellams J. Treatment outcome with clozapine in tardive dyskinesia, neuroleptic sensitivity and treatment-resistant psychosis. *J Clin Psychiatry* (1987) **48:** 263–7.

67. Conley R, Carpenter W, Tamminga C. Time to response and response-dose in an 12-month clozapine trial. *Am J Psychiatry* (1997) **154:** 1243–7.

68. Mallya A, Roos P, Roebuck-Colgan K. Restraint, seclusion and clozapine. *J Clin Psychiatry* (1992) **53:** 395–7.

69. Tamminga C, Thaker G, Moran M, Kakigi T, Gao X. Clozapine in tardive dyskinesia: observations from human and animal model studies. *J Clin Psychiatry* (1994) **55(Suppl B):** 102–6.

70. Meltzer H, Okayli G. Reduction of suicidality during clozapine treatment of neuroleptic-resistant schizophrenia: impact on risk–benefit assessment. *Am J Psychiatry* (1995) **152:** 183–90.

71. Buckley P, Donenwirth K, Bayer K et al. Risperidone for treatment-resistant schizophrenia: initial clinical experience in a state hospital. *J Pharm Tech* (1996) **12:** 271–5.

72. Keck P, Wilson D, Strakowski S et al. Clinical predictors of acute risperidone response in schizophrenia, schizoaffective disorder, and psychotic mood disorders. *J Clin Psychiatry* (1995) **56:** 455–70.

73. Chouinard G, Vainer J, Belanger M et al. Risperidone and clozapine in the treatment of drug-resistant schizophrenia and neuroleptic-induced supersensitivity psychosis. *Progr Neuropsychopharmacol Biol Psychiatry* (1994) **18:** 1129–41.

74. Smith R, Chua J, Lipetsker B. Efficacy of risperidone in reducing positive and negative symptoms in medication-refractory schizophrenia: an open prospective study. *J Clin Psychiatry* (1996) **57:** 460–6.

75. Lindenmayer J, Masual-Herne M, Simon F. Use of risperidone in neuroleptic refractory schizophrenics in a state psychiatric center. Abstracts of the 148th Annual Meeting of the American Psychiatric Association. *NR* (1995) **228:** 117.

76. Daniel D, Whitcomb S. Treatment of the refractory schizophrenic patient. *J Clin Psychiatry* (1998) **59(Suppl 1):** 13–19.

77. Tollefson G, Beasley C, Tran P et al. Olanzapine versus haloperidol in the treatment of schizophrenia, schizoaffective and schizophreniform disorders: results of an international collaborative trial. *Am J Psychiatry* (1997) **154:** 457–65.

78. Martín J, Gómez J-C, García-Bernardo E et al. Olanzapine in treatment-refractory schizophrenia: results of an open-label study. *J Clin Psychiatry* (1997) **58:** 479–83.

79. Harada T, Otsuki S, Sato M. Effectivity of zotepine in refractory psychosis: possible relationship between zotepine and non-dopamine psychosis. *Pharmacopsychiatry* (1987) **20(Suppl 1):** 47–51.

80. Harada T, Otsuki S, Fujiwara Y. Effectiveness of zotepine in therapy-refractory psychosis. An open multi-center study in 8 psychiatric clinics. *Fortschr Neurol Psychiatry* (1992) **59(Suppl 1):** 41–6.

81. Klieser E, Lehmann E, Kinzler E, Wurthmann C, Heinrich K. Randomized double-blind, controlled trial of risperidone versus clozapine in patients with chronic schizophrenia. *J Clin Psychopharmacol* (1995) **15(Suppl 1):** 45–51.

82. Still D, Dorson P, Crismon M, Pousson C. Effects of switching inpatients with treatment-resistant schizophrenia from clozapine to risperidone. *Psychiat Serv* (1996) **47:** 1382–4.

83. Lacey R, Preskorn S, Jerkovich G. Is risperidone a substitute for clozapine patients who do not respond to neuroleptics? *Am J Psychiatry* (1995) **152:** 1401 (letter).

84. Cavallaro C, Cordoba C, Smeraldi E. A pilot, open study on the treatment of refractory schizophrenia with risperidone and clozapine. *Hum Psychopharmacol* (1995) **10:** 231–4.

85. Daniel DG, Goldberg TE, Weinberger DR et al. Different side effect profiles of risperidone and clozapine in 20 outpatients with schizophrenia or schizoaffective disorder: a pilot study. *Am J Psychiatry* (1996) **153:** 417–19.

86. Lindenmayer J, Alexander A, Park M, Smith R, Apergi F-S,

Czobor P. Psychopathological and neuropsychological profile of clozapine vs. risperidone in refractory schizophrenics. *Schizophrenia Res* (1997) **24:** 195.

87. Flynn S, MacEwan G, Altman S et al. An open comparison of clozapine and risperidone in treatment-resistant schizophrenia. *Pharmacopsychiatry* (1998) **31:** 25–9.

88. Meyer-Lindenberg A, Gruppe H, Bauer U, Lis S, Krieger S, Gallhofer B. Improvement of cognitive function in schizophrenic patients receiving clozapine or zotepine: results from a double-blind study. *Pharmacopsychiatry* (1997) **30:** 35–42.

89. Wimmer P, Belmaker R, Scheidmann M, Treves I, Sapir M, Dossenbach M. Olanzapine in patients not responding to risperidone. *Schizophrenia Res* (1998) **29:** 148.

90. Baldacchino M, Stubbs H, Nevison-Andrews D. *Pharmacol J* (1997) **260:** 207–9.

91. Tran P, Shamir E, Poyorovski M et al. Olanzapine in the treatment of patients who failed to respond to or tolerate clozapine. *Psychopharmacol Bull* (1997) **33:** 599.

92. Small JG, Kellams JJ, Milstein V, Moore J. A placebo-controlled study of lithium combined with neuroleptics in chronic schizophrenic patients. *Am J Psychiatry* (1975) **132:** 1315–17.

93. Growe GA, Crayton JW, Klass DB, Evans H, Strizich M. Lithium in chronic schizophrenia. *Am J Psychiatry* (1979) **136:** 454–5.

94. Collins P, Larkin E, Shubsachs A. Lithium carbonate in chronic schizophrenia – a brief trial of lithium carbonate added to neuroleptics for treatment of resis-tant schizophrenic patients. *Acta Psychiatr Scand* (1991) **84:** 150–4.

95. Johns C, Thompson J. Adjunctive treatments in schizophrenia: pharmacotherapies and electroconvulsive therapy. *Schizophrenia Bull* (1995) **21:** 607–19.

96. Friedel R. The combined use of neuroleptics and ECT in drug-resistant schizophrenic patients. *Psychopharmacol Bull* (1986) **22:** 928–30.

97. Benatov R, Sirota P, Megged S. Neuroleptic-resistant schizophrenia treated with clozapine and ECT. *Convulsive Ther* (1996) **12:** 117–21.

98. Remington G, Kapur S, Zirpursky R. Pharmacotherapy of first-episode schizophrenia. *Br J Psychiatry* (1998) **172(Suppl 33):** 66–70.

99. McKenna P, Bailey P. The strange story of clozapine. *Br J Psychiatry* (1993) **162:** 32–7.

100. Meltzer H, Cola P, Way L et al. Cost effectiveness of clozapine in neuroleptic-resistant schizophrenia. *Am J Psychiatry* (1993) **150:** 1630–8.

101. Reid W, Mason M, Toprac M. Savings in hospital bed-days related to treatment with clozapine. *Hosp Commun Psychiatry* (1994) **45:** 261–4.

102. Chouinard G, Albright P. Economic and health state utility determinations for schizophrenic patients treated with risperidone or haloperidol. *J Clin Psychopharmacol* (1997) **17:** 298–307.

103. Finley P, Sommer B, Corbitt J, Brunson G, Lum B. Risperidone: clinical outcome predictors and cost-effectiveness in an naturalistic setting. *Psychopharmacol Bull* (1998) **34:** 75–81.

2
Treatment of tardive dyskinesia

Stephen R Marder

Overview of tardive dyskinesia

Tardive dyskinesia (TD) is a movement disorder that occurs in some patients who have received chronic treatment with antipsychotic medications. Patients demonstrate considerable variability in the type of abnormal movements they demonstrate as well as the severity of the movements. These frequently consist of mouth and tongue movements, such as lip smacking, sucking and puckering, as well as facial grimacing. Other movements may include irregular movements of the limbs, particularly choreoathetoid-like movements of the fingers and toes and slow, writhing movements of the trunk. Younger patients tend to develop slower athetoid movements of the trunk, extremities and neck. Although most individuals with TD have relatively mild movement disorders that do not affect their overall functioning, in a small proportion it may affect walking, breathing, eating and talking. Among the most disabling forms of tardive dyskinesia are tardive dystonias. These consist of sustained contractions of muscles, most commonly in the face and neck.

Jeste and Wyatt[1] and Schooler and Kane[2] used diagnostic criteria to produce similar definitions of TD that have been widely accepted by clinicians and researchers. The abnormal movements consist of choreiform, athetoid or rhythmic movements that are reduced by voluntary movements of the affected area and increased by movements of unaffected areas.[3] TD movements tend to increase when individuals are aroused, and they are not present during sleep. The criteria also require a history of at least 3 months of antipsychotic treatment and the presence of abnormal movements for at least 4 weeks.

Although orofacial dyskinesias have been found in patients who never received antipsychotics, the prevalence is greater in patients who have received these drugs. The prevalence of TD depends upon the patient mix and treatment practices. For example, Woerner et al. found a 13.3% prevalence of TD in a voluntary hospital and 36.1% in a state hospital.[4] Since TD can be suppressed by antipsychotics, the authors also studied TD rates after some patients' medications had been discontinued.

TD rates after drug discontinuation were 67% in the state hospital, 18% in the voluntary and 17% at the Department of Veterans' Affairs Hospitals.

Prospective studies indicate that approximately 5% of patients on a conventional dopamine receptor antagonist will develop TD each year.[3] The data suggest that the risk is stable during the first 4 years, with an incidence of 5% at 1 year, 10% at 2 years, 15% at 3 and 19% at 4. For the fifth year the risk is 23% and 26% for the sixth. Other studies have shown a similar risk.[5,6] A study by Glazer found that the risk of developing TD continues to rise, with 49% of antipsychotic-treated patients meeting criteria after 10 years and 68% after 25 years.[7]

The risk of developing TD increases with age, with elderly women being at particularly high risk. For example, Saltz et al. found that 31% of elderly patients developed TD after 43 weeks of antipsychotic exposure.[8] Other proposed risk factors include affective and organic mental illness, and diabetes.[9] Other factors that have been found to be associated with an increased risk of TD include a history of treatment with high doses of antipsychotics (in some, but not all studies) and a history of extrapyramidal side-effects (EPS) sensitivity.

The risk of developing TD on newer antipsychotics is not established at this time. There is convincing evidence that clozapine is associated with a reduced and, perhaps, a negligible risk.[10] Other evidence suggests that risperidone[11] and olanzapine[12] have a substantially lower risk of causing TD when compared with conventional dopamine receptor antagonists such as haloperidol. This lower risk is supported by evidence indicating that patients who develop EPS are at a greater risk of developing TD.[11] Since newer antipsychotics (also referred to as serotonin-dopamine receptor antagonists) are associated with fewer EPS, it follows that they may have a lower TD risk.

Strategies for the treatment of mild to severe TD?

At this time, there are no definitive treatments for TD. However, there are a number of approaches that may be effective under certain conditions. This chapter reviews a number of management strategies for patients who develop TD as well as the evidence supporting each strategy. This is followed by a section that focuses on the selection of the best approach, depending upon the severity of TD and the characteristics of the patient.

Educating patients and families

The diagnosis of TD should lead to a management strategy that is developed – whenever possible – with the involvement of both the patient and family members. In most cases, participation in these decisions will come after patients and families have been educated about the disorder, its natural course, the justification for the use of antipsychotics and potential management strategies. Materials are available to assist clinicians in this education process.[13]

Patients may have fears about TD that are not based on an understanding of the disorder. For example, some may believe that TD is inevitably progressive and irreversible. However, fewer than 10% of patients with TD have a moderately severe or severe form.[14] The most common course of TD appears to be one which includes mild to moderate symptoms that vary over many years.[9] Moreover, many patients experience a substantial improvement over time even when antipsychotics are continued. These observations suggest that the diagnosis of TD does not mean that patients are likely to deteriorate into a severe and disabling movement disorder. Most patients and their families will be relieved that the natural course of TD is usually more benign than they first believed.

Discontinuing antipsychotics

Discontinuing antipsychotics may be effective in reducing the severity of TD. The likelihood of improvement or remission depends on the severity of the disorder and its duration. However, the time course of improvement is likely to be slow, with some individuals requiring years before it is apparent. For example, one study found that a majority of patients improved after gradual discontinuation of drugs over 4 years.[15] Others have found substantially lower improvement rates when patients are monitored for a briefer period.[16] Also, TD may worsen during the weeks following the discontinuation of antipsychotics. After this initial period of worsening, there is usually a later period of improvement.[17,18] Younger patients were the most likely to improve or to demonstrate remissions.

Although most patients will improve following antipsychotic withdrawal, many will not experience a remission and some will not improve. For example, one study found improvement in only 13 of 22 patients.[19] However, in individuals with mild TD and without akathisia, 5 out of 8 achieved complete remission in 2–4 years. Another study found that only 2% of TD patients achieved remission, and only 20% actually improved.[16] Patients who are younger and those who have been treated with an antipsychotic for a briefer time period are the ones most likely to improve.[20]

Vitamin E for TD

One theory of the aetiology of TD proposes that antipsychotic activity leads to the production of free radicals. Free radicals are chemical species with an unpaired electron that have been implicated in a number of central nervous system disorders including Parkinson's disease and TD. The free radicals may lead to damage of dopamine neurons which, in turn, leads to the movement disorder in TD. Since vitamin E is an antioxidant and a free radical scavenger, it has been proposed as an agent for treating TD and as a means for preventing TD in patients receiving an antipsychotic.[21]

Egan et al. reviewed 11 double-blind comparisons of vitamin E and placebo.[9] These studies were all relatively small, the largest including 35 patients. Eight studies found a reduction of TD. Of the four studies that included more than 20 patients, three found positive results. The largest study found that 5 of the 17 patients (29%) who received vitamin E experienced a greater than 33% reduction in scores on the Abnormal Involuntary Movement Scale (AIMS).[22] Patients who had TD for 5 years or less tended to have the highest response rates. Although such results might encourage the use of vitamin E, these findings need to be confirmed in a larger study. A large co-operative study from the US Department of Veterans Affairs has recently completed data collection and the results are being analysed.

An interest in antioxidant treatment has also led to studies of selegiline – which is a selective monoamine oxidase B inhibitor as well as an antioxidant. Goff and colleagues compared selegiline to placebo in 33 patients with TD in a 6-week trial.[23] Selegiline did not appear to be effective in reducing abnormal movements.

Botulinum toxin

Botulinum toxin (BTX-a) is occasionally used for severe tardive dystonia. The drug is injected into the muscle that is dystonic, where it produces a chemical denervation. Tarsy and colleagues treated 34 patients, most of whom had cervical dystonias.[24] Twenty-nine of the 34 patients had marked or moderate improvement. In clinical practice, botulinum toxin is usually reserved for severe dystonias that fail to respond to other treatments.

Other pharmacological agents

Several studies have focused on the effectiveness of calcium channel blockers as a means of suppressing TD. One theory proposes that these agents may be effective in that they block postsynaptic D_2 receptors and inhibit presynaptic dopamine activity.[25] Unfortunately, there have been very few well-controlled studies that focused on the effectiveness of these agents. A review by Cates et al. found that studies were most encouraging for nifedipine.[26] One double-blind trial found significant improvement in TD with nifedipine.[27] There are also suggestions that this agent may improve cognitive function in patients with TD.[28] This is an area where further study is definitely indicated.

Dopamine-depleting (such as reserpine, tetrabenazine and alpha-methyldopa) have been proposed as drugs for suppressing TD movements. Reserpine may be the most prescribed of these drugs for TD, but double-blind studies are limited.[29,30] In open-label trials, Fahn found that reserpine was useful in managing patients with severe TD.[19] In a double-blind study, Huang and co-workers compared reserpine, alpha-methyldopa and placebo in 30 patients with TD.[31] Both active drugs were more effective than placebo for improving TD symptoms.

Tetrabenazine has received attention on account of its being both a dopamine depleter and a dopamine receptor blocker.[32] Jankovic and Beach followed over 400 patients with different hyperkinetic movement disorders.[33] Among patients with tardive dystonia, 80.5% demonstrated marked improvements. Jankovic also carried out a double-blind crossover comparison of tetrabenazine and placebo.[34] The four patients with TD demonstrated improvement on tetrabenazine.

Soni and co-workers found that oxypertine was initially effective in reducing abnormal movements in TD.[35] However, by 6 months improvements were no longer apparent. This study underlines the important principle that treatments for TD should demonstrate their effectiveness over long-term rather than short-term trials.

Dopamine agonists – including apomorphine, bromocriptine and levodopa – may downregulate dopamine receptors.[36] Since TD has been related to an overactivity of dopamine receptors, the downregulation of receptors should lead to improvement. On the other hand, since these agents stimulate dopamine receptors, they have the potential for worsening psychotic symptoms in schizophrenia and other psychotic disorders. With these limitations, dopamine agonists have been studied as treatments for TD. Double-blind studies of levodopa have shown mixed results,[37-39] although some case reports have been encouraging. Apomorphine has received relatively little attention, and its use would seem to be limited as a result of its side-effects.

The use of drugs that affect noradrenergic systems has developed from the theory that dopamine systems may be modulated by noradrenergic pathways. The most promising agent thus far has been clonidine, which is an alpha$_2$ agonist. Four studies found improvements in TD symptoms with clonidine.[40-43] The study by Nishikawa et al. was the largest ($n = 29$).[41] In this open label study (in which patients were observed for up to 4 years), 75% of clonidine patients showed at least moderate improvements and 50% demonstrated full remission.

Propranolol, a beta-adrenergic antagonist, has also received some attention in double-blind and open-label trials.[1,44-45] Unfortunately, all these trials used relatively small sample sizes, making it difficult to draw conclusions about the effectiveness of propranolol. Propranolol has also been found effective in some cases of tardive akathisia.[46] Since tardive akathisia is often viewed as a form of TD, these observations provide further support for the effectiveness of propranolol for TD.

Cholinergic drugs

During the 1970s there was considerable interest in the effectiveness of cholinomimetic drugs. This was based on the observation that there appeared to be a dynamic balance between dopamine and acetylcholine in the basal ganglia. This suggested that the proposed excessive dopamine activity of TD could be suppressed by increasing cholinergic activity with cholinomimetics. Studies focused on deanol, lecithin and choline. For all three drugs, a number of positive studies were balanced by negative studies. Moreover, even when effects were statistically significant, they were frequently not clinically meaningful.[1]

Clozapine for TD

The effectiveness of clozapine as a treatment for TD has been demonstrated in a number of open and controlled trials (reviewed in Lieberman et al.[47]). Its effectiveness has been best documented for cases of tardive dystonia.[48] Since conventional antipsychotics will often suppress TD, a critical question is whether clozapine is more effective than these agents. Although early double-blind studies[49,50] did not find that clozapine was helpful for TD, these studies lasted only 3–5 weeks. Tamminga and co-workers found that clozapine was more effective than haloperidol at suppressing motor symptoms.[51] It is important to note that this study lasted 12 months, indicating that the differences in effects were not a temporary suppression of motor movements but appeared to be an effective treatment.

There is also evidence that clozapine is associated with a lower risk of TD. This is important because, if clozapine suppresses TD, it is important that it does not cause the condition again at a later time. This is particularly so for individuals who are vulnerable to developing TD and who will need to receive an antipsychotic. The best data indicating risk for developing TD on clozapine come from prospective studies. Data from Kane et al. using survival analysis indicate that clozapine is associated with a substantially lower risk of causing TD when compared with conventional antipsychotics studied in the same setting.[10] The study included 28 patients who were followed for at least one year. Although two individuals had ratings of TD, both had borderline TD at the start of the study. The authors concluded that it was unclear if clozapine was associated with any risk of TD, but it appeared that risk of TD was lower than with conventional drugs.

Other serotonin–dopamine antagonists

Open-label studies have provided mixed results regarding the effects of risperidone on TD.[52,53] A double-blind study suggests that risperidone may suppress abnormal movements, although this study only lasted 8 weeks and would need to be replicated by a longer-term trial.[54] More encouraging is a review by Fleischhacker using the Janssen database, which indicated that the number of new cases of TD (the incidence) appears to be lower than would be expected with a conventional dopamine receptor antagonist.[55]

There is also evidence suggesting that olanzapine is associated with a lower risk of TD than conventional drugs. Tollefson and co-workers studied the incidence of TD in patients who received either olanzapine ($n = 707$) or haloperidol ($n = 197$).[12] Patients were participants in three long-term longitudinal studies that evaluated the effectiveness and safety of olanzapine. Individuals with a history of TD or those who met TD criteria at baseline were excluded from the study in order to ensure that true incidence was being measured. One per cent of olanzapine and 4.6% of haloperidol patients met TD criteria in the final two ratings, which occurred at a median duration of 237 days for olanzapine and 203 days for haloperidol ($p = 0.003$). Since studies by Kane et al.[14] have found an incidence of about 5% per year on conventional drugs such as haloperidol, these results support strongly a lower risk of TD for olanzapine.

Approaches to disabling TD

When TD is diagnosed clinicians should re-evaluate the indications for antipsychotic medications. Although discontinuing antipsychotics may be effective in some cases, it is usually not practical. In patients with schizophrenia, 75–85% are likely to relapse during the year following the drug discontinuation,[56] and nearly all will relapse by 5 years. Also, patients, who relapse will be treated with higher doses of antipsychotics when compared with those who are stable. As a result, drug discontinuation may lead to patients actually receiving higher medication doses. In other words, discontinuing drugs is only appropriate for a small proportion of patients on antipsychotics where the indications for medication are not well established.

For individuals with mood disorders and other psychotic illnesses, the need for antipsychotics may be less clear, and discontinuing antipsychotic medications may be a reasonable consideration. For first-episode patients, the development of TD after a relatively brief course of treatment with an antipsychotic is serious and requires the implementation of a strategy both to treat the disorder and to prevent recurrences. For these individuals, the choice may be between stopping antipsychotics and substituting an antipsychotic that is unlikely to cause TD.

If the abnormal movements are severe and disabling – particularly in individuals with tardive dystonia – treatment aimed at suppressing TD may be appropriate. As noted previously, nearly all the proposed treatments for TD are unproven and unreliable. Although treatments such as noradrenergic drugs, calcium channel blockers or cholinergic drugs appear to be helpful in some individuals, their effects are not likely to be substantial. Since vitamin E's effectiveness for TD is supported by a number of double-blind trials facilitated by its being relatively benign, it may be a worthwhile adjunct to other treatments. Botulinum toxin is an effective treatment that should be reserved for the individuals with severe tardive dystonia.

The antipsychotics may be the most reliable agents for suppressing TD. However, the conventional antipsychotics (the dopamine receptor antagonists) can only provide short-term symptomatic relief and may lead to an overall worsening of TD. Moreover, in some individuals TD movements may actually worsen as the dose of an antipsychotic is increased. For these two reasons, conventional antipsychotics should not be used for treating TD. On the other hand, the newer serotonin–dopamine antagonists (SDAs) may turn out to be the most effective agents for managing severe TD. The evidence supporting clozapine as an effective agent for suppressing abnormal movements is the strongest. Tardive dystonias – one of the potentially most serious forms of TD – seem to be particularly responsive to clozapine. Unfortunately, there are no studies to indicate the relative effectiveness of clozapine and other new antipsychotics for suppressing TD. At this stage clinical reports suggest that newer agents – particularly risperidone and olanzapine – can suppress TD movements. However, clozapine is the only agent that has been demonstrated to be effective in severe TD. Clinicians may choose SDAs other than clozapine because of its other side-effects (such as sedation, seizures and a risk of agranulocytosis).

Managing relatively mild tardive diskinesias

Most tardive diskinesias are mild and have minimal effects on the quality of life of patients who have the abnormal movements. Individuals with these mild symptoms may be concerned with the cosmetic effects of the abnormal movements (particularly when they affect the face) and may also be concerned that a mild TD will progress to a more severe disorder. For these individuals the choice of a strategy may depend on how long the TD has existed and the patient's age. If TD has been stable for years, the likelihood that a mild movement disorder will become severe is very small. For most of these individuals, TD may vary over time, but it is unlikely to progress to a disabling disorder.[57]

For these individuals and their treating clinicians, there are a number of options that can be considered. In some patients, it may be appropriate to continue the patient's pharmacotherapy with the understanding that the mild TD may not improve but that it is unlikely to worsen. There are suggestions that reducing the dose of the conventional antipsychotic may be helpful,[58] although a relationship between the dose of an anti-psychotic and the risk of TD has not been clearly demonstrated. Never-theless, it seems reasonable to manage patients with the lowest effective dose of an antipsychotic, since this may reduce EPS and the subsequent risk of the development of TD. A number of studies indicate that a sub-stantial proportion of stabilized patients with schizophrenia can be man-aged with relatively low doses of a conventional antipsychotic.[59-61] Strategies are also available to minimize the risk of patients who have had their dosages reduced.[62]

Patients with mild TD may also be candidates for other strategies that may minimize the risk that mild TD will worsen. For example, it has been proposed that vitamin E may reduce the risk that TD will progress.[63] Although this effect remains unproven, prescribing doses of 1200–1600 IU is not associated with any substantial risk.

Switching patients from a conventional DA to a newer serotonin dopamine antagonist (SDA) may also be reasonable for patients with milder TDs. As mentioned earlier, there is some evidence that drugs such as clozapine, risperidone and olanzapine are associated with a reduced risk of TD. Other new drugs with reduced EPS may have the same effect. Again, since there is no proven treatment for managing mild TD, clini-cians may consider prescribing a newer drug since there is a reasonable chance that it will reduce the likelihood of the abnormal movements wors-ening over time.

Summary

Although many medications have been tested in TD, none has distin-guished itself as being clearly effective. The most reliable drugs for sup-pressing abnormal movements may be the antipsychotics – the agents responsible for the disorder. The serotonin–dopamine antagonists (espe-cially clozapine) may have the advantage of being able to suppress the abnormal movements of TD without contributing to the progression of the illness.

The selection of a management strategy for TD is dependent upon the severity of the movement disorder. Patients who have severe and dis-abling TD may benefit from having their antipsychotics switched to cloza-pine or one of the other SDAs. Mild TDs are unlikely to progress to severe TD and may not require definitive treatment. However, patients with mild TD may also benefit from being switched to a newer SDA. Vitamin E, although not proven to be effective, is a benign treatment and may be considered for both mild and severe TD.

References

1. Jeste DV, Wyatt RJ. *Understanding and Treating Tardive Dyskinesia* (New York: Guilford Press, 1982).

2. Schooler NR, Kane JM. Research diagnostic criteria for tardive dyskinesia. *Arch Gen Psychiatry* (1982) **37:** 486–7.

3. Kane JM, Lieberman J. Tardive dyskinesia. In Kane JM, Lieberman JA (eds) *Adverse Effects of Psychotropic Drugs* (New York: Guilford Press, 1992): 235–45.

4. Woerner M, Kane JM, Lieberman JA et al. The prevalence of tardive dyskinesia. *J Clin Psychopharmacol* (1991) **11:** 34–42.

5. Yassa R, Nair V, Schwartz G. Tardive dyskinesia: a two-year followup study. *Psychosomatics* (1984) **25:** 852–5.

6. Chouinard G, Annable L, Mercier P, Ross-Chouinard A. A five-year follow-up study of tardive dyskinesia. *Psychopharmacol Bull* (1986) **22:** 259–63.

7. Glazer WM, Morgenstern H, Schooler NR et al. Predicting the long-term risk of tardive dyskinesia in outpatients maintained on neuroleptic medications. *J Clin Psychiatry* (1993) **54:** 133–9.

8. Saltz BL, Woerner M, Kane JM et al. Prospective study of tardive dyskinesia in the elderly. *JAMA* (1991) **266:** 2402–6.

9. Egan MF, Apud J, Wyatt RJ. Treatment of tardive dyskinesia. *Schizophrenia Bull* (1997) **23:** 583–609.

10. Kane JM, Woerner MG, Pollack S, Safferman AZ, Lieberman JA. Does clozapine cause tardive dyskinesia? *J Clin Psychiatry* (1993) **54:** 327–30.

11. Casey DE. Will the new antipsychotics bring hope of reducing the risk of developing extrapyramidal syndromes and tardive dyskinesia? *Int Clin Psychopharmacol* (1997) **12(Suppl):** S19–27.

12. Tollefson GD, Beasley CM Jr, Tamura RN, Tran PV, Potvin JH. Blind, controlled, long-term study of the comparative incidence of treatment-emergent tardive dyskinesia with olanzapine or haloperidol. *Am J Psychiatry* (1997) **154:** 1248–54.

13. Wyatt RJ. *Practical Psychiatric Practice: Clinical Interview Forms, Rating Scales and Patient Handouts.* (Washington, DC: American Psychiatric Press, 1995).

14. Kane JM, Woerner M, Lieberman JA et al. Tardive dyskinesia: prevalence, incidence, and risk factors. *J Clin Psychopharmacol* (1988) **8(Suppl 4):** 52–6.

15. Jus A, Jus K, Fontaine P. Long-term treatment of tardive dyskinesia. *J Clin Psychiatry* (1979) **40:** 72–7.

16. Glazer WM, Hafez HM. A comparison of masking effects of haloperidol versus molindone in tardive dyskinesia. *Schizophrenia Res* (1990) **3:** 315–20.

17. Gardos G, Cole JO, Rapkin RM et al. Anticholinergic challenge and neuroleptic withdrawal. *Arch Gen Psychiatry* (1984) **41:** 1030–5.

18. Glazer WM, Bowers MB, Charney DS et al. The effect of neuroleptic discontinuation on psychopathology, involuntary movements, and biochemical measures in patients with persistent tardive dyskinesia. *Biol Psychiatry* (1989) **26:** 224–33.

19. Fahn SA. A therapeutic approach to tardive dyskinesia. *J Clin Psychiatry* (1985) **464:** 19–24.

20. Smith JM, Baldessarini RJ. Changes in prevalence, severity and recovery in tardive dyskinesia. *Arch Gen Psychiatry* (1980) **37:** 1368–73.

21. Lohr JB. Oxygen radicals and neuropsychiatric illness. Some speculations. *Arch Gen Psychiatry* (1991) **48:** 1097–106 (review).

22. Lohr JB, Caliguri MP. A double-blind placebo controlled study of vitamin E treatment of tardive dyskinesia. *J Clin Psychiatry* (1996) **57:** 167–73.

23. Goff DC, Renshaw PF, Sarid-Segal O et al. A placebo-controlled trial of selegiline (L-deprenyl) in the treatment of tardive dyskinesia. *Biol Psychiatry* (1993) **33:** 700–6.

24. Tarsy D, Kaufman D, Sethi KD et al. An open-label study of botulinum toxin A for treatment of tardive dystonia. *Clin Neuropharmacol* (1997) **20:** 90–3.

25. Mena MA, Garcia MJ, Tabernero C et al. Effects of calcium antagonists on the dopamine system. *Clin Neuropharmacol* (1995) **18:** 410–26.

26. Cates M, Lusk K, Wells BG. Are calcium-channel blockers effective in the treatment of tardive dyskinesia? *Ann Pharmacother* (1993) **27:** 191–6.

27. Suddath RL, Straw GM, Freed WJ et al. A clinical trial of nifedipine in schizophrenia and tardive dyskinesia. *Pharmacol Biochem Behav* (1991) **39:** 743–5.

28. Schwartz BL, Fay-McCarthy M, Kendrick K et al. Effects of nifedipine, a calcium channel antagonist, on cognitive function in schizophrenic patients with tardive dyskinesia. *Clin Neuropharmacol* (1997) **20:** 364–70.

29. Duvoisin RC. Reserpine for tardive dyskinesia. *N Engl J Med* (1972) **286:** 611.

30. Sato S, Daly R, Peters H. Reserpine therapy of phenothiazine induced dyskinesia. *Dis Nerv Sys* (1971) **32:** 680–5.

31. Huang CC, Wang RI, Hasegawa A, Alverno L. Reserpine and alpha-methyldopa in the treatment of tardive dyskinesia. *Psychopharmacology* (1981) **73:** 359–62.

32. Kazamatsuri H, Chien CP, Cole JO. Long-term treatment of tardive dyskinesia with haloperidol and tetrabenazine. *Am J Psychiatry* (1973) **130:** 479–83.

33. Jankovic J, Beach J. Long-term effects of tetrabenazine in hyperkinetic movement disorders. *Neurology* (1997) **48:** 358–62.

34. Jankovic J. Treatment of hyperkinetic movement disorders with tetrabenzaine: a double-blind crossover study. *Ann Neurol* (1982) **11:** 41–7.

35. Soni SD, Freeman HL, Bamrah JS, Sampath G. Oxypertine in tardive dyskinesia: a long-term controlled study. *Acta Psychiatr Sand* (1986) **74:** 446–50.

36. Reches A, Wagner HR, Jiang D et al. The effect of chronic L-dopa administration on supersensitive pre- and postsynaptic dopaminergic receptors in rat brain. *Life Sci* (1982) **31:** 37–44.

37. Casey DE, Gerlach J, Bjorndal N. Levodopa and receptor sensitivity modification in tardive dyskinesia. *Psychopharmacology* (1982) **78:** 89–92.

38. Simpson GM, Yadalam KG, Stephanos MJ. Double-blind carbidopa/levodopa and placebo study in tardive dyskinesia. *J Clin Psychopharmacol* (1988) **8(Suppl 4):** 49S–51S.

39. Ludatscher JI. Stable remission of tardive dyskinesia by L-dopa. *J Clin Psychopharmacol* (1989) **9:** 39–41.

40. Freedman R, Kirch D, Bell J et al. Clonidine treatment of schizophrenia. Double-blind comparison to placebo and neuroleptic drugs. *Acta Psychiatr Scand* (1982) **65:** 35–45.

41. Nishikawa T, Tanaka M, Tsuda A et al. Clonidine therapy for tardive dyskinesia and related syn-

dromes. *Clin Neuropharmacol* (1984) **7:** 239–45.

42. Browne J, Silver H, Martin R et al. The use of clonidine in the treatment of neuroleptic-induced tardive dyskinesia. *J Clin Psychopharmacol* (1986) **6:** 88–92.

43. Tripodianakis J, Markianos M. Clonidine trial in tardive dyskinesia, therapeutic response, MHPG, and plasma DBH. *Pharmacopsychiatry* (1986) **19:** 365–7.

44. Perenyi A, Farkas A. Propranolol in the treatment of tardive dyskinesia. *Biol Psychiatry* (1983) **18:** 391–4.

45. Schrodt GR Jr, Wright JH, Simpson R et al. Treatment of tardive dyskinesia with propranolol. *J Clin Psychiatry* (1982) **43:** 328–31.

46. Sachdev P, Loneragan C. Intravenous benztropine and propranolol challenges in tardive akathisia. *Psychopharmacology* (1993) **113:** 119–22.

47. Lieberman JA, Saltz BL, Johns CA et al. The effects of clozapine on tardive dyskinesia. *Br J Psychiatry* (1991) **158:** 503–10.

48. Lamberti JS, Bellnier T. Clozapine and tardive dystonia. *J Nerv Ment Dis* (1993) **181:** 137–8.

49. Gerlach J, Koppelhus P, Helweg E, Monrad A. Clozapine and haloperidol in a single-blind crossover trial: therapeutic and biochemical aspects in the treatment of schizophrenia. *Acta Psychiatr Scand* (1974) **50:** 410–24.

50. Caine ED, Polinsky RJ, Kartzinel R et al. The trial use of clozapine for abnormal involuntary movement disorders. *Am J Psychiatry* (1979) **136:** 317–20.

51. Tamminga CA, Thaker GK, Moran M et al. Clozapine in tardive dyskinesia: observations from human and animal model studies. *J Clin Psychiatry* (1994) **55(Suppl B):** 102–6.

52. Meco G, Bedini L, Bonifanti V et al. Risperidone in the treatment of chronic schizophrenia with tardive dyskinesia: a single-blind crossover study versus placebo. *Curr Ther Res* (1989) **46:** 876–83.

53. Kopala LC, Honer WG. Schizophrenia and severe tardive dyskinesia responsive to risperidone. *J Clin Psychopharmacol* (1994) **14:** 430–1.

54. Chouinard G, Annable L, Ross-Chouinard A et al. Effects of risperidone in tardive dyskinesia: an analysis of the Canadian Risperidone Study. *J Clin Psychopharmacol* (1995) **15(Suppl 1):** 36–44.

55. Fleischhacker WW. The importance of EPS in the management of schizophrenia – the place of the newer antipsychotics. Paper presented at the 10th ECNP Congress, Vienna, Austria, September 1997.

56. Kissling W, Kane JM, Barnes TRE et al. Guidelines for neuroleptic relapse prevention in schizophrenia: towards a consensus view. In Kissling W (ed) *Guidelines for Neuroleptic Relapse Prevention in Schizophrenia* (Berlin: Springer-Verlag, 1991): 155–63.

57. Kane JM. Tardive dyskinesia: epidemiological and clinical presentation. In Bloom FE, Kupfer DJ (eds) *Psychopharmacology: The Fourth Generation of Progress* (New York: Raven Press, 1995): 1485–96.

58. Chakos MH, Alvir JM, Woerner MG et al. Incidence and correlates of tardive dyskinesia in first episode of schizophrenia. *Arch Gen Psychiatry* (1996) **53:** 313–19.

59. Kane JM, Rifkin A, Woerner M. Low dose neuroleptic treatment of outpatient schizophrenics. I. Preliminary results for relapse rates. *Arch Gen Psychiatry* (1983) **40:** 893–6.

60. Marder SR, Van Putten T, Mintz J et al. Low and conventional dose maintenance therapy with fluphenazine decanoate: two year outcome. *Arch Gen Psychiatry* (1987) **44:** 518–21.

61. Hogarty GE, McEvoy JP, Munetz M et al. Dose of fluphenazine, familial expression emotion, and outcome in schizophrenia: results of a two-year controlled study. *Arch Gen Psychiatry* (1988) **45:** 797–805.

62. Marder SR, Wirshing WC, Van Putten T et al. Fluphenazine versus placebo supplementation for prodromal signs of relapse in schizophrenia. *Arch Gen Psychiatry* (1994) **51:** 280–7.

63. Akar S, Jajor TR, Kumar S. Vitamin E in the treatment of tardive dyskinesia. *J Postgrad Med* (1993) **39:** 124–6.

3
Unstable manic-depressives

Michael Bauer

Introduction

The primary goal of prophylactic drug treatment in bipolar disorder is to modify and reduce the symptomatic expression of the illness with the result that fewer, shorter and milder phases occur. Modern mood-stabilizing drugs prevent the vast majority of patients from relapses and lead to interepisodic remission. Lithium can still be regarded as the first-choice substance in the prophylactic treatment of the 'classic' form of bipolar disorder. Valuable alternatives (carbamazepine and valproate) and other new agents have helped to circumvent refractoriness in those patients who do not respond to lithium monotherapy. However, even after introducing new agents about 10–20% of treated bipolar patients seem to remain refractory to prophylaxis. This chapter presents an overview of the prophylactic approaches and strategies applied in patients with refractory bipolar disorder, e.g. double and triple combinations of established mood stabilizers, adjunctive high-dose thyroid hormones, calcium channel antagonists, the addition of atypical neuroleptics and new anticonvulsants (e.g. lamotrigine and gabapentin). Conclusions for the optimization of prophylaxis in bipolar illness are given and available options are summarized in a treatment algorithm.

Epidemiology and course of manic-depressive illness

Manic-depressive illness (the modern diagnostic manuals prefer the term 'bipolar disorder') is a recurrent, long-term mood disorder characterized by the occurrence of both manic and depressive episodes or mixed episodes that appears in approximately 0.4–1.7% of the population.[1] It has been estimated that without adequate treatment the average patient experiencing the onset of bipolar disorder when aged 25 will suffer from a few episodes; however, 10–15% of patients will undergo more than 10 episodes. The most important progress in the treatment of bipolar disorder was the development of effective mood-stabilizing drugs, beginning with lithium (now more than 40 years ago).[2] However, despite the availability of drug alternatives to lithium in cases of refractoriness (the anticonvulsants carbamazepine and valproate), up to 10–20% of patients fail to improve satisfactorily with pharmacological prophylaxis. Patients with recurrent affective disorders who do not respond adequately to prophylactic treatment and remain treatment refractory are one of the challenging therapeutic issues in psychiatry today. Beside the problem of refractoriness to prophylaxis, interepisodic mood stabilization remains another important goal in the treatment of the disorder. Although the majority of individuals with bipolar disorder return to full recovery between affective episodes, approximately 20–30% continue to display interepisodic mood lability and interpersonal or occupational difficulties.[3]

Some pathophysiological considerations

In the study of the pathophysiology of manic-depressive illness, an unusual association has been described among gender, thyroid disease, affective illness and treatment with lithium–the major prophylactic drug in bipolar illness. Female gender and thyroid dysfunction have repeatedly been discussed as risk factors for the development of affective disorders. One of the most important associations (because of its clinical relevance) is the finding that female gender and hypothyroid states increase the risk that manic-depressive illness will become prophylaxis resistant and induce rapid cycling.[4]

Frequency and characteristics of rapid cycling

Rapid cycling disease (RCD), defined as the occurrence of at least four affective episodes during the previous 12 months, is the most malignant form of bipolar illness. This subpopulation is characterized by severe morbidity and a refractory clinical course.[5] Rapid cycling affects 10–15% of all bipolar patients with equal frequency in bipolar type I and type II patients.[6] Rapid cycling occurs predominantly in women, with 70–95% of rapid cycling patients being female.[5,7–10] This is in contrast to the even gender distribution found in studies of unselected bipolar patients.[1] Treatment is particularly problematic, as most patients with RCD are generally unresponsive to lithium therapy and at present there are no established treatment guidelines for this disease.[6,11,12]

Risk factors for rapid cycling

Antidepressants
Tricylic antidepressants (TCAs), and perhaps other drugs that affect monoaminergic neurotransmitter systems, have been implicated in triggering rapid mood cycling. The evidence for the association of anti-

depressants in the induction of rapid cycling has come from a number of studies designed to assess the efficacy of antidepressants in depressive disorders. Wehr and colleagues noted that continued administration of antidepressant drugs was responsible for rapid cycling in approximately 50% of 51 bipolar patients.[7] Kukopulos and colleagues demonstrated that antidepressant use caused an acceleration in the cycle frequency from 0.8 per year prior to treatment to 6.5 episodes per year following administration of these drugs.[13] Others have estimated that 20% of all cases of rapid cycling are caused by antidepressant treatment and that 95% of spontaneous rapid cycling patients may worsen with the use of antidepressants, mainly tricyclics.[9] However, this issue remains controverse and other authors stated that antidepressant-related switching and cycle acceleration are rare phenomena.[14] Because of their increasing use in clinical practice, the question has often been raised if the newer antidepressants have a lowered risk of inducing cycling acceleration. A meta-analysis by Peet of all available controlled trials of selective serotonin reuptake inhibitors (SSRIs) vs. TCAs revealed that the rate of manic switch in bipolar patients treated with SSRIs was significantly lower than in patients treated with TCAs.[15]

To summarize, it is generally recommended that antidepressants should be avoided in rapid cycling patients, particularly in cases where the rate of cycling or the length of the depressive phase are less than 4 weeks. If a patient with rapid cycling is on an antidepressant medication, the patient should be taken off this medication as soon as possible. The concomitant addition of a (second) mood stabilizer may then be necessary.

Female gender

Epidemiological data show that rapid cycling is more common among bipolar women.[6,10] In contrast to this clear association, the effects of reproductive system events (e.g. menstrual cycle, pregnancy, postpartum period, menopause, use of oral contraceptives and use of hormone replacement therapy) on the course of bipolar disorder have received little systematic study.[10] Uncontrolled observations have shown that estrogen may induce rapid cycling,[16] and that menstrually related mood changes may occur in some rapid cycling patients.[17] In addition, events associated with the reproductive cycle are capable of provoking affective changes in predisposed individuals. Examples include depression associated with oral contraceptives, the luteal phase of the menstrual cycle, the postpartum period and the menopause.[18] However, there has been no systematic study to explore the contributing role that female steroids may play in determining the specific interrelationship between female gender and RCD.[4]

Thyroid dysfunction

The lifetime prevalence of thyroid disease in women is some 4–10 times higher than estimates for men (e.g. women experience more goiter and autoimmune disease).[4] RCD is significantly associated with clinically overt hypothyroidism or grade I hypothyroidism.[8] Grade I hypothyroidism occurs disproportionally more frequently in RCD compared with nonrapid cycling bipolar disorder. Significantly, this association is independent of potential confounding factors such as lithium use. A high proportion of patients with RCD and hypothyroidism are women: approximately 58% of those experiencing 4–11 episodes a year are women, whereas virtually 100% of the individuals suffering 12 or more episodes are women.[4,6]

Lithium interference with thyroid axis

Lithium salts are drugs widely used in the acute and prophylactic treatment of affective disorders.[19] However, patients with RCD are particularly resistant to treatment with lithium.[5,6] Subsequently, a far higher incidence of peripheral thyroid disorder (mainly hypothyroidism) has been reported in those lithium-treated individuals who have a profile of rapid episodes when compared with patients with general bipolar disturbance.[8,20] Though various mechanisms, lithium interferes directly with thyroid hormone metabolism: its 'antithyroid' effects can cause goiter and hypothyroidism.[20,21] Preclinical studies report that lithium inhibits the conversion of thyroxine (T_4) to tri-iodothyronine (T_3) in the brain,[22] and it diminishes thyroid function by altering feedback mechanisms at several levels of the thyroid axis. Whybrow and co-workers (pers. comm.) have recently explored the response of the thyroid axis to lithium carbonate in rapid cycling male and female patients, comparing the response to one month with gender-and age-matched control groups. They found differences across the four groups: lithium challenge of the hypothalamic–pituitary–thyroid (HPT) axis tended to decrease thyroid functioning in patients with rapid cycling bipolar disorder more than in normal controls, an effect that was more prominent in female patients. It was concluded that rapid cycling female patients appeared to have a greater disturbance of their thyroid function regulation at the pituitary level compared with other groups.

In summary, it could be said that (adapted from ref.[4]):

- RCD is the most malignant form of bipolar illness, occurring predominantly in women;
- hypothyroidism is a major risk factor for RCD;
- women are at greater risk of thyroid disease than men;
- female gender increases the risk that bipolar illness will become prophylaxis resistant and develop into RCD;

- most patients with RCD are resistant to lithium;
- the therapeutic use of lithium in bipolar illness appears to play an important role in such associations because lithium is 'antithyroid'; and
- TCAs can increase episode frequency in rapid cycling.

Pharmacological treatment of bipolar disorder

In the management of bipolar illness the primary goals are the prevention of future affective episodes and the treatment of acute depressive and manic breakthrough episodes. Further goals are to deter patients making suicide attempts, to prevent the development of rapid cycling and to improve interepisodic mood lability. Bipolar morbidity and mortality can be significantly reduced by specific pharmacotherapy, if applied correctly. Lithium has been established as the clear first-choice drug for long-term maintenance treatment and for use in bipolar mania.[2,3,19,23] Beside its ability to prevent manic and depressive episodes, lithium has specific additional effects on mood and behaviour. Its value is underlined because of its proven effects against aggression, impulsivity[24] and suicidality.[24,25] However, a proportion of patients with bipolar illness fail to show adequate response to lithium. Failure rates for bipolar disorder with lithium prophylaxis have been estimated to be between 30 and 50%,[3,26] dependent upon the applied diagnostic criteria. New drugs and combination/augmentation strategies have therefore been introduced into mood-stabilizing treatments in the past 15 years (Table 3.1). However, empirical data on how to treat patients with prophylaxis-resistant and rapid cycling mood disorders are rare, and controlled trials are missing.[19]

Patterns affecting initial drug selection

To avoid and circumvent prophylaxis resistance in bipolar disorder, it is essential to take into account the differential efficacy of the various drugs used in maintenance treatment. Specific patterns and subgroups have been identified where the response to prophylactic drugs is either more favourable or poorer.

Lithium
A recent 2.5-year randomized multicentre study has shown that lithium is superior to carbamazepine in preventing hospitalizations and recurrences in bipolar patients with 'classical' clinical features (e.g. bipolar type I disorder without mood-incongruent delusions and without comorbidity.[27] Further clinical features associated with a good response to lithium include a family history of bipolar disorder and a personal history of a previous sequence of mania–depression euthymia.[28] The clinical features that predict a poorer outcome with lithium use in patients include

Table 3.1 Alternatives in the prophylactic pharmacotherapy of bipolar disorder.

	Treatment	Examples
Established mood stabilizers	Lithium salts	Lithium carbonate
	Classic anticonvulsants	Carbamazepine Valproate
Nonestablished mood stabilizers and drug combinations	Combination lithium + anticonvulsant (double combination)	Lithium + valproate Lithium + carbamazepine
	Combination anticonvulsant 1 + anticonvulsant 2	Valproate + carbamazepine
	Adjunctive thyroid hormones	High-dose levothyroxine (T_4)
	Triple combination of mood stabilizer	Lithium + valproate + carbamazepine
	Calcium channel antagonists (CCA)	Verapamil Nimodipine
	Adjunctive neuroleptics	Atypical (clozapine, olanzapine) Typical (haloperidol, perazine)
	New anticonvulsants	Lamotrigine Gabapentin
	Electroconvulsive therapy (ECT)	

- mixed or dysphoric mania;
- rapid cycling;
- mania with psychosis;
- a negative family history of affective illness in first-degree relatives;
- an occurrence of comorbid substance and alcohol dependency; and
- a pattern of illness with a direct switch from depression into mania.[29]

Carbamazepine and valproate

In contrast to the data available for lithium, there have been fewer studies of the clinical factors that predict a favourable response to carbamazepine and valproate.[30] *Carbamazepine* has been proven to be superior to lithium in bipolar patients with 'non classical' features – e.g. bipolar type II disorder (with hypomanic episodes), mood incongruent delusions, comorbidity and mixed states during the acute episodes.[27] In addition, Post and co-workers found that rapid cycling and a negative family history of mood disorder were associated with carbamazepine response.[31] The clinical factors associated with a good response to *valproate* maintenance treatment in bipolar patients include

- mixed mania;
- dysphoric mania;
- rapid cycling.[30]

An algorithmic approach to the pharmacological treatment of refractory bipolar illness

Systematic and treatment algorithms may help to prevent or overcome therapy refractoriness. Sequential treatment plans have been introduced in psychiatry, mainly in the treatment of refractory affective disorders.[32,33] The long-term and episodic course of bipolar affective disorder presents an excellent challenge to the physician who is conducting a systematic treatment plan. The bipolar patient who does not respond to treatment with a single mood stabilizer should, therefore, be managed using this systematic and procedural algorithmic approach (Table 3.2).

Optimizing prophylactic treatment

A substantial proportion of patients (approximately 30–50%) with recurrent affective disorders do not respond sufficiently to standard prophylactic drugs when these are administered as monotherapy. Such patients may be suitable candidates for a switch to different mood stabilizers or for a combination of two mood-stabilizing drugs (double combination).

Table 3.2   A systematic treatment algorithm for the maintenance treatment of refractory bipolar illness.

1	*Optimize the current treatment regimen according to the guidelines given in Table 3.3, and exclude 'pseudo-refractoriness'.*
2A	*Add a second established mood stabilizer (double combination, see Table 3.1)*
	or
2B	*Switch to another established mood stabilizer if*

- severe side-effects from the current medication endanger compliance;
- the course of the illness worsened during the use of the current prophylactic drug (e.g. an increase in the cycling pattern);

Note: Do not discontinue lithium without first reconsidering carefully its effect on the illness's previous course, including suicidal features.

3A	*Add a third established mood stabilizer (triple combination)*
	or
3B	*Change the double combination of the established mood stabilizer (see Table 3.1)*
	or
3C	*Add a neuroleptic drug* (in patients with predominantly manic episodes)
	or
3D	*Augment with thyroid hormones* (augment levothyroxine (T_4) in supraphysiological doses and aim for TSH suppression).
4	*Use new drugs*

- Calcium channel blockers (e.g. for ultra-rapid cycling patterns);
  or
- new anticonvulsants (lamotrigine or gabapentine).

The question of which procedure is to be recommended in such a situation cannot at present be satisfactorily answered from the available data-bases. Controlled data do not exist to guide the psychiatrist in choosing whether to replace one monotherapy with another or when to add a second drug. The unanswered question is whether the second drug may potentiate the actions of the first – even if the first drug initiated an inadequate response. A review of the literature and experience reveal that adding a second mood stabilizer rather than switching to a different drug seems to be the method of choice.[19] However, before combination treatment is initiated prophylactic monotherapy should be optimized (Table 3.3).

The first step in the selection of an appropriate alternative treatment is to illustrate graphically any history of a previous course of illness (the frequency, amplitude and duration of affective episodes, and hospitaliza-

Table 3.3 Guidelines for the optimization of prophylaxis in unstable manic-depressives.

- Use the appropriate systematic life-chart methodology (the graphical reconstruction of the previous course of the illness and its medication).
- Verify the diagnosis 'bipolar illness' with respect to the subtypes and specifiers of illness (e.g. rapid cycling, seasonal pattern, psychotic features).
- Check compliance more frequently (blood drug levels).
- Exclude occult somatic illness (e.g. endocrine dysfunctions, neurological and autoimmune diseases).
- Exclude psychiatric comorbidity (e.g. substance dependency).
- Explore for underlying interpersonal and social problems.
- Treat somatic and psychiatric comorbidity.
- Increase the blood levels of mood-stabilizing drugs to their upper limits (if side-effects allow):
  — lithium up to 1.0 mmol/l
  — carbamazepine up to 10–12 mg/l
  — valproate up to 100–120 mg/l
- Discontinue drugs that induce rapid cycling (tricyclics, psychostimulants).
- Add low-dose L-thyroxine (50–125 µg/d) if basal TSH is elevated (grade II or subclinical hypothyroidism).

tions) and subsequent medication (the life-chart methodology[34]). This will establish cycling patterns, treatment failures and intolerance, and possible refractoriness after the discontinuation of prophylaxis (a typical case of such graphic representation is given in Figure 3.1). This figure provides a rapid overview of the longitudinal course of an illness and it clarifies the medication (non-)responsiveness of a female, rapid cycling bipolar type II patient. The patient was unresponsive to amitriptyline, lithium and carbamazepine, given alone or in combination; cycling was finally stopped after the addition of high-dose thyroxine (300 µg/day) to lithium (for treatment with high-dose thyroxine – see below).

It is clear that treatment intolerance secondary to side-effects that are left untreated will lead to poor treatment compliance; other factors that frequently lead to noncompliance are the patient's illness concepts and treatment expectations when these differ from those of the treating physician. A lack of sufficient information about the course and treatment of the illness may be resolved by restating the instructions and through programmes of education. Recommending suitable books to read will help patients and their relatives to understand the disorder more fully and will also help them to comply with the required treatments (excellent books have been written by Schou,[35] Greil et al.[36] and Whybrow[37]).

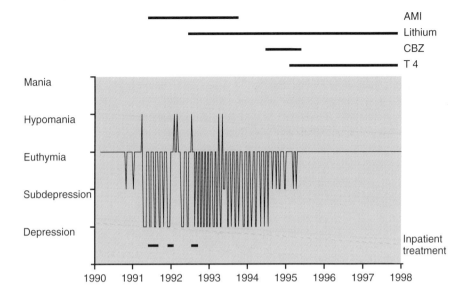

Figure 3.1

Graphing the course of illness of a 44-year-old female bipolar patient with rapid cycling. The affective status is plotted on the ordinate, the time course on the abscissa. The bars at the top indicate prophylactic medication. The time of hospitalization is indicated at the bottom of the diagram.

AMI = amitriptyline; CBZ = carbamazepine; T4 = high-dose levothyroxine.

In the second step of diagnosis, the condition itself should be reconsidered. Diagnostic classification should be assessed carefully with regard to clinical subtypes (e.g. dysphoric subtypes, mixed affective states and atypical features) and the specifiers of the disorder (e.g. the occurrence of rapid cycling, seasonal patterns and psychotic features).[38] Somatic and mental comorbidity should be excluded by appropriate investigations and, if detected, treated adequately. Endocrine (thyroid dysfunction) and neurological disorders, as well as substance dependencies (alcohol, benzodiazepines and psychostimulants), are frequently underlying diseases that cause 'pseudo-refractoriness' to prophylactic treatment. The blood levels of mood stabilizers may be increased to the upper end of the usual therapeutic range.[39,40]

Empirical evidence for combining mood stabilizers

A number of observations have been conducted into patients' beneficial responses to combined mood-stabilizer treatment. These observations have been made from case reports, retrospective studies and open clinical trials. To date, no controlled study has been undertaken to prove the efficacy of a combined treatment strategy. However, clinical practice has shown that a substantial part of those who are nonresponders to monotherapy improves when two or more mood stabilizers are used concurrently.

Choice of a second mood stabilizer

If a patient needs to be maintained on more than one mood-stabilizing drug, the choice of the second drug may be made according to the clinical characteristics that have been identified as correlating with a higher rate of response (see above). The combination that has been most extensively studied in series of open trials is the combination of lithium and carbamazepine.[41-44] Lithium and carbamazepine have additive therapeutic effects in refractory bipolar illness, particularly in patients who are unresponsive to either drug used alone. Coadministration has usually been found to be safe, but some patients have suffered from an increase in neurological side-effects. In open trials, lithium and valproate have been described as effective,[45] and this combination has the advantage that each does not interfere with the metabolism of the other.[46] Some pharmacokinetic interactions have been identified between carbamazepine and valproate (e.g. carbamazepine may lower valproate levels).[47,48] Serum monitoring is therefore necessary more frequently when the two anticonvulsants are used in combination.[46]

Alternatives to established mood stabilizers – adjunctive and new drugs

Thyroid hormone augmentation
It has long been recognized that the state of the thyroid can have a profound effect on mental function. A large corpus of literature has accumulated that shows an association between disturbances of the hypothalamic–pituitary–thyroid (HPT) axis and mood disorders. Studies have also demonstrated a high incidence of psychiatric illness in patients with both hyper- and hypothyroidism.[49] In open studies, the use of high-dose thyroxine as an adjunct to prophylactic agents, such as lithium and the anticonvulsants, has recently been shown to induce clinical remission in prophylaxis-resistant bipolar illness, particularly in women.[50-52] In a study of 11 patients with rapid cycling disorder, adjunctive treatment with TSH-suppressive doses of T_4 reduced the manic and depressive phases in both their amplitude and frequency, and even led to remission in some patients.[50] Open trials have shown the efficacy of high-dose levothyroxine (between 300 and 600 µg/day) in prophylaxis-resistant mood disorder,[51,52]

and in refractory-depressed unipolar and bipolar patients.[53] For inclusion in the prophylaxis study,[52] patients had to have failed two or more standard, adequately conducted, prophylactic treatments. High-dose thyroxine was added in an open fashion to the stable baseline medication (e.g. lithium, carbamazepine or a combination of both). Since 1990, 20 patients with recurrent mood disorder have been included in the study, and the overall clinical outcome has been favourable: the mean number of relapses during the follow-up period of each patient declined significantly in the respective periods prior to the institution of high-dose T_4 (evaluation was by the so-called 'mirror method': the decline of mean recurrences was from 4.6 to 1.5). Nine patients (45%) were full responders (no more relapses after T_4 institution); 7 patients (35%) were partial responders (episodes milder, rare and/or shorter); and 4 patients (20%) did not respond. Tolerability of high T_4 doses was good, and side-effects occurred only rarely (some patients had no side-effects at all).[52] However, it must be emphasized that these favourable adjunctive thyroid hormone observations need to be confirmed through controlled studies.

Benzodiazepines

Benzodiazepines play a minor role in the prophylaxis of bipolar disorder because of their potential risk of creating dependency. However, in the acute manic phase and on a short-term basis, a benzodiazepine is often helpful when given with a primary mood-stabilizing agent. Benzodiazepines are effective in the rapid sedation of the acutely hyperactive and excited manic patient. Further, benzodiazepines may reduce the requirement for antipsychotics. The two benzodiazepines commonly used in bipolar disorder are lorazepam and clonazepam. These are also effective in improving sleep in manic or depressed patients.[54]

Neuroleptics

Long-term neuroleptic treatment should be avoided in the maintenance treatment of affective disorders, as these are likely to cause tardive dyskinesia.[55] However, an adjunctive trial with a neuroleptic is justified in refractory bipolar patients who have predominantly manic episodes. Clozapine (an atypical neuroleptic with antagonism of dopamine (D_1-D_4) and serotonin ($5-HT_2$) receptors) is a potent mood stabilizer that has been used effectively in the treatment of affectively ill patients who were refractory to standard treatments. The anti-manic and prophylactic effects of clozapine have been described at a dose of up to 500 mg/d. The efficacy of clozapine has been shown in case series and open trials in patients who have bipolar disorder with psychotic features, bipolar rapid cycling and dysphoric mania.[56-59] Because of its similar pharmacological receptor profile, the new antipsychotic drug, olanzapine, seems to be an interesting alternative to clozapine. However, systematic studies have not yet been published.

Calcium channel antagonists

The calcium channel antagonists (CCAs), or calcium channel blocking agents, comprise a class of medications that are usually administered for the treatment of cardiovascular disorders, such as hypertension and cardiac arrhythmias. Evidence from basic research that links disturbed calcium ion metabolism to affective disorders has led to the use of CCAs in various indications for bipolar disorder.[54,60] The clinical efficacy of verapamil in the treatment of acute mania has been shown in open and placebo-controlled trials.[61] In a controlled double-blind trial, nimodipine had positive effects on rapid-cycling patients.[62]

New anticonvulsants

Among a group of new, approved anticonvulsants that have few side-effects are lamotrigine and gabapentin – two anticonvulsants that have recently been studied in case series and open trials in the treatment of bipolar disorders. Evidence from these trials suggest that lamotrigine[63,64] and gabapentin[65,66] possess a broad spectrum of efficacy in refractory bipolar disorder, including depression, mania and mixed states. Until these observations are confirmed by controlled trials, these new anticonvulsants should be applied only to refractory patients.

Treatment of depressive breakthrough episodes

Although lithium has been established as a first-line prophylactic medication in recurrent affective disorders, and especially in bipolar disorder, patients on lithium prophylaxis may still experience a depressive relapse. In general, all antidepressants that have been shown to be effective in treating major depression are also effective in treating bipolar depression, and it is reasonable to assume that this applies to breakthrough episodes of major depression during lithium prophylaxis. However, few controlled studies have been reported that specifically address the issue of the adjunctive psychopharmacologic treatment of acute depressive episodes during lithium prophylaxis.[67] Treatment of the depressive phase is often complicated by the potential risks of a rapid change to mania which is caused by the use of antidepressant drugs (for discussion, see above). Paroxetine represents the more recently developed class of SSRI antidepressants that have gained wide acceptance in clinical and general practice because of improved tolerability and relative safety in overdose as compared with the TCAs. The results from a number of recent controlled and naturalistic studies provide evidence that many physicians combine an SSRI (citalopram, fluoxetine, fluvoxamine, paroxetine or sertraline) and lithium to treat depressive episodes. A 6-week randomized, double-blind study has recently been completed to compare the efficacy and safety of antidepressant augmentation (paroxetine vs. amitriptyline) in lithium-maintained patients suffering from a depressive breakthrough episode.[68] After 4 weeks, a significantly greater proportion of patients in the paroxetine group had achieved a 50% reduction in depressive symptoms, and the mean improvement in the Clinical Global Impression (CGI) severity of illness was significantly greater in the paroxetine group at week 3–5. The type and number of emergent events occurring during study treatment corresponded to the known side-effect profiles of paroxetine and amitriptyline. It was proposed that the more rapid improvement demonstrated by the group receiving the combination of lithium and SSRI may be due to the synergistic serotonergic effects of these two medications.[68] In cases of severe and refractory depressive breakthrough episodes, electroconvulsive therapy (ECT) is recommended on the grounds of its proven strong antidepressant efficacy, especially in patients with delusions.[23,67]

Treatment of manic breakthrough episodes

If a bipolar patient suffers from a manic breakthrough episode, specific-manic therapies should be implemented as early as possible.[54] As a first step, the current mood stabilizer should be elevated to the maximum tolerated blood level. Manic patients frequently need larger lithium doses in the acute manic episode to achieve higher blood levels. The established mood stabilizers (lithium, carbamazepine and valproate) have good antimanic properties. However, they all have a lag phase until they show their specific effects. One of the reasons for this is that it takes several days until adequate serum drug levels are achieved. In hyperactive and aggressive patients, therefore, it is unavoidable but to administer tranquillizing doses of benzodiazepines (e.g. lorazepam 2–6 mg/day) or neuroleptics to control agitation and sleep.[23,69] Delusional patients should additionally be treated with high-potency neuroleptics (e.g. haloperidol). Patients with milder forms of mania may be treated with an additional anticonvulsant (e.g. carbamazepine or valproate). Dysphoric and mixed manic patients will benefit especially from valproate.[30,32]

Modalities and consequences of lithium discontinuation

In the course of bipolar illness the treating physician often faces the problem of deciding how long prophylactic treatment should be maintained. Patients frequently discontinue lithium on their own because of side-effects, from a feeling of loss of creativity or because of a longing for (hypo-)manic episodes. On medical advice lithium is often discontinued for its lack of efficacy, for signs of toxicity, severe adverse events and before a planned pregnancy. Discontinuation of long-term lithium maintenance therapy in bipolar patients has been associated with a significant short-term increase in the risk of recurrence.[70] After discontinuation as a result of 'unresponsiveness', the patient and the physician often realize that the lithium medication was necessary when the patient experiences a recurrence after having stopped prophylaxis. There is strong clinical evidence that, if discontinuation becomes necessary, lithium should be discontinued gradually whenever possible: abrupt discontinuation seems to be associated with an increased risk of recurrence, whereas gradual discontinuation may reduce a high risk of early relapse.[71] The recommendation is to taper the lithium dose over a period of weeks (or preferably months) and to look carefully for any signs that might indicate a new episode.[19] This strategy is also recommended for the discontinuation of other prophylactic agents.

Loss of efficacy after lithium discontinuation?

After discontinuation of lithium prophylaxis, affective morbidity and subsequently risk of suicide increase,[73] particularly after abrupt removal of the drug. Potential loss of efficacy after discontinuation and reinstitution of lithium prophylaxis has been reported but this issue remains controversial. Some authors have described the phenomenon of 'lithium-discontinuation-induced refractoriness'[73,74] and have noted that non-response to reinstituted lithium maintenance should be considered among the possible risks of interrupting effective lithium prophylaxis.[75,76] Other authors conclude from an analysis of the life-charts of bipolar patients that such a phenomenon appears to be very rare and may be caused by inappropriate patient selection for long-term lithium treatment.[77] More recently, Post and co-workers have proposed that the therapeutic loss of drug efficacy may also occur in the course of long-term treatment with valproate and carbamazepine.[78]

Summary

Drugs that stabilize mood are the most important tool in the treatment of patients with manic-depressive (bipolar) illness. The primary goal of prophylactic drug treatment is to modify and reduce the symptomatic expression of the illness, with the result that fewer, shorter and milder phases occur. Modern mood-stabilizing drugs prevent the vast majority of patients from relapsing and lead to interepisodic remission. Most experts still regard lithium as the drug of first choice in the prophylaxis of this recurrent long-term mood disorder. Valuable alternatives (carbamazepine and valproate) and other new agents and strategies (e.g. double and triple combinations of established mood stabilizers, adjunctive high-dose thyroid hormones, calcium channel antagonists, atypical neuroleptics – i.e. clozapine – and new anticonvulsants) have assisted in circumventing refractoriness in those patients who do not respond to lithium monotherapy. However, even after the introduction of new agents and the optimization of treatment, about 10–20% of treated bipolar patients seem to remain refractory to prophylaxis, and some develop rapid cycling. Skilful (poly-)pharmacological interventions and algorithmic treatment approaches are therefore needed to improve the course of the most malignant forms of manic-depressive illness. Further criteria for resistance to prophylactic treatment have to be established, and it is suggested that at least two adequate trials of more than 12 months' duration (6 months' in rapid cycling) at sufficient drug blood levels should be performed before refractoriness is discussed.

References

1. Robins LN, Regier DA (eds). *Psychiatric Disorders in America* (New York: Free Press, 1991).

2. Schou M. Forty years of lithium treatment. *Arch Gen Psychiatry* (1997) **54:** 9–13.

3. Goodwin FK, Jamison KR. *Manic-Depressive Illness* (New York: Oxford University Press, 1990).

4. Whybrow PC. Sex differences in thyroid axis function: relevance to affective disorder and its treatment. *Depression* (1995) **3:** 33–42.

5. Dunner DL, Fieve RR. Clinical factors in lithium carbonate prophylaxis failure. *Arch Gen Psychiatry* (1974) **30:** 229–33.

6. Bauer MS, Whybrow PC. Rapid cycling bipolar disorder: clinical features, treatment, and etiology. In Amsterdam JD (ed) *Advances in Neuropsychiatry and Psychopharmacology. Vol. 2. Refractory Depression* (New York: Raven Press, 1991): 191–208.

7. Wehr T, Sack D, Rosenthal N et al. Rapid cycling affective disorder: contributing factors and treatment responses in 51 patients. *Am J Psychiatry* (1988) **145:** 179–84.

8. Bauer MS, Whybrow PC, Winokur A. Rapid cycling bipolar affective disorder. I. Association with grade I hypothyroidism. *Arch Gen Psychiatry* (1990) **47:** 427–32.

9. Bauer MS, Calabrese J, Dunner DL et al. Multisite data reanalysis of the validity of rapid cycling as a course modifier for bipolar disorder in DSM-IV. *Am J Psychiatry* (1994) **151:** 506–15.

10. Leibenluft E. Women with bipolar illness: clinical and research issues. *Am J Psychiatry* (1996) **153:** 163–73.

11. Sharma V, Persad E. Pharmacotherapy of rapid cycling bipolar disorder: a review. *Lithium* (1994) **5:** 117–25.

12. Krüger S, Bräunig P, Young LT. Biological treatment of rapid-cycling bipolar disorder. *Pharmacopsychiatry* (1996) **29:** 167–75.

13. Kukopulos A, Reginaldi D, Laddomada P et al. Course of the manic-depressive cycle and changes caused by treatments. *Pharmakopsychiatrie-Neuropsychopharmacol* (1980) **13:** 156–67.

14. Coryell W, Endicott J, Keller M. Rapidly cycling affective disorder. Demographics, diagnosis, family history, and course. *Arch Gen Psychiatry* (1992) **49:** 126–31.

15. Peet M. Induction of mania with selective serotonin re-uptake inhibitors and tricyclic antidepressants. *Br J Psychiatry* (1994) **164:** 549–50.

16. Oppenheim G. A case of rapid

mood cycling with estrogen: implications for therapy. *J Clin Psychiatry* (1984) **45:** 34–5.

17. Price W, DiMarzio L. Premenstrual tension syndrome in rapid-cycling bipolar affective disorder. *J Clin Psychiatry* (1986) **47:** 415–17.

18. Parry BL. Mood disorders linked to the reproductive cycle in women. In Bloom FE, Kupfer DJ (eds) *Psychopharmacology: The Fourth Generation of Progress* (New York: Raven Press, 1995): 1029–42.

19. Bauer M, Ahrens B. Bipolar disorder. A practical guide to drug treatment. *CNS Drugs* (1996) **6:** 35–52.

20. Cho JT, Bone S, Dunner DL et al. The effect of lithium treatment on thyroid function in patients with primary affective disorder. *Am J Psychiatry* (1979) **136:** 115–16.

21. Bschor T, Bauer M. Thyroid function and treatment with lithium. *Nervenarzt* (1998) **69:** 189–95.

22. St Germain D. Regulatory effect of lithium on thyroxine metabolism in murine neural and anterior pituitary tissue. *Endocrinology* (1987) **120:** 430–8.

23. American Psychiatric Association. Practice guideline for the treatment of patients with bipolar disorder. *Am J Psychiatry* (1994) **151(Dec Suppl):** 1–36.

24. Sheard MH, Marini JL, Bridges CI et al. The effect of lithium on impulsive aggressive behavior in man. *Am J Psychiatry* (1976) **133:** 1409–13.

25. Müller-Oerlinghausen B, Ahrens B, Grof E et al. The effect of long-term lithium treatment on the mortality of patients with manic-depressive or schizo-affective illness. *Acta Psychiatr Scand* (1992) **86:** 218–22.

26. Vestergaard P. Treatment and prevention of mania: a Scandinavian perspective. *Neuropsychopharmacology* (1992) **7:** 249–60.

27. Greil W, Kleindienst N, Erazo N et al. Differential response to lithium and carbamazepine in the prophylaxis of bipolar disorder. *J Clin Psychopharmacol*, in press.

28. Grof P, Alda M, Grof E et al. The challenge of predicting response to stabilising lithium treatment. *Br J Psychiatry* (1993) **163(Suppl 21):** 16–19.

29. Frye MA, Altshuler LL. Selection of initial treatment for bipolar disorder, manic phase. In Rush AJ (ed) *Mood Disorders. Systematic Medication Management* (Basel: Karger, 1997): 88–113.

30. Keck PE, McElroy SL. Outcome in the pharmacological treatment of bipolar disorder. *J Clin Psychopharmacol* (1996) **16(Suppl 1):** 15S–23S.

31. Post RM, Uhde TW, Roy-Byrne PP et al. Correlates of antimanic response to carbamazepine. *Psychiatry Res* (1987) **21:** 71–83.

32. Sachs GS. Bipolar mood disorder: practical strategies for acute and maintenance phase treatment. *J Clin Psychopharmacol* (1996) **16(Suppl 1):** 32–47.

33. Berghöfer A, Müller EB, Bauer M et al. Sequentielle Behandlungsstrategien zur Vermeidung und Überwindung von Therapieresistenz bei depressiven Erkrankungen. In Bauer M, Berghöfer A (eds) *Therapieresistente Depressionen* (Berlin, Heidelberg and New York: Springer-Verlag, 1997): 235–43.

34. Post RM, Roy-Byrne PP, Uhde TW. Graphic representation of the life course of illness in patients with affective disorder. *Am J Psychiatry* (1988) **145:** 844–8.

35. Schou M. *Treatment of Manic-Depressive Illness: A Practical Guide* (5th edn) (New York: Karger Verlag, 1993).

36. Greil W, Sassim N, Ströbel-Sassim C. *Manic-Depressive Illness:*

Therapy with Carbamazepine (Stuttgart and New York: Thieme Verlag, 1996).

37. Whybrow PC. *A Mood Apart. Depression, Mania, and Other Afflictions of the Self* (New York: Basic Books, 1997).

38. American Psychiatric Association. *Diagnostic and Statistical Manual: DSM-IV* (4th edn) (Washington, DC: American Psychiatric Press, 1994).

39. Gelenberg AJ, Kane JM, Keller MB et al. Comparison of standard and low serum levels of lithium for maintenance treatment of bipolar disorders. *N Engl J Med* (1986) **321:** 1489–93.

40. Simhandl Ch, Denk E, Thau K. The comparative efficacy of carbamazepine low and high serum level and lithium carbonate in the prophylaxis of affective disorders. *J Affect Disorders* (1993) **28:** 221–31.

41. Nolen WA. Carbamazepine, a possible adjunct or alternative to lithium in bipolar disorder. *Acta Psychiatr Scand* (1983) **67:** 218–25.

42. Di Constanzo E, Schifano F. Lithium alone or in combination with carbamazepine for the treatment of rapid-cycling bipolar affective disorder. *Acta Psychiatr Scand* (1991) **83:** 456–9.

43. Peselow ED, Fieve RR, Difiglia C et al. Lithium prophylaxis of bipolar illness. The value of combination treatment. *Br J Psychiatry* (1994) **164:** 208–14.

44. Bocchetta A, Chillotti C, Severino G et al. Carbamazepine augmentation in lithium-refractory bipolar patients. A prospective study on long-term prophylactic effectiveness. *J Clin Psychopharmacol* (1997) **17:** 92–6.

45. Sharma V, Persad E, Mazmanian D et al. Treatment of rapid cycling bipolar disorder with combination therapy of valproate and lithium. *Can J Psychiatry* (1993) **38:** 137–9.

46. Bowden CL. Role of newer medications for bipolar disorder. *J Clin Psychopharmacol* (1996) **16(Suppl 1):** 48S–55S.

47. Ketter TA, Pazzaglia PJ, Post RM. Synergy of carbamazepine and valproic acid in affective illness: case report and review of the literature. *J Clin Psychopharmacol* (1992) **12:** 276–81.

48. Tohen M, Castillo J, Pope HG et al. Concomitant use of valproate and carbamazepine in bipolar and schizoaffective disorders. *J Clin Psychopharmacol* (1994) **14:** 67–70.

49. Whybrow PC. The therapeutic use of triiodothyronine and high dose thyroxine in psychiatric disorder. *Acta Med Austriaca* (1994) **21:** 44–7.

50. Bauer MS, Whybrow PC. Rapid cycling bipolar affective disorder. II. Treatment of refractory rapid cycling with high-dose levothyroxine: a preliminary study. *Arch Gen Psychiatry* (1990) **47:** 435–40.

51. Baumgartner A, Bauer M, Hellweg R. Treatment of intractable non-rapid cycling bipolar affective disorder with high-dose thyroxine: an open clinical trial. *Neuropsychopharmacology* (1994) **10:** 183–9.

52. Bauer M. High-dose thryoxine in prophylaxis resistant affective disorder. *Biol Psychiatry* (1997) **42:** 78S–79S.

53. Bauer M, Hellweg R, Gräf KJ et al. Treatment of refractory depression with high-dose thryoxine. *Neuropsychopharmacology* (1998) **18:** 444–55.

54. Post RM, Denicoff KD, Frye MA et al. Algorithms for bipolar mania. In Rush AJ (ed) *Mood Disorders. Systematic Medication Management* (Basel: Karger, 1997): 114–45.

55. Mukherjee S, Rosen AM, Caracci G et al. Persistent tardive dyskinesia in bipolar patients. *Arch Gen Psychiatry* (1996) **43:** 342–6.

56. Calabrese JR, Meltzer HY, Markovitz PJ. Clozapine prophylaxis in rapid cycling bipolar disorder. *J Clin Psychopharmacol* (1991) **11:** 396–7.

57. McElroy SL, Dessain EC, Pope HG Jr et al. Clozapine in the treatment of psychotic mood disorders: schizoaffective disorder, and schizophrenia. *J Clin Psychiatry* (1991) **52:** 411–14.

58. Banov MD, Zarate CA, Tohen M et al. Clozapine therapy in refractory affective disorders: polarity predicts response in long-term follow-up. *J Clin Psychiatry* (1994) **55:** 295–300.

59. Suppes T, Phillips KA, Judd CR. Clozapine treatment of non-psychotic rapid cycling bipolar disorder: a report of three cases. *Biol Psychiatry* (1994) **36:** 338–40.

60. Dubovsky SL, Buzan R. The role of calcium channel blockers in the treatment of psychiatric disorders. *CNS Drugs* (1995) **4:** 47–57.

61. Garza-Trevino ES, Overall JE, Hollister LE. Verapamil versus lithium in acute mania. *Am J Psychiatry* (1992) **149:** 121–2.

62. Pazzaglia PJ, Post RM, Ketter TA et al. Preliminary controlled trial of nimodipine in ultra-rapid cycling affective dysregulation. *Psychiatry Res* (1993) **49:** 257–72.

63. Calabrese JR, Bowden CL, McElroy SL et al. Lamotrigine in bipolar disorder: preliminary data. *American Psychiatric Association Annual Meeting, Syllabus & Proceedings Summary* 1997 (abstract no. 33B).

64. Sporn J, Sachs G. The anticonvulsant lamotrigine in treatment-resistant manic-depressive illness. *J Clin Psychopharmacol* (1997) **17:** 185–9.

65. Bennett J, Goldman WT, Suppes T. Gabapentin for treatment of bipolar and schizoaffective disorders. *J Clin Psychopharmacol* (1997) **17:** 141–2.

66. Schaffer CB, Schaffer LC. Gabapentin in the treatment of bipolar disorder. *Am J Psychiatry* (1997) **154:** 291–2.

67. Zornberg GL, Pope Jr HG. Treatment of depression in bipolar disorder: new directions for research. *J Clin Psychopharmacol* (1993) **13:** 397–408.

68. Bauer M, Zanninelli R, Müller-Oerlinghausen B et al. Paroxetine and amitriptyline augmentation of lithium in the treatment of major depression: a double blind study. *J Clin Psychopharmacol* (1999) (in press).

69. Sachs GS, Weilburg JB, Rosenbaum JF. Clonazepam vs neuroleptics as adjuncts to lithium maintenance. *Psychopharmacol Bull* (1990) **26:** 137–43.

70. Suppes T, Baldessarini RJ, Faedda GL et al. Risk of recurrence following discontinuation of lithium treatment in bipolar disorder. *Arch Gen Psychiatry* (1991) **48:** 1082–8.

71. Faedda GL, Tondo L, Baldessarini RJ et al. Outcome after rapid vs. gradual discontinuation of lithium treatment in bipolar disorders. *Arch Gen Psychiatry* (1993) **50:** 448–55.

72. Müller-Oerlinghausen B, Ahrens B, Glaenz T et al. Mortality of patients who dropped out from regular lithium prophylaxis: a collaborative study by the International Group for the Study of Lithium-Treated Patients. *Acta Psychiatr Scand* (1996) **94:** 344–77.

73. Post RM, Leverich GS, Altshuler L. Lithium-discontinuation-induced refractoriness: preliminary observations. *Am J Psychiatry* (1992) **149:** 1727–9.

74. Bauer M. Refractoriness induced by lithium-discontinuation despite adequate serum lithium levels. *Am J Psychiatry* (1994) **151:** 1522.

75. Maj M, Pirozzi R, Magliano L. Non-response to reinstituted lithium prophylaxis in previously responsive bipolar patients: prevalence and predictors. *Am J Psychiatry* (1995) **152:** 1810–11.

76. Tondo L, Baldessarini RJ, Floris G et al. Effectiveness of restarting lithium treatment after its discontinuation in bipolar I and bipolar II disorders. *Am J Psychiatry* (1997) **154:** 548–50.

77. Berghöfer A, Müller-Oerlinghausen B. No loss of efficacy after discontinuation and reinstitution of long-term lithium treatment? In Gallicchio VS, Birch NJ (eds) *Lithium: Biochemical and Clinical Advances* (Cheshire, CT: Weidner Publishing Group, 1996): 39–46.

78. Post RM, Denicoff KD, Frye MA et al. A history of the use of anticonvulsants as mood stabilizers in the last two decades of the 20th century. *Neuropsychobiology* (1998) **38:** 152–66.

4

Treatment-resistant unipolar depression

Graham D Burrows and Trevor R Norman

Introduction

The prognosis for unipolar depression is relatively favourable, with psychological well-being and high functioning usually being restored by an adequate course of antidepressant medications or other forms of therapy (e.g. cognitive behaviour therapy). In those patients for whom pharmacotherapy is deemed appropriate, it is well recognized that perhaps as many as 30–40% do not respond to the first course of drug treatment chosen. Many (perhaps a further 10–15%) are helped by a course of another antidepressant from a different chemical class or by electroconvulsive therapy (ECT). There remains a residual group of patients (about 5–10%) for whom multiple interventions are unhelpful and who remain depressed and do not achieve a satisfactory level of functioning.[1] This group of patients has been referred to as treatment-resistant, refractory depression or intractable depression.[2]

Treatment-resistant depression: a review of definitions

A number of authors have reviewed the concept of treatment-resistant depression and commented on the lack of uniformity of diagnostic criteria.[1-3] Clearly the absence of agreement hinders empirical research into aetiology and treatment. One simple definition of treatment-resistant depression proposed by Fava and Davidson[1] is the failure to achieve and sustain euthymia with an adequate antidepressant treatment. Helmchen[4] proposed a failure to respond to two successive courses of pharmacologically different antidepressants given in adequate dosage and for a sufficient period. Each of these definitions, while apparently useful, has some inherent weaknesses, not the least of which is what constitutes an adequate treatment trial. A high proportion of patients referred to tertiary settings for evaluation and management of resistant depression have clearly not received an adequate antidepressant trial. Many general practitioners do not use recommended doses or are reluctant to exceed these doses of antidepressant drugs.[5] Such cases of inadequate treatment do not constitute treatment resistance.

Adequacy of treatment remains a vexed question. The issues of both dose and compliance with treatment are inherent in any such definition. There is no correct dosage for an individual antidepressant. Interindividual differences in drug handling and factors such as age, sex, weight, physical condition and the presence or absence of concomitant medications will determine how well a patient will tolerate a particular agent. Less problematic is the question of compliance, where plasma-level monitoring may ensure that patients at least achieve steady state. More contentious is the issue of the relationship of plasma concentration and clinical efficacy. While for some antidepressants therapeutic ranges have been reported, for many tricyclic antidepressants (TCAs) and for the newer agents in particular, the data are too sparse to be reliable. Adequacy of treatment cannot be ensured merely from the attainment of steady-state plasma levels.

Assessment of what constitutes an acceptable response to treatment varies substantially among clinical investigators.[6] In controlled clinical evaluations standardized rating scales, such as the Hamilton Depression Rating scale, are used to assess response. A frequently used criterion of full remission is a decrease in the initial Hamilton score of >50%. For many patients who meet the 50% decline only, this represents at best a partial response to medication, particularly where their initial depression score is high. More stringent criteria, such as a decline in Hamilton score to a range within that observed in normal subjects, can be regarded as a complete remission.

An adequate length of treatment is an important variable for the assessment of antidepressant response. Several studies have established that trials of short duration (4 weeks or less) are inadequate to establish the efficiency of antidepressant treatments.[7–10] For example, after 5 weeks, response to high doses of imipramine was shown to occur in only 25% of patients, whereas by 17 weeks 75% of patients treated had responded.[7] In elderly depressed patients, 12 weeks of treatment was necessary for a response to either phenelzine or nortriptyline.[11] While failure to respond to continuous therapy of a single antidepressant for 12 weeks might constitute one definition of treatment resistance, this has some practical limitations. First, there are the ethical considerations of a patient being inadequately treated for such a long period. Secondly, there are questions of patient tolerance and compliance with a drug regimen which may produce side-effects and pose a risk of toxicity in overdose.

Resistance, relapse and recurrence

Further confounding the diagnosis of treatment resistance is the failure to distinguish resistance from relapse or recurrence.[12] In this context relapse or recurrence can be taken to mean the return of symptoms to the point of meeting the criteria for major depression after having made an initial response to treatment. Clearly the distinction between these labels for an individual patient needs to be made on the basis of a longitudinal history, as clinical features are unlikely to distinguish them. Patient recall biases may underestimate the efficacy of previous drug treatments so that recurrence, relapse and resistance become indistinguishable. Thus the term 'treatment resistant depression' is properly reserved for patients whose depression is nonresponsive despite at least two treatment trials with drugs from pharmacologically different classes, each used in adequate doses for adequate time periods.[2,4] In order to define more precisely the notion 'treatment resistance' the staging of patients according to past treatment history has been proposed[2] (see Table 4.1). Typically, patients move through the stages according to the number and classes of antidepressants to which they have failed to respond. While such a staging approach has merit for producing a uniform classification, the reliability of data on which it might be based is limited by the accuracy of patient recall and medical records.

While treatment-resistant depression is well recognized as a significant clinical problem, an agreement on uniform diagnostic criteria has been difficult to achieve. Pragmatically the definitions offered by Thase and Rush[2] and Helmchen,[4] notwithstanding the caveats discussed here, would appear to be acceptable to most.

Table 4.1   Staging of depression based on past treatment responses.[a]

Stage	Treatment response
0	No adequate medication trials
1	One adequate medication trial but not responsive
2	Two different adequate trials of monotherapy from different classes (such as TCAs, SSRIs), but not responsive
3	Stage 2 with the addition of failure to respond to one augmentation strategy (such as lithium) of a monotherapy
4	Stage 3 with the addition of failure to respond to a second augmentation
5	Stage 4 with the addition of failure to respond to ECT

Note:
[a]Staging criteria are those of Thase and Rush.[2]

Treatment strategies for resistant depression

Despite the lack of adequate criteria for defining treatment resistance, numerous controlled and uncontrolled pharmacological management strategies have been published.[2,6,13] Critical to the evaluation of the usefulness of any such strategy must be the authors' criteria for the definition of treatment resistance. To overcome this potential difficulty, Thase and Rush[2] advocate a conservative approach, namely, to extend the duration of the ineffective medication treatment for another 2–4 weeks at an optimized dose. Failure to respond under these circumstances will necessitate discontinuation of the ineffective agent and substitution of an alternative medication. Switching between TCAs is frequently employed in clinical practice but there is little empirical evidence to suggest that such a strategy is useful, while the use of other heterocyclic antidepressants apparently fares just as poorly in clinical studies (see Table 4.2). In cases of nonresponse to a course of TCAs, better empirical evidence is available to support the use of specific serotonin reuptake inhibitors (SSRIs) as the next line of treatment (see Table 4.2). Whether this represents a strategy for 'treatment resistance' is a moot point as it could be argued that, in the course of 'normal' treatment, where one agent has failed, it would be prudent to utilize drugs from other classes. Given the range of antidepressants currently available and their putatively different

Table 4.2   Efficacy of antidepressants used following treatment failure.[a]

Antidepressant	Population[b]	Prior treatment	% responders	Reference
Desipramine	UP (n = 11)	TCAs[c]	9	80
Imipramine	UP (n = 27)	TCAs	30	81
Imipramine	UP (n = 15)	Paroxetine	73	82
Imipramine	UP (n = 22)	Phenelzine	41	83
Nomifensine	UP (n = 10)	TCAs	10	84
Nomifensine	UP, BP (n = 20)	TCAs	20	85
Trazodone	UP, BP (n = 25)	TCAs	56	86
Oxaprotiline	UP (n = 64)	TCAs, fluvoxamine	33	87
Fluoxetine	UP (n = 40)	TCAs	43	81
Fluoxetine	UP (n = 35)	TCAs	51	88
Fluvoxamine	UP (n = 56)	TCAs, oxaprotiline	4	87
Fluvoxamine	UP (n = 28)	TCAs	28	89
Fluvoxamine	UP (n = 12)	Desipramine	75	90
Paroxetine	UP (n = 10)	Imipramine	50	82
Paroxetine	UP (n = 28)	TCAs	64	91

Notes:
[a]Modified from Thase and Rush.[2]
[b]UP = unipolar depression; BP = bipolar depression.
[c]TCAs = tricyclic antidepressants.

mechanisms of action, criteria for treatment resistance could be readily met without exhausting all the 'pharmacologically different' drugs. Much of the literature reporting medication trials in 'treatment-resistant patients' reflects a contemporary confusion between increasing the rate of response in depressed patients and increasing the proportion of patients who respond. This distinction is important in the context of evaluating the efficacy of combinations of medications in treatment resistance. Increasing the speed of onset of medication does not equate to increasing the proportion of patients who respond to a drug combination. This confusion has arisen where some combinations of medications, e.g. lithium and tricyclics, pindolol and SSRIs, have been used both in the context of increasing the proportion of previously unresponsive patients who respond to the medication (i.e. quasi-treatment-resistant patients) and to speed the onset of action of the drug in patients who may or may not have been unresponsive to previous drug treatments. For many studies this distinction is not clear and a precise definition of the term 'treatment resistance' is lacking. As far as possible the present review is of studies in which patients have been shown to be unresponsive to previous medication trials. There is no lack of approaches that have been applied to treatment-resistant patients. By far the most advocated strategies have relied upon combinations of medications, some of which would be usually regarded as contraindicated.

Lithium augmentation

Addition of lithium to an existing antidepressant regimen has been recommended in treatment-resistant depression.[14] Table 4.3 summarizes some studies examining lithium augmentation of antidepressants. The efficacy of the strategy has been well documented.[15–17] Enhanced response to a lithium–TCA combination was reported based on case studies,[18] and subsequently confirmed in a placebo-controlled, double-blind study.[19] In eight patients who had failed to respond to at least 3 weeks of antidepressant treatment, addition of lithium was reported to decrease depressive symptoms significantly within 48 hours.[20] Using a double-blind placebo-controlled study, the efficacy of lithium addition to patients nonresponsive to 3 weeks' treatment with TCAs or mianserin could be confirmed, but the rapid response could not.[21] Sustained reduction in depression scores has been noted in some studies within 7 days of commencing lithium[22,23] while other studies suggest that up to 6 weeks may be required for response.[24] Meta-analysis of placebo-controlled studies of lithium augmentation in resistant depression showed nearly 40% response to this strategy.[25]

Addition of lithium to the monoamine oxidase (MAO) inhibitors isocarboxazid and tranylcypromine has also been shown to be of benefit in treatment-resistant depression.[26,27] In patients previously unresponsive to

Table 4.3 The effect of lithium augmentation of antidepressants in treatment-resistant depression: representative data.

Study design	Definition of resistance	No. patients (age range)	Drugs used (dosage)	Efficacy	Reference
Open evaluation	1) Failure to respond to 3 weeks' TCA 2) HAM-D (Hamilton Depression Rating Scale) decreased <40% of baseline	34 (27–66 years)	AMI 217 mg/day $n = 16$ IMI[a] 225 mg/day $n = 12$ TRI[a] 204 mg/day $n = 6$ DMI[a] 237 mg/day $n = 4$ DOX[a] 181 mg/day $n = 4$ Li[a] 900 mg/day	30/42 trials resulted in 50% improvement in 48 hours Side-effects: tremor, abdominal pain, pruritis ($n = 3$) Lithium plasma level 0.4–1.2 mmol/l	20
Placebo-controlled, double-blind comparative study	1) Failure to respond to 3 weeks' TCA 2) HAM-D decreased <50% of baseline	15 (23–68 years)	DMI 150–250 mg/day $n = 6$ AMI 150–300 mg/day $n = 5$ MIA 90–120 mg/day $n = 4$ Li 900–1200 mg/day	Lithium induced a significant improvement mostly after 5–8 days Crossover of patients in the initial placebo addition group produced rapid improvement Lithium plasma level 0.5–1.1 mmol/l	21
Open evaluation	1) No response to 4 weeks' TCA 2) No response to lithium augmentation 3) Minimal improvement on clinical scales	12 (20–68 years)	TRANYL 30–60 mg/day Li 600–1200 mg/day	Global ratings showed 67% response rate; 8/12 patients much or very much improved Side-effects: orthostatic hypotension, no major adverse effects Lithium plasma level 0.6–1.3 mmol/l	29

Design	n (age)	Criteria	Drug/dose	Results	Ref.
Blind study	15 (24–60 years)	No response to chronic CARBAM therapy	CARBAM 200–1600 mg/day Li 1116 mg/day	8/15 (53%) patients were ratec improved following lithium addition Side-effects: 7 patients weakness, tiredness, headache, diarrhoea, nausea, dizziness Lithium plasma level 0.7–1 2 mmol/l	92
Open evaluation	9 (65–93 years)	No response to adequate courses of TCA	LOF 140–210 mg/day $n = 8$ AMI 150 mg/day $n = 1$ Li 400 mg/day	7/9 patients made good recovery at follow-up over 20 months Lithium plasma level 0.4–1.1 mmol/l	93
Random assignment	41 (39.6 ± 9.9 years)	No response to 8 weeks' FLX	FLX 40–60 mg/day $n = 15$ FLX 20 mg/day + DMI 20–25 mg/day $n = 14$ FLX 20 Li 300–600 mg/day $n = 12$	4/14 patients on Li + FLX recovered Lithium plasma level 0.21 mmol/l	31
Placebo-controlled, double-blind comparative study	51 (37.4 ± 11.2 years)	Failure to respond to DMI or IMI at 2.5 mg/kg for 5 weeks	T_3 37.5 µg/day $n = 17$ Li 900 mg/day $n = 17$ Placebo $n = 16$ DMI, IMI 150–300 mg/day	10/17 responded to T_3; 9/17 to lithium; 3/16 to placebo Lithium plasma level >0.55 mmol/l	94

Notes:
AMI = amitriptyline; CARBAM = carbamazepine; DMI = desipramine; DOX = doxepin; FLX = fluoxetine; IMI = imipramine; Li = lithium; LOF = lofepramine; MIA = mianserin; T_3 = L-tri-iodothyronine; TCA = tricyclic antidepressant; TRANYL = tranylcypromine; TRI = trimipramine.

phenelzine, lithium addition was able to increase the therapeutic benefits.[28] An open evaluation of tranylcypromine and lithium in severely depressed inpatients resistant to other treatments produced sufficient improvement for all 12 patients to be discharged.[29] Augmentation by lithium of the responses to SSRIs has been described in some open and double-blind evaluations.[22,30–33] Response rates were generally similar to those observed in trials with other antidepressants, while the onset of action was also similar.

Lithium augmentation appears to be most successful when steady-state plasma concentrations are maintained within the usual therapeutic range, while a period of 3–4 weeks would seem to be an adequate length of time in which to judge clinical response.[34] Factors predicting outcome in lithium augmentation were investigated in a series of inpatients.[35] Bipolar diagnosis, improvement within 1 week and less-severe illness indicated a better prognosis. Similarly in 105 patients with resistant depression, response to lithium addition was predicted by significant weight loss, psychomotor retardation and poor control of cortisol secretion (high post-dexamethasone cortisol levels).[36] Severe depression appears to respond less frequently to lithium addition and is associated with a poor prognosis.[15] A 5-year follow-up of responders to augmentation with lithium indicated that they were less likely to have recurrent episodes of depression, while suicide attempts, completed suicide and hospitalizations were more frequent in nonresponders.[37,38]

Augmentation by lithium of TCAs is generally well tolerated. The side-effects of the various combinations are those that would be anticipated from the use of either drug alone. Serotonin syndrome has been reported when lithium is administered with SSRIs or TCAs with significant serotonergic activity.[39,40] Absence seizures have also been reported.[41]

Thyroid hormone augmentation

Potentiation of the effects of antidepressant drugs by thyroid hormones has been demonstrated in a number of clinical studies (see Table 4.4). A diminished latency period for the onset of action of imipramine by the addition of T_3 (25 µg/day) was first demonstrated by Prange and co-workers.[42] This observation was confirmed for both amitriptyline and imipramine independently[43,44] but not by all investigators.[45] This approach was extended to patients with resistant depression and early studies suggested that T_3 augmentation might be effective in as many as 50–90% of patients. Thyroid hormone addition was successful in 14 of 25 unipolar and bipolar depressed patients unresponsive to the TCA, imipramine.[46] In a double-blind study, T_3 (25 µg or 50 µg) was added to 12 hospitalized patients with major depressive disorder who failed to respond to a minimum of 4 weeks' treatment with amitriptyline or imipramine.[47] Significant declines in depression scores were noted in 75% of patients over the

Table 4.4 Potentiation of TCA response by tri-iodothyronine in treatment-resistant patients: a selection of studies.

Patient population	Medications and design of study	Results	Reference
25 UP/BP outpatients	IMI, AMI, PT + T_3 25 µg daily; open evaluation	Response in 14 patients	46
44 UP/BP	TCA + T_3 open evaluation	Response in 29 patients	95
49 UP/BP	AMI + T_3 20–40 µg vs. AMI; open evaluation	Response in 23 of 33 on T_3 vs. alone 4 of 16 on AMI	96
12 UP/BP	IMI, AMI + 25 or 50 µg T_3; double-blind, crossover	Response in 12 patients	47
11 depressed	TCA + 5–25 µg T_3; open evaluation	Response in 10 patients	48
16 UP	IMI + 25 µg T_3; double-blind, placebo-controlled crossover	T_3 = placebo	49
20 UP	IMI + 25 µg T_3 vs. IMI alone	Response in 5 of 20 on T_3 vs. 4 of 20 on IMI alone	50
38 UP	DMI, IMI + 37.5 µg T_3 vs. 150 µg T_4	Response in 10 of 17 on T_3 vs. 4 of 21 on T_4	51
21 UP	TCA + 25 µg T_3 or 100 µg T_4; open evaluation	Response in 7 patients (5 of 6 hypothyroid, 2 of 15 euthyroid)	52
51 UP outpatients	DMI, IMI + 37.5 µg T_3 vs. 900 mg Li vs. placebo	Response 10 of 17 on T_3; 9 of 17 on Li; 3 of 16 on placebo; T_3 = Li > PBO	94

Notes:
AMI = amitriptyline; BP = bipolar; DMI = desipramine; IMI = imipramine; Li = lithium; PBO = placebo; PT = protriptyline; T_3 = L-tri-iodothyronine; TCA = tricyclic antidepressant; T_4 = thyroxine; UP = unipolar.

ensuing 21 days. Response was generally rapid (within 3 days) and side-effects were minimal. While some open evaluations have reported improvement in 90% of patients,[48] not all trials have had such impressive responses.[49,50] In a 4-week open evaluation of T_3 (25 μg/day) added to 20 inpatients who had not responded to 3 months of imipramine, response rates were 25% compared with 20% in historic controls not receiving T_3.[50] Similarly, 4 weeks of T_3 (25 μg/day) was no more effective than placebo in a double-blind comparison in male nonresponders to TCAs.[49]

Differential responses have been noted for different thyroid hormones. In patients unresponsive to tricyclics, augmentation with T_3 gave a higher response rate than augmentation with T_4.[51] Furthermore, thyroid function status may also determine the responsiveness to augmentation. The effectiveness of either T_3 or T_4 augmentation was shown to be limited to the group of patients with exaggerated thyroid-stimulating hormone (TSH) responses to infusion of thyrotropin-releasing hormone, i.e. to those patients with an indicator of early thyroid dysfunction.[52]

To date there have been few studies investigating potentiation of the antidepressant responses of monoamine oxidase inhibitors (MAOIs) or SSRIs. Case studies suggest that the response to both phenelzine[53] and fluoxetine[54–56] can be potentiated by T_3.

Combined antidepressant drugs

Combining two antidepressants in treatment-resistant patients remains a controversial practice, although enthusiastically embraced by some. Although the combination of a TCA and SSRI has been shown to be effective in resistant patients,[57,58] the general observation of increased plasma levels of the tricyclics could theoretically lead to an increased propensity for cardiac arrhythmias,[59] while grand mal seizure has been reported.[60] Preclinical studies have shown that the combination of desipramine and an SSRI produces a rapid downregulation of post-synaptic β_1-adrenoceptors.[61] An open evaluation of combined desipramine–fluoxetine noted a rapid, robust clinical effect.[62] High response rates (~90%) were reported for the combination in other open evaluations of patients with minimal response to various heterocyclic drugs.[58] On the other hand, in a double-blind study augmentation of fluoxetine (20 mg/day) with low-dose (25–50 mg/day) desipramine was not as effective as 40–60 mg/day fluoxetine alone.[31]

The combination of MAOIs and TCAs has generally been regarded as contraindicated. Nevertheless, it has been claimed that fatal or serious reactions are usually the result of overdoses: combining several drugs or using imipramine or clomipramine in combination with the MAOI.[63] For some patients previously resistant to antidepressants, recovery on an MAOI–TCA combination has been claimed.[64] Response in 62% of 157 depressed outpatients previously unresponsive to one or more antidepressant therapies has been reported.[65] In a trial of 20 patients who had failed to maintain improvement after ECT and an antidepressant drug, 70% were reported to do well on the combination of an MAOI and TCA.[66] Similarly, 9 out of 10 patients who were unresponsive to a TCA, MAOI or ECT became symptom-free on a combination of phenelzine and amitriptyline.[67] While these trials suggest the usefulness of the combination, their open-label design requires that caution is exercised in accepting the findings uncritically. Further double-blind comparisons are needed before this potentially dangerous combination could be recommended for widespread use.

Pindolol augmentation

Recent electrophysiological and microdialysis studies have implicated inhibition of the 5-HT_{1A} receptor as intimately involved in the delayed onset of action of antidepressants.[68] The combination of a 5-HT_{1A} antagonist with an antidepressant has been shown in preclinical studies to increase serotonin concentrations in the hypothalamus and hippocampus.[69] Increased serotonin availability, it was reasoned, would both speed the onset of the action of antidepressants and convert nonresponsive patients to responders. Thus Artigas et al. demonstrated rapid response (within one week) in 5 out of 8 patients receiving SSRIs or MAOIs to the addition of pindolol (2.5 mg three times a day) where previously they had been treatment resistant.[70] A similar rapid response was noted in 10 of 19 treatment-resistant patients within 1 week of pindolol addition.[71] Less-impressive results were noted in another open trial where only 3 of 13 patients, who had failed to respond to an SSRI, had made significant clinical progress by 12 days after the addition of pindolol.[72] While some double-blind placebo-controlled studies have shown pindolol augmentation to be effective in nonresistant depression, only one methodologically rigorous study has examined response in treatment-resistant patients.[73] Both pindolol (2.5 mg tds) and fluoxetine (20 mg) were superior to placebo in augmenting the response to 100 mg/day trazodone.

The pindolol strategy holds promise for treatment-resistant depression. Further controlled comparisons in well-defined patients are necessary to judge its usefulness, while a detailed understanding of the mechanism of action may potentially improve the onset of action of antidepressants. The use of 5-HT_{1A} antagonists more specific than pindolol may also prove beneficial and lead to the development of drugs with greater efficacy than those currently in use.

Other strategies

Several other augmentation strategies have been applied in treatment-resistant depression, including the addition of mood stabilizers (such as carbamazepine or valproate, sex hormones, tryptophan, psychostimulants, buspirone and antipsychotic drugs).[2,13,17] While each of these augmentation approaches has been shown to be effective for individual patients or has been evaluated in a small series of patients in open trials, large-scale, double-blind, placebo-controlled trials are usually lacking. Such approaches are at best experimental and most are associated with a high risk of pharmacokinetic and pharmacodynamic interaction potential.

Electroconvulsive therapy (ECT)

For treatment-resistant depression, ECT still remains the most important and perhaps the most consistently effective form of treatment.[74] The response rate for ECT is at least equivalent to lithium augmentation and may even be better. At least 50% of patients who did not improve on imipramine treatment were responders to ECT,[75] while 6 of 9 amitriptyline nonresponders made a good response to ECT.[76] A study of 153 endogenously depressed patients who failed to respond to imipramine found that 78% were ECT responders.[77] Similarly patients with intractable and serious depression were found to respond favourably to ECT in the majority of cases.[78] ECT represents an alternative to augmentation strategies when treatment resistance ensues.

Psychosurgery

Limbic surgery may be considered for a minority of patients with treatment-resistant depression. The question needs to be asked whether the cure is worse than the disease. Clearly the efficacy of psychosurgery needs to be considered. A number of nonblind trials have shown that frontal leucotomy is more effective than a sham operation, while up to 89% of refractory patients made marked or moderate improvement following psychosurgery.[79] The procedure is usually recommended only for patients whose illness has lasted more than 2 years, with the majority of patients being constantly depressed for many more years.

The risks of psychosurgery are low, particularly with limited stereotactic techniques. Mortality is about 0.17% while the risk of epilepsy is around 0.6%. Personality changes may ensue but, after perhaps 20 years of constant depressed mood, this might be regarded as a cure. Clearly psychosurgery is a treatment of very last resort when extensive medication and other trials have been shown to fail categorically.

Conclusions

While modern treatment of depressive illness is satisfactory for the majority of patients, a small group, perhaps 10% or so, are not helped by monotherapy. In this group of 'treatment-resistant' patients strategies based on the addition of another agent may be indicated in order to enhance response. The strategy for which the greatest empirical evidence exists is the addition of lithium at the usual therapeutic doses. Other augmentation strategies, although used in some clinical practices, are not as strongly supported by controlled clinical trials. All combinations of medications add to the potential for drug–drug interactions arising either from pharmacokinetic or pharmacodynamic mechanisms. Such combinations of agents, where they are used, require careful clinical judgements to be made for individual patients and an awareness of the side-effects and any special precautions to be exercised in their use. ECT is a viable and effective alternative to augmentation strategies, with empirical evidence suggesting that it is at least as effective as lithium augmentation.

Summary

A small group of depressed patients, up to 10%, are not helped by multiple drug interventions and remain depressed. This group of patients has been termed 'treatment resistant'. While a precise clinical definition of treatment resistance remains elusive, it is well recognized that such patients represent a difficult problem in clinical practice. Recent attention has focused on this group with a view to improving treatment outcomes by the use of combinations of medications. The addition of lithium to an existing regimen of antidepressant drug has the largest body of empirical evidence of support for its efficacy. Meta-analysis of placebo-controlled studies of lithium augmentation suggest that about 40% of treatment-resistant patients respond to this strategy. The best results are obtained when lithium concentrations are maintained within the usual therapeutic range. While, in some studies, alleviation of the depressive symptoms has been reported as commencing within 48 hours of the addition of lithium, this is not the case in all studies; a period of 2 to 3 weeks would appear to be necessary to judge the response to lithium augmentation properly. While the combination of lithium and an antidepressant is generally well tolerated, side-effects and toxicity can occur even at the low doses used for augmentation.

A similar body of empirical data attests to the efficacy and safety of thyroid hormone addition for treatment resistance. The addition of T_3 (25 µg/day) to an existing antidepressant regimen has been shown to produce significant therapeutic gains within 3 weeks. After that time few patients, if any, will respond. The use of thyroid hormone demands additional laboratory testing for the management of patients, though some evidence exists for the usefulness of combining two antidepressant drugs in treatment-resistant depression. Combinations of SSRIs and tricyclic antidepressants generally lead to raised plasma levels of the latter with an increased propensity for side-effects, particularly cardiac arrhythmias. The combination of a MAOI with TCA, while reported as effective in some studies, is generally regarded as contraindicated. If such combinations of antidepressants are to be attempted they are best reserved for inpatients, where careful monitoring for adverse events can occur.

A recent augmentation strategy has been to use pindolol augmentation of antidepressants, principally SSRIs. Although a β-blocker, pindolol is believed to exert its effects due to its $5HT_{1A}$ antagonist properties. The combination has been reported to both speed the onset of action of antidepressants as well as convert nonresponsive patients to responders. The evidence for the efficacy of this combination remains controversial.

Many other strategies for treatment-resistant patients have been proposed but the evidence for their efficacy is mainly anecdotal. Controlled clinical trials are lacking for the addition of mood stabilizers (apart from lithium), sex hormones, tryptophan, buspirone and psychostimulants; many of these combinations have a high risk of drug–drug interaction. Also, electroconvulsive therapy is an often neglected but highly effective form of treatment for patients who fail to respond to medications. For severe intractable forms of depression limbic surgery may be an option for a minority of patients.

References

1. Fava M, Davidson KG. Definition and epidemiology of treatment-resistant depression. *Psychiat Clin N Am* (1996) **19:** 179–200.

2. Thase M, Rush AJ. Treatment-resistant depression. In Bloom FE, Kupfer DJ (eds) *Psychopharmacology: The Fourth Generation of Progress* (New York: Raven Press, 1995): 1081–97.

3. Scott J. Epidemiology, demography and definitions. *Int Clin Psychopharmacol* (1991) **6(Suppl 1):** 1–12.

4. Helmchen H. Therapy resistance in depression. In Gaspar M, Kielholz P (eds) *Problems in Psychiatry in General Practice* (Lewiston, NY: Hogrefe & Huber, 1991): 97–106.

5. Thompson C, Thompson CE. Treatment resistant or irresolutely treated? *Int Clin Psychopharmacol* (1991) **6(Suppl 1):** 31–9.

6. Nierenberg AA, Amsterdam JD. Treatment-resistant depression: definition and treatment approaches. *J Clin Psychiatry* (1990) **51(Suppl 6):** 39–47.

7. Greenhouse JB, Kufer DJ, Frank E et al. Analysis of time to stabilisation in the treatment of depression: biological and clinical correlates. *J Affect Disorders* (1987) **13:** 259–66.

8. Donovan S, Quitkin F, Stewart J et al. Duration of antidepressant trials: clinical and research implications. *J Clin Psychopharmacol* (1994) **14:** 64–6.

9. Quitkin F, Rabkin J, Ross D et al. Duration of antidepressant drug treatment: what is an adequate trial. *Arch Gen Psychiatry* **41:** 238–45.

10. Schweizer E, Rickels K, Amsterdam J et al. What constitutes an

adequate antidepressant trial of fluoxetine? *J Clin Psychiatry* (1990) **51:** 8–11.

11. Georgotas A, McCue RE, Cooper GL et al. Factors affecting the delay of antidepressant effect in responders to nortriptyline and phenelzine. *Psychiatry Res* (1989) **28:** 1–9.

12. Wilhelm K, Mitchell P, Boyce P et al. Treatment resistant depression in an Australian context. I. The utility of the term and approaches to management. *Aust & NZJ Psychiatry* (1994) **28:** 14–22.

13. Burrows GD, Norman TR, Judd FK. Definition and differential diagnosis of treatment-resistant depression. *Int Clin Psychopharmacol* (1994) **9(Suppl 2):** 5–10.

14. Cowen PJ. Depression resistant to tricyclic antidepressants. *Br Med J* (1988) **297:** 435–6.

15. Nemeroff CB. Augmentation strategies in patients with refractory depression. *Depression and Anxiety* (1996/1997) **4:** 169–81.

16. De Montigny C. Lithium addition in treatment-resistant depression. *Int Clin Psychopharmacol* (1994) **9(Suppl 2):** 31–5.

17. Schweitzer I, Tuckwell V, Johnson G. A review of the use of augmentation therapy for the treatment of resistant depression: implications for the clinician. *Aust & NZ J Psychiatry* (1997) **31:** 340–52.

18. O'Flanagan P. Clomipramine infusion and lithium carbonate: a synergistic effect? *Lancet* (1963) **2:** 974.

19. Lingjaerde O, Edlund AH, Gormsen CA et al. The effect of lithium carbonate in combination with tricyclic antidepressants in endogenous depression. *Acta Psychiatr Scand* (1974) **50:** 233–42.

20. De Montigny C, Crunberg P, Mayer A et al. Lithium induces rapid relief of depression in tricyclic antidepressant drug non-

responders. *Br J Psychiatry* (1981) **138:** 252–6.

21. Heninger GR, Charney DS, Sternberg DE. Lithium carbonate augmentation of antidepressant treatment: an effective prescription for the treatment of refractory depression. *Arch Gen Psychiatry* (1983) **40:** 1335–42.

22. Dinan TG. Lithium augmentation in sertraline-resistant depression: a preliminary dose response study. *Acta Psychiatr Scand* (1993) **88:** 300–1.

23. Schopf J, Baumann P, Lemarchand T et al. Treatment of endogenous depressions resistant to tricyclic antidepressants or related drugs by lithium addition: results of a placebo controlled, double-blind study. *Pharmacopsychiatry* (1989) **22:** 183–7.

24. Thase ME, Kupfer DJ, Frank E et al. Treatment of imipramine-resistant recurrent depression. II. An open clinical trial of lithium augmentation. *J Clin Psychiatry* (1989) **50:** 413–17.

25. Austin MPV, Souza FGM, Goodwin GM. Lithium augmentation in antidepressant-resistant patients. A quantitative analysis. *Br J Psychiatry* (1991) **159:** 510–14.

26. Zall H. Lithium carbonate and isocarboxazid – an effective drug approach in severe depression. *Am J Psychiatry* (1971) **127:** 1400–3.

27. Himmelhoch JM, Detre T, Kupfer DJ et al. Treatment of previously intractable depressions with tranylcypromine and lithium. *J Nerv Ment Dis* (1972) **155:** 216–20.

28. Nelson JG, Byck R. Rapid response to lithium in phenelzine non-responders. *Br J Psychiatry* (1982) **142:** 111–19.

29. Price LH, Charney DS, Heninger GR. Efficacy of lithium–tranylcypromine treatment in refractory

depression. *Am J Psychiatry* (1985) **142:** 619–23.

30. Pope HG, McElroy SL, Nixon RA. Possible synergism between fluoxetine and lithium in refractory depression. *Am J Psychiatry* (1988) **145:** 1292–4.

31. Fava M, Rosenbaum JF, McGrath PJ et al. Lithium and tricyclic augmentation of fluoxetine treatment for resistant major depression: a double-blind, controlled study. *Am J Psychiatry* (1994) **151:** 1372–4.

32. Ontiveros A, Fontaine R, Elie R. Refractory depression: the addition of lithium to fluoxetine or desipramine. *Acta Psychiatr Scand* (1991) **83:** 188–92.

33. Katona CLE, Abou-Saleh MT, Harrison DA et al. Placebo-controlled trial of lithium augmentation of fluoxetine and lofepramine. *Br J Psychiatry* (1995) **166:** 80–6.

34. Stein G, Bernadt M. Lithium augmentation therapy in tricyclic-resistant depression: a controlled trial using lithium in low and normal doses. *Br J Psychiatry* (1993) **162:** 634–40.

35. Rybakowski J, Matkowski K. Adding lithium to antidepressant therapy: factors related to therapeutic potentiation. *Eur Neuropsychopharmacol* (1992) **2:** 161–5.

36. Alvarez E, Perezsola V, Peresblanco J et al. Predicting outcome of lithium added to antidepressants in resistant depression. *J Affect Disorders* (1997) **42:** 179–86.

37. Nierenberg AA, Price LH, Charney DS et al. After lithium augmentation: a retrospective follow-up of patients with antidepressant-refractory depression. *J Affect Disorders* (1990) **18:** 167–75.

38. Joffe RT, Levitt AJ, Bagby RM et al. Predictors of response to lithium and tri-iodothyronine augmentation of antidepressants in tricycle non-responders. *Br J Psychiatry* (1993) **163:** 574–8.

39. Kojima H, Terao T, Yoshimura R. Serotonin syndrome during clomipramine and lithium treatment. *Am J Psychiatry* (1993) **150:** 1897.

40. Muly EC, McDonald W, Stefens D et al. Serotonin syndrome produced by a combination of fluoxetine and lithium. *Am J Psychiatry* (1993) **150:** 1565.

41. Sacristan JA, Iglesias C, Arellana F et al. Absence seizures induced by lithium: possible interaction with fluoxetine. *Am J Psychiatry* (1991) **148:** 146–7.

42. Prange A, Wilson I, Rabon A et al. Enhancement of imipramine antidepressant activity by thyroid hormone. *Am J Psychiatry* (1969) **126:** 457–60.

43. Coppen A, Whybrow PC, Noguera R et al. The comparative antidepressant value of tryptophan and imipramine with and without attempted potentiation by liothyronine. *Arch Gen Psychiatry* (1972) **26:** 234–41.

44. Wheatley D. Potentiation of amitriptyline by thyroid hormone. *Arch Gen Psychiatry* (1972) **26:** 229–33.

45. Feighner JP, King W, Schuckit MA et al. Hormonal potentiation of imipramine and ECT in primary depression. *Am J Psychiatry* (1972) **128:** 50–8.

46. Earle BV. Thyroid hormone and tricyclic antidepressants in resistant depression. *Am J Psychiatry* (1970) **126:** 143–5.

47. Goodwin F, Prange A, Post R et al. Potentiation of antidepressant effects by L-triiodothyronine in tricyclic non-responders. *Am J Psychiatry* (1982) **139:** 34–8.

48. Tsutsui S, Yamazaki Y, Namba T et al. Combined therapy of T_3 and antidepressants in depression. *J Int Med Res* (1979) **7:** 138–46.

49. Gitlin MJ, Weiner H, Fairbanks L et

al. Failure of T_3 to potentiate tricyclic antidepressant response. *J Affect Disorders* (1987) **13:** 267–72.

50. Thase ME, Kupfer DJ, Jarrett DB. Treatment of imipramine-resistant recurrent depression. I. An open clinical trial of adjunctive L-triiodothyronine. *J Clin Psychiatry* (1989) **50:** 385–8.

51. Joffe RT, Singer W. A comparison of triiodothyronine and thyroxine in the potentiation of tricyclic antidepressants. *Psychiatry Res* (1990) **31:** 241–51.

52. Targum SD, Greenberg RD, Harmon RL et al. Thyroid hormone and the TRH stimulation test in refractory depression. *J Clin Psychiatry* (1984) **45:** 345–6.

53. Hillet FJ, Bidder TG. Phenelzine plus triiodothyronine combination in a case of refractory depression. *J Nerv Ment Dis* (1983) **171:** 318–20.

54. Gupta S, Masand P, Tanquary S. Thyroid hormone supplementation of fluoxetine in the treatment of a major depression. *Br J Psychiatry* (1991) **159:** 866–7.

55. Joffe RT. T_3 potentiation of fluoxetine. *Can J Psychiatry* (1992) **37:** 48–50.

56. Barak Y, Stein D, Levine J et al. Thyroxine augmentation of fluoxetine treatment for resistant depression in the elderly – an open trial. *Human Psychopharmacol* (1996) **11:** 463–7.

57. Weilburg JB, Rosenbaum JF, Meltzer-Brody S et al. Tricyclic augmentation of fluoxetine. *Ann Clin Psychiatry* (1991) **3:** 209–13.

58. Weilburg JB, Rosenbaum JF, Biderman J et al. Fluoxetine added to non-MAOI antidepressants converts non-responders to responders: a preliminary report. *J Clin Psychiatry* (1989) **50:** 447–9.

59. Sloman JG, Norman TR, Burrows GD. Clinical studies of antidepressant cardiotoxicity. In Burrows GD, Norman TR, Davies BM (eds) *Drugs in Psychiatry. Vol. 1. Antidepressants* (Amsterdam: Elsevier Science, 1983): 173–86.

60. Preskorn SH, Beber JH, Faul JC et al. Serious adverse effects of combining fluoxetine and tricyclic antidepressants. *Am J Psychiatry* (1990) **147:** 532.

61. Baron BM, Ogden AM, Siegel BW et al. Rapid down regulation of β-adrenoceptors by co-administration of desipramine and fluoxetine. *Eur J Pharmacol* (1988) **153:** 125–34.

62. Nelson JG, Mazure CM, Bowers MB et al. A preliminary, open study of the combination of fluoxetine and desipramine for rapid treatment of major depression. *Arch Gen Psychiatry* (1991) **48:** 303–7.

63. Pare CMB. The present status of monoamine oxidase inhibitors. *Brit J Psychiatry* (1985) **146:** 576–84.

64. Dally PJ. Combining antidepressant drugs. *Br Med J* (1965) **1:** 384.

65. Gander DR. Combining the antidepressant drugs. *Br Med J* (1965) **1:** 521.

66. Winston F. Combined antidepressant therapy. *Br J Psychiatry* (1971) **118:** 301–4.

67. Sethna E. A study of refractory cases of depressive illness and their response to combined antidepressant treatment. *Br J Psychiatry* (1974) **123:** 265–72.

68. Artigas F, Romero L, DeMontigny C et al. Acceleration of the effect of selected antidepressant drugs in major depression by $5HT_{1A}$ antagonists. *Trends Pharmacol Sci* (1996) **19:** 378–83.

69. Dreshfield LR, Wong DT, Perry KW et al. Enhancement of fluoxetine dependent increase of extracellular serotonin (5HT) levels by (−) pindolol, an antagonist at $5HT_{1A}$

receptors. *Neurochem Res* (1996) **21:** 557–62.

70. Artigas F, Perez V, Alvarez E. Pindolol induces a rapid improvement of depressed patients treated with serotonin reuptake inhibitors. *Arch Gen Psychiatry* (1994) **51:** 248–51.

71. Blier P, Bergeron R. Effectiveness of pindolol with selected antidepressant drugs in the treatment of major depression. *J Clin Psychopharmacol* (1995) **15:** 217–22.

72. Dinan TG, Scott LV. Does pindolol induce a rapid improvement in depressed patients resistant to serotonin reuptake inhibitors? *J Serotonin Res* (1996) **3:** 119–21.

73. Maes M, Vandoolaeghe E, Desnyder R. Efficacy of treatment with trazodone in combination with pindolol or fluoxetine in major depression. *J Affect Disorders* (1996) **41:** 201–10.

74. Devanand DP, Sackheim HA, Prudic J. Electroconvulsive therapy in the treatment resistant patient. *Psychiat Clin Am* (1991) **14:** 905–23.

75. Clinical Research Committee of the British Medical Research Council. Clinical trial of the treatment of depression. *Br Med J* (1965) **1:** 881–6.

76. Browne MW, Kreeger LG. A clinical trial of amitriptyline in depressive illness. *Br J Psychiatry* (1963) **109:** 692–4.

77. Avery D, Lubrano A. Depression treated with imipramine and ECT: the DeCardis study reconsidered. *Am J Psychiatry* (1979) **136:** 559–62.

78. Paul SM, Extein I, Calil HM et al. Use of ECT with treatment-resistant depressed patients at the NIMH. *Am J Psychiatry* (1981) **138:** 486–9.

79. Kiloh LE. The treatment of refractory depression. In Johnson GFS (ed) *Recent Trends in the Treatment of Depression* (Sydney: Boots Company, 1986): 53–6.

80. Charney DS, Price LH, Heninger GR. Desipramine–yohimbine combination treatment of refractory depression. *Arch Gen Psychiatry* (1986) **43:** 1155–61.

81. Reimherr FW, Woods DR, Byerley B et al. Characteristics of responders to fluoxetine. *Psychopharmacol Bull* (1984) **20:** 70–2.

82. Peselow ED, Filippi AM, Goodnick P et al. The short- and long-term efficacy of paroxetine HCl: B. Data from a double-blind crossover study and year long trial vis imipramine and placebo. *Psychopharmacol Bull* (1989) **25:** 272–6.

83. McGrath PJ, Stewart JW, Nunes EV et al. A double-blind crossover trial of imipramine and phenelzine for outpatients with treatment-refractory depression. *Am J Psychiatry* (1993) **250:** 118–23.

84. Nolen WA, VanDePutte JJ, Dijken WA et al. Treatment strategy in depression. II. MAO inhibitors in depression resistant to cyclic antidepressants: two controlled crossover studies with tranylcypromine versus L-5-hydroxytryptophan and nomifensine. *Acta Psychiatr Scand* (1988) **78:** 676–83.

85. Schmauss M, Laakmann G, Dieterle D. Nomifensine: a double-blind comparison of intravenous versus oral administration in therapy-resistant depressed patients. *Pharmacopsychiatry* (1985) **18:** 88–90.

86. Cole JO, Schatzberg AF, Sniffin C et al. Trazodone in treatment-resistant depression. An open study. *J Clin Psychopharmacol* (1981) **1(Suppl):** 49–54.

87. Nolen WA, Van De Putte JJ, Dijken WA et al. Treatment strategies in depression. I. Nontricyclic and selective reuptake inhibitors in resistant depression: a double-blind partial crossover study on the effects of oxaprotiline and flu-

voxamine. *Acta Psychiatr Scand* (1988) **78:** 668–75.

88. Beasley CM, Sayler ME, Cunningham GE et al. Fluoxetine in tricyclic refractory major depressive disorder. *J Affect Disorders* (1990) **20:** 193–200.

89. Delgado PL, Price LH, Charney DS et al. Efficacy of fluvoxamine in treatment-refractory depression. *J Affect Disorders* (1988) **15:** 55–60.

90. White K, Wykoff W, Tynes LL et al. Fluvoxamine in the treatment of tricyclic-resistant depression. *Psychiatr J Univ Ottawa* (1990) **15:** 156–8.

91. Gagiano CA, Muller PGM, Gourie J et al. The therapeutic efficacy of paroxetine: (a) an open study in patients with major depression not responding to antidepressants; (b) a double-blind comparison with amitriptyline in depressed outpatients. *Acta Psychiatr Scand* (1993) **80:** 130–1.

92. Kramlinger KG, Post RM. The addition of lithium to carbamazepine: antidepressant efficacy in treatment resistant depression. *Arch Gen Psychiatry* (1989) **46:** 794–800.

93. Finch EJL, Katona CLE. Lithium augmentation in the treatment of refractory depression in old age. *Int J Ger Psychiatry* (1989) **4:** 41–6.

94. Joffe RT, Singer W, Levitt AJ et al. A placebo-controlled comparison of lithium and tri-iodothyronine augmentation of tricyclic antidepressants in unipolar refractory depression. *Arch Gen Psychiatry* (1993) **50:** 387–93.

95. Ogura G, Okuma T, Uchida Y et al. Combined thyroid (tri-iodothyronine)-tricyclic antidepressant treatment in depressive states. *Folia Psychiatr Neurol Jpn* (1975) **28:** 179–86.

96. Banki CM. Cerebrospinal fluid amine metabolites after combined amitriptyline tri-iodothyronine treatment of depressed women. *Eur J Clin Pharmacol* (1977) **11:** 311–15.

5
Treatment of the difficult panic patient

Antoine Pélissolo and Jean-Pierre Lépine

Panic disorder with and without agoraphobia is a common, debilitating psychiatric condition that will afflict about 1.5–2.5% of the general population at some time in their lives. Since it was classified in 1980 in the DSM-III (*Diagnostic and Statistical Manual of Mental Disorder* – 3rd edn), an impressive profusion of clinical, epidemiological, biological and therapeutic research about panic disorder has been published. The ability of clinicians to identify the symptoms of the disorder has increased and, during the same period of time, specific and effective treatments have been developed, including pharmacotherapy and psychotherapy. The most critical problems for the clinician confronted by patients are, at present, choosing from among the various therapeutic strategies available the most adequate one and managing many difficult patients – who may be nonresponders to first-line treatment or who create some particularly difficult clinical problems. After a brief general overview of panic disorder, this chapter presents an outline of the current knowledge on the pharmacotherapy and psychotherapy of panic disorder and then discusses some specific points for the treatment of difficult patients.

Main features of panic disorder

Panic disorder is characterized by the spontaneous occurrence of panic attacks that consist of short-lived (usually less than one hour) periods of intense fear, anxiety or discomfort. The symptoms include various physiological and cognitive signs of anxiety, and can be accompanied by behavioural disorders. The diagnostic criteria for a panic attack are listed in Table 5.1.

In panic disorder, attacks are recurrent and unexpected, and are followed by at least one month of persistent fear of having other panic attacks (anticipatory anxiety), worry about their possible implications or consequences, or a significant behavioural change related to the attacks. Attacks due to the direct effects of a substance or a general medical condition must not be taken into account for the diagnosis of panic disorder, and it must be differentiated from other disorders that may include

Table 5.1   Diagnostic criteria for panic attack.

A discrete period of intense fear or discomfort, in which four (or more) of the
following symptoms developed abruptly and reached a peak within 10 minutes:

- Palpitations, pounding heart or accelerated heart rate
- Sweating
- Trembling or shaking
- Sensations of shortness of breath or smothering
- Feeling of choking
- Chest pain or discomfort
- Nausea or abdominal distress
- Feeling dizzy, unsteady, light-headed or faint
- Derealization (feelings of unreality) or depersonalization (being detached from
  oneself)
- Fear of losing control or going crazy
- Fear of dying
- Paraesthesias (numbness or tingling sensations)
- Chills or hot flushes

Source:
American Psychiatric Association.[1]

panic attacks or share similar clinical features, such as major depression,
phobia, obsessive-compulsive disorder or post-traumatic stress
disorder.[1]

Two forms of panic disorder are codified in DSM-IV: with or without
agoraphobia. In the case of panic disorder with agoraphobia, the patient
has an anxiety of, avoids or endures with marked distress, places or situations from which escape might be difficult or embarrassing or in which
help might not be available in the event of a panic attack (busy streets,
crowded stores, closed-in spaces such as tunnels, bridges and eleva-
tors, or an enclosed vehicle such as a subway, bus or airplane). The
degree of phobic avoidance may vary from mild to severe, condemning
the patient to an extremely constricted lifestyle, with the need for some
agoraphobics to be accompanied every time they leave the house.

The lifetime prevalence rate has been found in many worldwide epidemiologic studies to range between 1.5 and 2.5%, with an annual
prevalence of about 1%.[2] Women are two to three times more likely to be
affected than are men. The age at onset of panic disorder is generally in
the early to middle 20s, but it has been reported to occur at any age (for
example, in children and adolescents). To date, the limited findings

about the long-term course of panic disorder suggest that it is a chronic disorder, with a waxing-and-waning course of severity.

Even if the diagnosis of panic disorder with or without agoraphobia is relatively clear in most cases, the differential diagnosis for a patient with this disorder includes a large number of general medical conditions and psychiatric disorders.[3] Medical differential diagnosis includes cardiovascular diseases (angina, hypertension, paradoxical atrial tachycardia, mitral valve prolapse), pulmonary diseases (asthma), neurological diseases (epilepsy, migraine, Ménière's disease), endocrine diseases (hyperthyroidism, pheochromocytoma, hypoglycaemia) and drug intoxication or withdrawal. Concerning psychiatric disorders, the clinician has to determine whether the panic is unexpected, situationally bound or situationally predisposed.[1] The latter generally indicates another diagnosis, such as social phobia or specific phobia (when exposed to the phobic situation), obsessive-compulsive disorder (when trying to resist a compulsion) or a depressive disorder. However, difficult patients commonly have comorbid disorders, such as panic disorder associated with social phobia. Other psychiatric differential diagnoses include post-traumatic stress disorder, depersonalization disorder and somatoform disorders.

The severity of panic disorder can be related to the intensity and the frequency of panic attacks, the degree of intrusiveness of anticipatory anxiety and the impairment associated with avoidance behaviours. Demoralization, depressive symptoms or major depression are often present in patients with panic disorder and agoraphobia, and studies have found that the lifetime risk of suicide attempts is increased.[2,3] Other frequent psychiatric comorbid conditions are all the other anxiety disorders, alcohol or other substance use disorders and personality disorders. General medical conditions that are frequently associated with panic disorder include atypical chest pain, asthma, migraine and irritable bowel syndrome.[4]

Pharmacotherapy of panic disorder

Which drugs are effective?

Three categories of drugs have been proposed as first-line treatment for panic disorder, on the basis of controlled studies (Table 5.2): tricyclic antidepressants (TCAs), selective serotonin reuptake inhibitors (SSRIs) and high-potency benzodiazepines (BZDs).

The earliest reports on the anti-panic properties of TCAs appeared in the 1960s, especially with Klein's studies using imipramine.[5] Five large recent studies have definitely demonstrated imipramine efficacy in panic disorder, with doses ranging between 150 and 250 mg/d (for a review

Table 5.2   Drug treatment for panic disorder.

Effective treatments

- SSRIs:

  fluvoxamine (150–300 mg/d)
  paroxetine (40–60 mg/d)
  sertraline (50–200 mg/d)
  citalopram (20–30 mg/d)
  fluoxetine (20–60 mg/d)

- Tricyclic antidepressants:

  clomipramine (75–150 mg/d)
  imipramine (150–250 mg/d)

- High-potency benzodiazepines:

  alprazolam (4–6 mg/d)
  clonazepam (2–3 mg/d)

- MAOI:

  phenelzine (45–90 mg/d)

Management

- Very slow increase of the doses at the beginning
- Dosage adjustment according to side-effects and outcome
- Acute phase: 6–8 weeks
- Continuation phase: 6–12 months
- Long-term treatment: 2 years or more
- Slow tapering with a close supervision at the end

see Pélissolo and Lépine[6]). In phase II of the Cross-National Collaborative Panic Study,[7] conducted in 391 patients with panic disorder, the efficacy of imipramine (155 mg/d) compared to placebo and alprazolam was apparent by week 4 and was maintained throughout the four following weeks of the trial. The efficacy of clomipramine has also been demonstrated in controlled studies, but generally with lower dosages (between 75 and 150 mg/d). Interestingly, agoraphobic patients may require higher doses of clomipramine or imipramine than depressed patients.[8]

A growing number of controlled trials have recently been conducted with SSRIs in panic disorder, with significant improvement obtained when compared with placebo. In six different studies, fluvoxamine (100–300 mg/d) was found to be superior to placebo and to maprotiline, superior or equal to imipramine and equivalent to brofaromine.[9] Overall, improvement in panic symptoms was reported for 50–61% of patients on fluvoxamine, compared with 20–42% of patients on placebo. Two studies found fluvoxamine to be superior to cognitive-behavioural therapy.[10,11] Three controlled studies have been conducted with paroxetine in panic patients, which found this SSRI to be superior to placebo at doses between 20 and 60 mg/d.[12–14] Paroxetine was as effective as clomipramine (50–150 mg/d), but with a more rapid onset of action (by weeks 4–6 compared with 10–12 for imipramine) and with a better tolerance in a 48-week continuation phase of treatment.[14,15] Other favourable controlled studies have been conducted with the SSRIs sertraline,[16,17] fluoxetine and citalopram,[18] but several have not yet been published.[8,9] The target dose for citalopram seems to be 20–30 mg/d and, as yet, there is no evidence suggesting any particular dosage range with fluoxetine, most clinicians utilizing 20–80 mg/d.[8] Lastly, a recent placebo-controlled study conducted with venlafaxine in a small sample of panic patients showed encouraging results.[19]

High-potency BZDs constitute another class of drugs with a demonstrated efficacy in panic disorder. This is especially the case for alprazolam, with two large controlled studies having shown that high dosages of this drug (5–6 mg/d) were superior to placebo and equivalent to imipramine in treating panic disorder.[7,20] Other high-potency BZDs have been shown to be effective in panic disorder in controlled studies: clonazepam and adinazolam.[6]

Short-term management of drug therapy

The first question to solve concerning a patient who meets the criteria for panic disorder is to determine if a pharmacological treatment is indicated. Schatzberg and Ballenger proposed guidelines for acute therapy requirements:[21]

- A primary diagnosis of panic disorder, and not attacks that are superimposed on another, more primary, underlying disorder, such as alcoholism or major depression.
- The existence of severe or frequent panic attacks, or severe generalized anticipatory anxiety.
- The existence of clear morbidity signs: a marked limitation of functioning at work or socially, development of demoralization or suicidal idealization, marked avoidance behaviour or alcohol usage.
- The development of disorders secondary to the panic, such as alcohol abuse or major depression.

The choice of the drug, among the three pharmacological classes already cited, is the second question to consider. There are few data suggesting that a given patient might be especially responsive to one class of drug.[22] However, before the recent extension of SSRIs use in anxious disorders, some authors reported that patients with prominent respiratory symptoms (shortness of breath, choking, fear of dying) in the acute phase and more spontaneous panic attacks appeared to respond better to TCAs (imipramine), while patients with prominent cardiovascular symptoms (palpitations, dizziness, nausea) and more situational panic attacks appeared to respond better to a BZD such as alprazolam.[23,24]

However, these data have not been confirmed fully, and the choice should be orientated pragmatically, depending on the clinical condition of a particular patient and based on the advantages and disadvantages of each of these drugs.[25] The high-potency BZDs have a rapid onset of action, tend to be well tolerated and are effective for reducing anticipatory anxiety. However, they require multiple daily dosing (especially alprazolam), have sedative and negative cognitive effects, and are associated with a significant risk of dependence and withdrawal syndromes. This risk is particularly striking with high dosages and long duration of treatment, as habitually required in patients with panic disorder.[26]

Among the antidepressants, the most recent expert consensus statements and meta-analyses concluded that SSRIs represent the best choice for the first-line treatment of panic disorder.[8,9,25,27–29] Indeed, TCAs produce numerous side-effects, including orthostatic hypotension, anticholinergic effects, sexual dysfunction, weight gain and activation or jitteriness, and they have a limited safety margin in overdoses.[21] The potent side-effects of SSRIs are also notable (nausea, diarrhoea, insomnia, somnolence, nervousness, sexual dysfunction), but with a better benefit/risk ratio.

There are no trials comparing SSRIs in panic disorders. They can be partially differentiated in their side-effect profiles and on their potent interactions based on differences in the oxidative metabolic processes involving the P-450 enzymes in the liver, even if the clinical implications of these differences are still unclear. For example, fluvoxamine has been observed to increase the levels of TCAs, carbamazepine and propranolol; fluoxetine increases TCAs, carbamazepine and the BZDs; paroxetine increases the levels of TCAs and digoxin; sertraline has been observed to increase desipramine; and citalopram seems only to increase the levels of phenothiazines.[8]

One of the important rules when prescribing the SSRIs in panic disorder (as well as for the TCAs) is to titrate the dosage very slowly at the beginning of treatment in order to avoid the 'hyperstimulation/jitteriness syndrome', most frequently observed with fluoxetine, clomipramine and fluvoxamine.[8] The dose may be, for example, 10 mg/d of paroxetine or 25 mg/d of fluvoxamine during the first week. The dosage can be doubled in the second week, with the same titration rate during the following weeks, in order to reach the recommended dosages of 40 mg/d of paroxetine or 150–200 mg/d of fluvoxamine, if tolerated. On the other hand, a fixed-dose study on sertraline showed that higher doses were no more effective than the 50 mg/d dose,[16] while other available evidence suggested that a range of 100–150 mg/d is probably best.[8] Treatment efficacy cannot be assessed before a sufficient period of administration (about 6–8 weeks). The goal of panic disorder treatment is to achieve the triple suppression of panic attacks, anticipatory anxiety and phobic avoidance. Once this therapeutic objective has been obtained, a several-week plateau with the same dosage should be observed in order to stabilize an asymptomatic state. The persistence of limited-symptom attacks must be taken into account in the efficacy assessment, as well as subtle avoidance behaviours.

There are to date no clearly defined early predictors of final outcome for any medications used in panic disorder. The analysis of a multicentre trial of alprazolam, imipramine and placebo in 1010 patients showed that early improvement within the first week of treatment in the number of spontaneous panic attacks predicted outcome (after 8 weeks of treatment) in the alprazolam but not the imipramine group.[30] Thus, a rapid panic-blocking action seems to be a relevant outcome for alprazolam, but a longer period of action is necessary for imipramine and presumably for other antidepressant effects.

Duration of treatment and long-term pharmacotherapy

Even if punctuated by remissions and relapses of varying duration, the clinical natural history of panic disorder is commonly found to be chronic.[31] Two naturalistic studies conducted in the follow-up of clinical trials showed that 47–70% of patients were still receiving a drug treatment 2.5 years after their inclusion.[32,33] However, there are few experimental data on the optimal duration of treatment; from a clinical point of view, length of treatment should be adapted to the severity of the panic disorder and agoraphobia. For mild disorder or for an illness of less than 6 months' duration, 6 months' treatment may be appropriate. However, severe and persistent panic disorders need at least 12 months' treatment, and probably up to 2 years. In all cases, discontinuation of medication can only be considered when full, sustained remission is achieved, when anxiety management skills are acquired and when patients have a stable life situation.[34] The drug must be tapered very slowly at the end of the treatment over a period of 2–6 months, with close supervision because of the risk of rebound and relapse.[35]

Most controlled trials on the pharmacotherapy of panic disorder have been short-term studies, but long-term efficacy data are available for the TCAs (clomipramine and imipramine), paroxetine and alprazolam, for about a 9-month period of maintenance treatment.[36] Further, some data indicate that improvement can continue with the prolonged administration of anti-panic therapy.[15,37] On the other hand, rates of relapse at the end of short-term treatment are estimated to be at between 30 and 40%.[34] Since patients may be concerned about long-lasting treatment, they should be reassured that panic disorder is a condition that generally requires therapy that continues for several years, with a positive benefit/risk ratio for this chronic and disabling condition.[35]

The question of long-term dosing schedules has been addressed in only a few studies. In a very select group of patients, Mavissakalian and Perel suggested that (after an initial 6-month period with imipramine), slowly reducing the dose from 168 mg/d to 83 mg/d for a 12-month continuation phase led to a relapse rate of only 7%.[37] A study with imipramine[38] and trials with alprazolam seem to indicate there is no observed loss of efficacy in lowering the dose during the maintenance phase. This is especially important for short- and long-term compliance to TCAs and BZDs because of their side-effects.

Alternative drug treatments

If no improvement is achieved with the first drug treatment, and if the maximum tolerated dose has been used and continued for long enough, the second-line recommendation is to switch the medication to one of another class, i.e. an SSRI, TCA or high-potency BZD.[25,28] If the first treatment used is an SSRI, one consensus group has suggested trying another SSRI if there were no tolerance problems and some indication of partial response.[35] However, to date, no controlled studies have been conducted to support these views, even if they fit with current clinical practice. Another choice in the case of partial response is a combination of anti-panic medications: patients taking a TCA or an SSRI may have a BZD added and, conversely, patients on a BZD could have an antidepressant added even if pharmacological data on this issue are controversial.

When several first or second-line treatments have been prescribed and have been found to be not fully effective, monoamine oxidase inhibitors (MAOIs) may be considered[22,25] because their efficacy in panic disorder has been suggested by several controlled studies – especially for phenelzine and tranylcypromine. One of their advantages should be a better anti-phobic action than for other drugs. However, their well-known side-effect profile (cardiovascular effects requiring restricted diet and insomnia and weight gain) limits the routine use of this class in anxious patients. Moreover, a washout period must be observed between SSRI withdrawal and the introduction of an MAOI drug.

Other alternative propositions are essentially based on isolated case reports or on open-study findings. Various drugs such as buspirone, nefazodone, valproate, carbamazepine, verapamil, propranolol, baclofen, ondansetron and inositol, have been proposed as effective, either in monotherapy or in combination with the many anti-panic agents.[39–41] Their use may be justified only in multidrug-resistant patients.

Psychotherapy of panic disorder

The concept of panic disorder has been, in part, inherited directly from Freud's 'anxiety-neurosis' concept,[42] and current psychoanalytic views of anxiety may be compatible with the application of some forms of psychodynamic therapy.[43] The efficacy of cognitive-behavioural therapy (CBT) has been extensively demonstrated in this disorder and is recommended by most authors. The CBT model, based on the hypothesis that a subject's erroneous cognitive processing may be a basic factor involved in anxious mood and behaviour, incorporates the possible aetiological roles of other factors – genetic, temperamental, neurobiological, traumatic events, psychodynamic processes – and, thus, may be combined with other treatments (i.e. pharmacological) for the treatment of anxiety disorders.[44]

Depending on the patient and therapist, the emphasis can be placed on behavioural or cognitive techniques but, in practice, the approaches are combined (Table 5.3). In a small sample of patients, Salkovskis et al. showed that cognitive techniques alone (without exposure or breathing retraining) may diminish the frequency and intensity of panic attacks, but that a combination of these behavioural interventions improves global outcome.[45] Exposure behavioural techniques seem to be almost imperative (i.e. a central ingredient) when agoraphobic avoidance is deeply

Table 5.3   Ingredients of cognitive-behavioural therapy for panic disorder.

- Detailed behaviour analysis of panic attacks, anticipatory anxiety, positive and negative reinforcements, agoraphobic behaviours and comorbid affective or anxiety disorders
- Self-monitoring techniques (e.g. daily record of panic attacks and behaviours)
- Relaxation techniques, including respiratory control and applied relaxation
- Exposure techniques with gradual densitization to external stimuli
- Exposure to anxiogenic internal sensations (hyperventilation and breathing retraining)
- Cognitive restructuration with special attention focused on catastrophic misinterpretations of bodily and mental experiences

installed, as is commonly the case in difficult panic patients.

The first step of all CBT for panic disorder with agoraphobia is to use a self-monitoring technique, giving the patient instructions to keep a daily record, for example, of the number of panic attacks and/or of his or her limitations in certain activities. This technique is used to define the baseline level of the disorder's severity so that progress may be assessed; however, it also has some therapeutic value. It has been noted frequently that a careful monitoring of these kinds of data can improve the patient's level of mindfulness and comprehension about the maladaptive behaviour and, thus, may decrease it.[44] This may be helpful for the development of practice exercises and may facilitate recognition of the distorted cognitions.

Behavioural strategies

As already mentioned, a major aspect of CBT for the treatment of panic disorder is exposure technique. This has the objective of supporting all the patient's encounters with external or internal anxiogenic cues (e.g. enclosed spaces or vehicles, sensations of losing control or physical sensations). Numerous techniques have been proposed that can be used to help the patient when he or she confronts these situations, but gradual desensitization (as typically employed in many cases of phobia) is the most common. The patient is gradually exposed to anxiety-provoking situations that have been organized into a hierarchy of severity by the patient him or herself. Using actual situations or images of these situations, exposure exercises of increasing difficulty are scheduled, beginning with the least anxiogenic situations and moving on to the next item only when an extinction (spontaneous or with relaxation techniques) of the anxious response is obtained. Other forms of exposure techniques that have a less or non-graduated course (such as flooding) can be effective but may be difficult to apply to most patients.[46] Effective procedures generally involve clearly planned, specified goals, repeated and prolonged exposure (with a progression from low to high-stress situations) and the patient's active rather than passive participation.[47]

Learning a relaxation technique is often a cornerstone in the treatment of panic. Various methods can be used. In progressive muscle relaxation, the objective is to lower the level of tension associated with physiological arousal. Instructions are given to the patient to tense and relax specific muscle groups actively in a sequence of, for example, about 5 seconds for tension and 10 seconds for relaxation. The patient practises these exercises during sessions and daily as homework.

The second important method is diaphragmatic breathing. Indeed, respiratory control is a major aspect of panic management, especially to control hyperventilation.[48] The aim of this technique is to reduce the rate and depth of the breathing and to promote abdominal rather than supradiaphragmatic breathing.

In a nonspecific manner, relaxation training methods are helpful in reducing a continuous or subcontinuous level of generalized anxiety and in facilitating the exposure exercises as described above. They are also very useful in managing spontaneous or in-situation panics. Specific techniques have been developed with this objective in mind. In applied relaxation, patients learn to identify the first signs of tension and anxiety (especially small bodily sensations) and to cope as soon as possible with anxiety in an active, positive manner before the symptoms develop into a complete panic attack.[49,50] After learning monitoring techniques and after having had training in progressive relaxation, patients are instructed to apply these on a specific command, which leads to cue-controlled relaxation. Patients have to apply their relaxation skills in daily life (such as in a meeting or when travelling by train) and in fear-provoking situations.

Some authors have developed complex cognitive-behaviour protocols designed to target panic attacks directly, such as panic control treatment.[51] This technique includes a cognitive therapy component and coping strategies as well as breathing retraining, and it is useful in the control of feared and anxiogenic internal sensations (e.g. palpitations, paraesthesia, shortness of breath, dizziness and sensations of depersonalization and derealization). Using hyperventilation exercises, this technique is employed when the patient is exposed to internal stimuli.[52] Griez and van den Hout have even developed repeated CO_2 inhalation techniques for use in therapeutic exposure to interoceptive anxiogenic cues.[53]

Cognitive therapy

Cognitive therapy is, hence, the last technique to use in treating panic disorder. It can be employed as an isolated method but also in treatment packages, as in panic control treatment or in combination with drug therapy. The efficacy of cognitive therapy for panic disorder has been demonstrated in several controlled trials, with results showing that between 74 and 95% of patients became panic-free after 3 months of treatment, and that benefits were maintained on follow-up periods lasting up to one year.[54-56] The objective of the cognitive therapy of panic disorder is to help patients identify and change their misinterpretations of harmless bodily sensations. According to the cognitive model, these misinterpretations are conceived as the centre of a positive feedback loop that culminates in a panic attack. Physical sensations (such as palpitations) are misinterpreted as indications of a physical or psychological catastrophe (such as a heart attack) and thus they produce extensions of the anxiety that, in turn, intensify the sensations.[54] Cognitive therapy in a programme of about 12 weekly sessions aims to change these misinterpretations, using the classical methods employed in dealing with depressive or anxiety disorders: identifying and recording automatic thoughts and cognitive distortions with a guided discovery and a Socratic style of questioning and, subsequently, modifying these thoughts, distortions and underlying schemas through such procedures as examining the evidence and developing rational alternatives.[44,57,58] There is preliminary evidence that maintained improvement (i.e. 15 months after the end of the treatment) can be predicted by the patient's changing perceptions of his or her bodily sensations as acquired during the course of treatment.[54]

Other forms of psychosocial treatments

Addressing the agoraphobic's interpersonal system, in combination with exposure treatment, can be useful, particularly with difficult patients.[59] Some investigators have included the patient's spouse as co-therapist in educational and treatment interventions, with the spouse helping the agoraphobic patient to carry out exposure homework exercises.[47,60] Arnow et al. have shown that some forms of marital therapy (such as couples' communication and problem-solving training), in addition to exposure therapy, may have positive effects on outcome.[61]

Comparison of drugs with psychological treatments

Drug therapy and psychological treatment have different goals and can be applied to different types of patient. As already mentioned, both appear to be clinically efficient and helpful in treating panic patients. Numerous studies have been conducted to compare their effectiveness even if outcome assessment methods are difficult to apply in the same manner for both psychological and pharmacological therapies. A comprehensive review of all the studies was published in 1990 (i.e. before the use of SSRIs in panic disorder) that included an assessment of the comparative effect of various acute treatments on four clinical variables: panic, agoraphobia, depression and anxiety.[62] The study's main conclusions were that a placebo effect was not consistently effective for any of the variables; that classical BZDs (such as diazepam) had a pronounced effect on the anxiety variable but not on the panic dimension; that alprazolam and imipramine had similar positive effects on anxiety, panic and agoraphobia; and that exposure in vivo was associated with a pronounced effect on agoraphobia and the panic variables. A significant effect on the agoraphobia measurement was found for exposure in vivo in comparison with both imipramine and alprazolam. Other studies have confirmed that cognitive therapy is as effective as drug treatment.[54]

Some studies have concluded that drug treatment can be effective in patients who are resistant to psychological therapy. For example, Hoffart et al. demonstrated the short-term efficacy of clomipramine in panic agoraphobic patients who had not responded to previous behavioural treatment.[63]

Efficacy of combined treatments

In clinical practice, a combination of drug therapy and psychological treatment is often proposed for panic patients,[69] especially for severe patients. However, data from controlled studies of these combinations are inconclusive. Most comparative studies have found a better clinical improvement of panic disorder when drug and psychological treatments were combined.[65,66] For example, in a meta-analysis, Mattick et al. showed that a combination of imipramine and exposure in vivo had extra value compared with each treatment separately (i.e. the superiority of the combination over imipramine alone for the scale of agoraphobia).[62] However, this is not always the case for a combination of BZDs with CBT, as has been shown for alprazolam and diazepam, as there is a probable negative interference between these medications and exposure therapy.[65,66]

The short-term benefit of combined treatment has not been found to persist at long-term follow-up, as has been shown by Cohne et al.[67] and Mavissakalian and Michelson[68] in studies that included a 2-year follow-up after an acute phase of combined treatments compared with CBT alone. Based on the limited available data, Telch and Lucas recommended therapists to use CBT alone in a first-line decision for the panic disorder patient and to add drug therapy if CBT is either unavailable, unacceptable or (probably) inefficient (e.g. the presence of severe depression or substance abuse).[65] However, these recommendations were made without data about the efficacy of SSRIs in combined treatment, as well as without data about recent specific cognitive or CBT procedures that target panic directly. Thus it is difficult at the moment to assess evidence about precise recommendations for combined treatment, at least as a first-line decision. For severe forms of illness or for resistant patients, a combination of psychological and pharmacological treatments is clearly necessary, as discussed later.

Special recommendation for the management of difficult patients

Even if the majority of panic patients can be improved adequately by drug and/or psychological treatment, a significant number will be partial or complete non-responders to the first-line treatment prescribed. For example, 30–40% of patients fail to benefit completely from exposure therapy, 65% stop short of recovery and many continue to seek pharmacological or psychological help after exposure therapy.[59] As in the treatment of major depression, about 60% of patients are responders to antidepressants in control trials (i.e. about 40% need an augmentation or an alternative strategy).[8,9] Noyes et al., in a 7-year follow-up study of outcome in panic disorder, analysed the illness variables that were predictive of poor outcome.[69] Most of these variables reflected the severity of the illness at inclusion: more severe panic and agoraphobic symptoms, psychiatric hospitalization and longer duration of the illness. Other variables associated with poor outcome were comorbid depression, high personality sensitivity and a number of significant life events or environmental factors (separation from a parent by death or divorce, low social class, unmarried status). It is probably important to recognize these poor outcome factors early on in the course of treatment in order to decide as soon as possible on the most adequate therapeutic strategy.

As a general rule, educating the patient is a key issue in managing anxiety, and especially in panic disorder. All the explanations that can be given about the definition, symptomatology, physiopathology, course and associated features of panic will improve the patient's comprehension about his or her sensations and behaviours, and may reduce the demoralization tendencies that are frequently associated with this long-lasting condition; hence they may improve the patient–physician alliance. When the clinician considers that there is a choice between various therapeutic strategies (i.e. between drug and psychological therapy), selection should be based on patient preference. The patient with panic disorder needs to be an active, fully informed participant in the treatment process, and demystification about the features of therapy is frequently needed.[4] Compliance to treatment (i.e. accurate drug intake and/or adequate exposure exercises) will be enhanced by any information that is given about the goals of the treatment, on the medication's mechanisms of action and on the treatment's benefit/risk ratio. The management of the medication's side-effects is of considerable importance as panic patients are particularly sensitive to these effects and because of the long duration of most of the treatments required. Critical to successful outcome is not stopping medication abruptly (BZDs as with other drugs) without consulting the physician. This will avoid rebound or withdrawal effects, even if the treatment has not been entirely effective.

Another important point in the management of panic disorder is an awareness of a possible residual symptomatology that can persist for a long period of time even if the more dramatic symptoms seem to be under control. These subtle signs might be limited panic attacks (such as brief, but not severe or recurrent, periods of dizziness), minor phobic avoidance tendencies or moderate but long-lasting anticipatory anxiety. The tenacious persistence of these symptoms can contribute to the patient maintaining a high level of impairment or distress, which in turn can lead to demoralizing counteractions that disrupt full compliance with the treatment and hence facilitate relapse.

As already mentioned, comorbidity is of crucial importance in the treatment of panic disorder. A history of or the presence of a comorbid condition can alter the validity of the diagnosis, influence the patient's compliance and modify treatment efficacy. A complete psychological assessment and medical examination are needed as about 70% of patients with panic disorder may have a comorbid condition that will need to be taken into account in planning therapy.[4] Even patients who are demoralized secondary to their suffering panic attacks will need treatment for their panic attacks first, and other, severe, conditions may require concurrent treatment: major depression, bipolar mood disorder, dissociative disorder, eating disorder and all the anxiety disorders (such as post-traumatic stress disorder, social phobia or obsessive–compulsive disorder). Moreover, a careful assessment of substance abuse or dependence is also needed, including alcohol, cannabis, opiates, hallucinogens, cocaine, benzodiazepines, caffeine and over-the-counter drugs (such as nasal sprays or diet pills).[4]

Most of these comorbid disorders will influence, in part, the choice of the treatment for panic. For example, the treatment must be an antidepressant if major depression is detected. Similarly, a current or past history of addictive disorder will discourage the use of a BZD because of the increased risk of dependence or abuse in such patients. Personality disorders may also affect treatment responses,[70] and so the choice of pharmacological treatment and psychological therapy must take the patient's personality profile into account. Hence, borderline personality disorder takes on a special importance because of the behavioural and emotional instability and the high risk of suicide attempts associated with this condition.

Medical conditions that may affect the treatment schedule and that may need to be treated concurrently with the panic disorder are, first, conditions with a prominent component of chronic or acute anxiety (such as thyroid disease, polycythaemia, lupus and pulmonary insufficiency); secondly, conditions that may affect the safety or efficacy of psychopharmacological treatment (such as some specific cardiovascular, pulmonary, gastrointestinal or endocrine disease, pregnancy and lactation); and, thirdly, conditions requiring medications that may cause or exacerbate anxiety (such as vasoconstrictors, bronchodilatators or steroids).[4]

Lastly, panic disorder is rare in elderly subjects but can be more difficult to manage in these patients, at least with pharmacological treatments. Elderly patients are often more vulnerable to certain antidepressant side-effects (such as anticholinergic, orthostatic and sedative effects) than are younger patients. Thus, TCAs and MAOIs should be used with caution, while SSRIs are safer and well tolerated. Elderly subjects are also particularly susceptible to the unwanted effects of BZDs such as ataxia, amnesia and confusion (see Table 5.4).

Table 5.4   Key points for the management of difficult panic patients.

- Diagnostic issues: careful assessment of somatic (especially cardiovascular, pulmonary and endocrine diseases) and psychiatric comorbidity (affective, anxiety and personality disorders, as well as alcohol and substance abuse risks)
- Educational interventions in the disorder and the treatment used
- Combined psychological and drug therapy if possible
- High doses, and a combination of drug therapy (e.g. SSRI plus BZD) (if tolerated) in cases of resistance
- Special attention paid to residual symptomatology and to environmental contingencies that may maintain the problem
- Alternative drug therapy and other forms of psychosocial treatments

Conclusions

Various efficient treatments are now available for treating panic disorder. These are chiefly pharmacological treatments (with the SSRIs being the first line) and CBT. The choice of the treatment should be guided by clinical features (e.g. history, course, previous responses) and by clinician and patient preferences. Drugs and psychological treatment can be combined. After an acute response, long-term therapy is recommended, in most cases lasting up to 1–2 years. The main concerns in the management of difficult panic patients are comorbidity issues, compliance (and thus education) and relapse prevention.

References

1. American Psychiatric Association. *Diagnostic and Statistical Manual of Mental Disorders* (4th edn) (Washington, DC: American Psychiatric Association, 1994).

2. Pélissolo A, Lépine JP. Epidemiology of depression and anxiety disorders. In Montgomery SA, den Boer JA (eds) *SSRIs in Depression and Anxiety* (Chichester: Wiley, 1998): 1–21.

3. Kaplan HI, Sadock BJ, Grebb JA. *Synopsis of Psychiatry* (7th edn) (Baltimore, MD: Williams & Wilkins, 1994).

4. Wolfe BE, Maser JD. *Treatment of Panic Disorder. A Consensus Development Conference* (Washington, DC: American Psychiatric Press, 1994).

5. Klein DF. Delineation of two drug-responsive anxiety syndromes. *Psychopharmacologia* (1964) **5:** 397–408.

6. Pélissolo A, Lépine JP. Psychopharmacological approaches to the treatment of anxiety disorders: a critical review and practical guidelines. In den Boer JA (ed) *Clinical Management of Anxi-*

ety: Theory and Practical Applications (New York: Marcel Dekker, 1997): 249–94.

7. Cross-National Collaborative Panic Study, Second Phase Investigators. Drug treatment of panic disorder. Comparative efficacy of alprazolam, imipramine, and placebo. *Br J Psychiatry* (1992) **160:** 191–202.

8. Ballenger JC. Treatment of panic disorder with serotonin reuptake inhibitors (SSRIs). In Montgomery SA, den Boer JA (eds) *SSRIs in Depression and Anxiety: Perspective in Psychiatry. Vol. 7* (Chichester: Wiley, 1998): 115–34.

9. Bell CJ, Nutt DJ. Serotonin and panic. *Br J Psychiatry* (1998) **172:** 465–71.

10. de Beurs E, van Balkom A, Lange A et al. Treatment of panic disorder with agoraphobia: comparison of fluvoxamine, placebo and psychological panic management combined with exposure and of exposure in vivo alone. *Am J Psychiatry* (1995) **152:** 683–91.

11. Black DW, Wesner R, Bowers W et al. A comparison of fluvoxamine, cognitive therapy and placebo in the treatment of panic disorder. *Arch Gen Psychiatry* (1993) **50:** 44–50.

12. Dunbar G, Steiner M, Oakes R et al. A fixed dose study of paroxetine (10 mg, 20 mg, 40 mg) and placebo in the treatment of panic disorder. *Eur Neuropsychopharmacol* (1995) **5:** 361.

13. Oehrberg S, Christiansen PE, Behnke K et al. Paroxetine in the treatment of panic disorder. A randomized, double-blind, placebo-controlled study. *Br J Psychiatry* (1995) **167:** 374–9.

14. Lecrubier Y, Bakker A, Dunbar G et al. A comparison of paroxetine, clomipramine and placebo in the treatment of panic disorder. *Acta Psychiatr Scand* (1997) **95:** 145–52.

15. Lecrubier Y, Judge R, Collaborative Paroxetine Panic Study Investigators. Long-term evaluation of paroxetine, clomipramine and placebo in panic disorder. *Acta Psychiatr Scand* (1997) **95:** 153–60.

16. Londborg PD, Wolokow R, Smith WT et al. Sertraline in the treatment of panic disorder. A multisite, double-blind, placebo-controlled, fixed-dose investigation. *Br J Psychiatry* (1998) **173:** 54–60.

17. Rapaport MH, Wolkow RM, Clary CM. Methodologies and outcomes from the sertraline multicenter flexible-dose trials. *Psychopharmacol Bull* (1998) **34:** 183–9.

18. Wade A, Lepola U, Koponen H et al. The effect of citalopram in panic disorder. *Br J Psychiatry* (1997) **170:** 549–53.

19. Pollack MH, Worthington JJ, Otto MW et al. Venlafaxine for panic disorder: results from a double-blind, placebo-controlled study. *Psychopharmacol Bull* (1996) **32:** 667–70.

20. Ballenger JC, Burrows GD, Dupont RL et al. Alprazolam in panic disorder and agoraphobia: results from a multicenter trial. I. Efficacy in short-term treatment. *Arch Gen Psychiatry* (1988) **45:** 413–22.

21. Schatzberg AF, Ballenger JC. Decisions for the clinician in the treatment of panic disorder: when to treat, which treatment to use, and how long to treat. *J Clin Psychiatry* (1991) **52(Suppl 2):** 26–31.

22. Ballenger JC. Overview of the pharmacotherapy of panic disorder. In Wolfe BE, Maser JD (eds) *Treatment of Panic Disorder. A Consensus Development Conference* (Washington, DC: American Psychiatric Press, 1994): 59–81.

23. Briggs AC, Stretch DD, Brandon S. Subtyping of panic disorder by

symptom profile. *Br J Psychiatry* (1993) **163:** 201–9.

24. Klein DF. Commentary: the treatment of panic. *Psychopharmacol Bull* (1998) **34:** 197.

25. Lépine JP, Aschauer H, van den Broek WA et al. Treatment of panic disorder: algorithms for pharmacotherapy. *Int J Psychiatry Clin Pract* (1997) **1(Suppl 1):** S13–S15.

26. Salzman C. Benzodiazepine treatment of panic and agoraphobic symptoms: use, dependence, toxicity, abuse. *J Psychiatr Res* (1993) **27(Suppl 1):** 97–100 (review).

27. Boyer W. Serotonin uptake inhibitors are superior to imipramine and alprazolam in alleviating panic attacks: a meta-analysis. *Int Clin Psychopharmacol* (1995) **10:** 45–9.

28. Jobson KO, Davidson JRT, Lydiard RB et al. Algorithm for the treatment of panic disorder. *Psychopharmacol Bull* (1995) **31:** 483–5.

29. Westenberg HGM. Developments in the drug treatment of panic disorder: what is the place of the selective serotonin reuptake inhibitors? *J Affect Disorders* (1996) **40:** 85–93.

30. Albus M, Lecrubier Y, Maier W et al. Drug treatment of panic disorder: early response to treatment as a predictor of final outcome. *Acta Psychiatr Scand* (1990) **82:** 359–65.

31. Pollack MH, Smoller JW. The longitudinal course and outcome of panic disorder. *Psychiatr Clin N Am* (1995) **18:** 785–801.

32. Noyes R Jr, Garvey MJ, Cook BL et al. Problems with tricyclic use in patients with panic disorder or agoraphobia: results of a naturalistic follow-up study. *J Clin Psychiatry* (1989) **50:** 163–9.

33. Nagy LM, Krystal JH, Charney DS et al. Long-term outcome of panic disorder after short-term imipramine and behavioral group treatment: 2.9-year naturalistic follow-up study. *J Clin Psychopharmacol* (1993) **13:** 16–24.

34. Davidson JRT. The long-term treatment of panic disorder. *J Clin Psychiatry* (1998) **59(Suppl 8):** 17–21.

35. Ballenger JC, Davidson JRT, Lecrubier Y et al. Consensus statement on panic disorder from an international consensus group on depression and anxiety. *J Clin Psychiatry* (1998) **59(Suppl 8):** 47–54.

36. Den Boer JA. Pharmacotherapy of panic disorder: differential efficacy from a clinical viewpoint. *J Clin Psychiatry* (1998) **59(Suppl 8):** 30–6.

37. Mavissakalian M, Perel JM. Clinical experiments in maintenance and discontinuation of imipramine therapy in panic disorder with agoraphobia. *Arch Gen Psychiatry* (1992) **49:** 318–23.

38. Noyes R Jr, Perry P. Maintenance treatment with antidepressants in panic disorder. *J Clin Psychiatry* (1990) **51(Suppl 12):** 24–30.

39. Rosenberg R. Drug treatment of panic disorder. *Pharmacol Toxicol* (1993) **72:** 344–53.

40. Brawman-Mintzer O, Lydiard RB. Psychopharmacology of anxiety disorders. *Psychiatr Clin N Am* (1994) **1:** 51–79.

41. Coplan JD, Pine DS, Papp LA, Gorman JM. An algorithm-oriented approach for panic disorder. *Psychiatr Ann* (1996) **26:** 192–201.

42. Frances A, Miele GM, Widiger TA et al. The classification of panic disorders: from Freud to DSM-IV. *J Psychiatry Res* (1993) **27(Suppl 1):** 3–10.

43. de Jonghe F. Current psychoanalytical views on anxiety: consequences for therapy. In den Boer JA (ed) *Clinical Management of*

Anxiety: Theory and Practical Applications (New York: Marcel Dekker, 1997): 179–96.

44. Schrodt GR Jr, Wright JH, Breen KJ. Practical application of cognitive-behavioral therapy in anxiety disorders. In den Boer JA (ed) *Clinical Management of Anxiety: Theory and Practical Applications* (New York: Marcel Dekker, 1997): 151–77.

45. Salkovskis P, Clark DM, Heckman A. Treatment of panic attacks using cognitive therapy without exposure or breathing retraining. *Behav Res Ther* (1991) **29:** 161–6.

46. Marks IM, Boulougouris UR, Marset P. Flooding versus densitization in the treatment of phobic patients: a crossover study. *Br J Psychiatry* (1971) **144:** 1160–5.

47. Barlow DH, O'Brien GT, Last CG. Couples treatment of agoraphobia. *Behav Ther* (1984) **15:** 41–58.

48. Clark DM, Salkovskis PM, Chalkley AJ. Respiratory control as a treatment for panic attacks. *J Behav Ther Exp Psychiatry* (1985) **16:** 23–30.

49. Ost LG. Applied relaxation: description of a coping technique and review of controlled studies. *Behav Res Ther* (1987) **25:** 397–410.

50. Emmelkamp PMG, Scholing A. Behavioral strategies for panic disorder, social phobia, and obsessive-compulsive disorder. In den Boer JA (ed) *Clinical Management of Anxiety: Theory and Practical Applications* (New York: Marcel Dekker, 1996): 79–108.

51. Barlow DH. Effectiveness of behavior treatment for panic disorder with and without agoraphobia. In Wolfe BE, Maser JD (eds) *Treatment of Panic Disorder: A Consensus Development Conference* (Washington, DC: American Psychiatric Press, 1994): 105–20.

52. Barlow DH, Craske M, Cerny J, Klosko J. Behavioral treatment of panic disorder. *Behav Ther* (1989) **20:** 261–82.

53. Griez E, van den Hout MA. CO_2 inhalation in the treatment of panic attacks. *Behav Res Ther* (1986) **24:** 145–50.

54. Clark DM. Cognitive therapy for panic disorder. In Wolfe BE, Maser JD (eds) *Treatment of Panic Disorder: A Consensus Development Conference* (Washington, DC: American Psychiatric Press, 1994): 121–32.

55. Margraf J, Schneider S. Outcome and active ingredients of cognitive-behavioral treatment for panic disorders. Paper presented at annual meeting of the Association for Advance of Behavior Therapy, New York, 26 November 1991.

56. Beck AT, Sokol J, Clark DA et al. A crossover study of focused cognitive therapy for panic disorder. *Am J Psychiatry* (1992) **147:** 778–83.

57. Beck AT, Emery GD, Greenberg RL. *Anxiety Disorders and Phobias: A Cognitive Perspective* (New York: Basic Books, 1985).

58. Barlow DH, Cerny JA. *Psychological Treatment of Panic* (New York: Guilford Press, 1988).

59. Chambless DL, Gillis MM. A review of psychological treatments for panic disorder. In Wolfe BE, Maser JD (eds) *Treatment of Panic Disorder. A Consensus Development Conference* (Washington, DC: American Psychiatric Press, 1994): 149–73.

60. Cobb JP, Mathews AM, Childs-Clarke A et al. The spouse as co-therapist in the treatment of agoraphobia. *Br J Psychiatry* (1984) **144:** 282–7.

61. Arnow BA, Taylor CB, Agras WS et al. Enhancing agoraphobia treatment outcome by changing couple communication patterns. *Behav Ther* (1985) **16:** 452–67.

62. Mattick RP, Andrews G, Hadzi-Pavlovic D, Christensen H. Treatment of panic and agoraphobia: an integrative review. *J Nerv Ment Dis* (1990) **178:** 567–76.

63. Hoffart A, Due-Madsen J, Lande B et al. Clomipramine in the treatment of agoraphobic inpatients resistant to behavioral therapy. *J Clin Psychiatry* (1993) **54:** 481–7.

64. Taylor CB, King R, Margraf J et al. Use of medication and in vivo exposure in volunteers for panic disorder research. *Am J Psychiatry* (1989) **146:** 1423–6.

65. Telch MJ, Lucas RA. Combined pharmacological and psychological treatment of panic disorder: current status and future directions. In Wolfe BE, Maser JD (eds) *Treatment of Panic Disorder. A Consensus Development Conference* (Washington, DC: American Psychiatric Press, 1994): 177–97.

66. Van Dyck R, van Balkom JLM. Combination therapy for anxiety disorders. In den Boer JA (ed) *Clinical Management of Anxiety: Theory and Practical Applications* (New York: Marcel Dekker, 1997): 109–36.

67. Cohen SD, Monteiro W, Marks IM. Two-year follow-up agoraphobics after exposure and imipramine. *Br J Psychiatry* (1984) **144:** 276–81.

68. Mavissakalian M, Michelson L. Two-year follow-up of exposure and imipramine treatment of agoraphobia. *Am J Psychiatry* (1986) **143:** 1106–12.

69. Noyes R, Clancey J, Woodman C et al. Environmental factors related to the outcome of panic disorder. A seven-year follow-up study. *J Nerv Dis* (1993) **181:** 529–38.

70. Reich JH, Vasile RG. Effect of personality disorders on the treatment outcome of axis I conditions: an update. *J Nerv Ment Dis* (1993) **181:** 475–84.

6
Treatment of the difficult obsessive–compulsive disorder patient

Dan J Stein and Robin A Emsley

Introduction

In recent years there have been dramatic advances in our understanding and management of obsessive–compulsive disorder (OCD). OCD has long been considered a relatively uncommon disorder, caused by unconscious conflicts, and rather unresponsive to treatment. However, studies have now demonstrated that OCD is one of the most prevalent psychiatric disorders,[1,2] that it has important neurobiological underpinnings[3,4] and that it responds well to specific medications and psychotherapies.[5,6] Media attention and the formation of strong advocacy groups have helped translate these advances into concrete benefits for thousands of people with OCD.

Despite these advances, there are many patients with OCD who may continue to be characterized as 'difficult' by the treating clinician. Patients may be difficult to diagnose or may have complicating diagnoses, factors contributing to the pathogenesis of the OCD may be complex and problematic, and standard anti-OCD treatments may be completely or partially unsuccessful. In this chapter these various kinds of difficulties are discussed. Current clinical guidelines for the management of the difficult OCD patient are provided and areas for future research are outlined.

Diagnostic difficulties

The hallmark of OCD are obsessions and compulsions.[7] Obsessions are recurrent and persistent thoughts, impulses or images the person typically regards as intrusive and inappropriate. Compulsions are repetitive behaviours or mental acts the person feels driven to perform in response to an obsession, or according to rules that must be followed rigidly. Common obsessions and compulsions, such as contamination obsessions and hand-washing compulsions, or thoughts about harm and repetitive checking, are usually easily recognized by clinicians when described by patients.

An immediate difficulty, however, is that patients may not describe the presence of obsessions and compulsions unless specific inquiries are made about these symptoms. Several possible reasons for this exist, including the belief that such phenomena are personality traits rather than treatable symptoms, or shame and embarrassment about symptoms (e.g. blasphemous thoughts in a religious person).[8] Occasionally certain obsessions interfere with help-seeking (e.g. a patient of ours had obsessions that she might in fact be psychotic and avoided doctors on the grounds they might label her insane). In general, however, this difficulty can be overcome by routinely including questions about intrusive thoughts and repetitive actions in the psychiatric history.

In children it is particularly important to inquire about the presence of obsessions and compulsions given that such patients are relatively unlikely to disclose their symptoms spontaneously to a clinician. Young children with OCD may be distressed by their symptoms and may have clearly observable motoric compulsions. Nevertheless, they may have difficulty in articulating the underlying obsessions (if these are present) that lead to rituals, or in describing the intrusive nature of symptoms. It is of course important also to interview family members or other caregivers in such cases.

Some OCD patients have unusual symptoms that delay or confuse diagnosis. Obsessions such as intrusive tunes, olfactory concerns or obsessional jealousy may not be recognized initially as obsessions.[9,10] Compulsions may be entirely mental (e.g. mental checking or mental reviewing), making them less obvious and harder to describe. The subgroup of OCD patients with obsessional slowness is sometimes difficult to recognize as having OCD. OCD patients with poor insight may be misdiagnosed as psychotic. Nevertheless, a careful psychiatric history and a high index of suspicion for OCD are usually sufficient to determine whether symptoms conform to the general form of obsessions and compulsions. Furthermore, in many patients there is also a history of more classical OCD symptoms.

Conversely, some patients who do not in fact have OCD may be misdiagnosed with this disorder. Possible errors include the misdiagnosis of ruminations in depression, worries in generalized anxiety disorder and intrusive symptoms in post-traumatic stress disorder as obsessions. Perfectionistic traits in obsessive–compulsive personality disorder and stereotyped symptoms in schizophrenia and other disorders may mimic compulsions. Finally, of course, it is important to determine whether obsessions and compulsions are due to an underlying medical condition, such as Sydenham's chorea.

The recent notion of obsessive–compulsive spectrum disorders, which includes conditions that have phenomenological and neurobiological similarities with OCD, may be helpful in making accurate diagnoses.[11] For example, it is increasingly recognized that patients with body dysmorphic disorder (where there are obsessive and compulsive symptoms relating to imagined ugliness) or hypochondriasis (where there are obsessive and compulsive symptoms relating to imagined illness) have much in common with OCD.[12,13] Certainly, diagnosis of these disorders suggests the use of pharmacotherapeutic and psychotherapeutic interventions that are useful in OCD.

Nevertheless, there are may also be important dissimilarities between symptoms in OCD and in spectrum disorders. For example, there are differences in the kinds of obsessive and compulsive symptoms usually experienced in patients with and without Tourette's disorder.[14] Similarly, there may be important differences in the management of OCD and spectrum disorders such as trichotillomania. Thus, the notion of an obsessive–compulsive spectrum may best be viewed currently as providing a useful clinical and research heuristic, rather than as comprising a well-validated nosological construct.

Complicating diagnoses

Many patients with OCD have comorbid diagnoses, including mood and anxiety disorders. Certain comorbid illnesses impact negatively on treatment. For example, a number of personality disorders have been associated with relatively poor outcome of OCD to standard psychotherapy and pharmacotherapy,[15–17] and the total number of abnormal personality disorder traits has been associated with worse outcome in some studies.[18] On the other hand, comorbid disorders in OCD, including comorbid personality disorder traits, may also respond during standard anti-OCD management. Thus, OCD treatment should be vigorously pursued whether or not comorbid disorders are present.

A number of authors have described the phenomenon of OCD patients with comorbid schizotypal personality disorder. These patients may be less motivated to seek treatment, and may respond more poorly to both behaviour therapy[15] and pharmacotherapy.[16] It is possible that in addition to the serotonergic dysfunction that may play a role in their OCD, these patients also display the dopaminergic abnormalities thought to be present in patients with schizotypal personality disorder. The combination of serotonin reuptake blockers and dopamine blockers, which is useful in some treatment-refractory OCD patients (see below), should therefore be considered. In addition, help from the family in maintaining compliance with treatment may well be needed.

Obsessive–compulsive symptoms have been included in the wide range of mood and anxiety symptoms suffered by patients with borderline personality disorder (BPD).[17] While abnormal personality disorder traits may improve during successful treatment of OCD,[19,20] both disorders may well require ongoing attention in patients with OCD and BPD. Such patients may display behaviours that are characteristic of BPD patients, including setting practitioners at odds with one another, devaluing suggested interventions and displaying symptoms, such as impulsivity, which can interfere with treatment. In addition to anti-OCD treatment, a psychotherapy focused on interpersonal issues may well be indicated.

OCD may be complicated by a range of more 'impulsive' diagnoses, including conduct disorder, antisocial personality disorder or substance abuse. Indeed, a reanalysis of the epidemiological catchment area data demonstrated that OCD patients had increased rates of childhood conduct symptoms, adult antisocial personality disorder problems and suicide attempts compared with patients with no or with other psychiatric disorders.[21] During treatment of OCD, there may, however, be a decrease in impulsive symptoms.[22] In patients with OCD and comorbid substance dependence, this latter diagnosis must clearly be addressed if management of OCD is to be successful.

Some OCD patients may have serious comorbid psychopathology, such as schizophrenia. It has been noted that certain antipsychotic agents, such as clozapine, may initiate or exacerbate OCD symptoms in patients with schizophrenia.[23] On the other hand, there is also increasing evidence that the combination of antipsychotics and serotonin reuptake blockers is useful in patients with comorbid schizophrenia and OCD.[24] In addition, serotonin reuptake inhibitors (SRIs) may initiate or exacerbate manic or hypomanic symptoms in some OCD patients. Again, however, such patients may respond to the combined use of antidepressants and mood stabilizers, including lithium.

Complications in pathogenesis

The pathogenesis of OCD is at present not entirely understood. Current theory suggests that genetic factors and environmental factors (including bacterial infections) play an important role.[25] Certainly, there is good evidence that OCD symptoms are mediated by cortico-striatal circuits.[4] Nevertheless, a range of different factors may contribute to the pathogenesis of the disorder, leading to various clinical difficulties.

In families where different members have subclinical OCD or frank obsessive–compulsive behaviour, for example, obsessions and compulsions in one person may be further exacerbated. A male patient of ours who had contamination obsessions and compulsive hand-washing married a woman who was extremely fastidious and neat in their new home. Rather than recognizing his symptoms as pathological, she reinforced them as appropriate behaviours. During the initial years of the marriage his symptoms become more and more time-consuming. When he did seek treatment, his wife was reluctant to encourage exposure and response prevention.

At times, a similar role may be played by the patient's cultural group. For example, certain religious movements may encourage the performance of rituals. More commonly, however, the patient worries that the actions must be done because of religious beliefs, but the symptoms are in fact recognized as pathological within his or her religious peer group. In our practice we have not infrequently met with the patient and his or her religious leader in order to determine the boundaries of religion and psychopathology and in order to encourage the religious leader to 'coach' the person in exposure and response prevention techniques. Such leaders often support the implementation of this kind of treatment.

We mentioned earlier that patients with Tourette's syndrome or with chronic motor tics may have symptoms of OCD. It is possible that such patients have subtle differences in underlying neurobiology when compared to other patients with OCD. Certainly, while pharmacological challenge and pharmacotherapeutic dissection studies show good evidence for the specific involvement of the serotonin system in OCD,[3] similar kinds of studies indicate involvement of the dopamine system in tic disorders. It is important to ask all patients with OCD about history of tics. Furthermore, studies showing that OCD patients with tics may have a poorer response to SRI treatment, but may respond to augmentation of SRIs with dopamine blockers, suggest that this treatment strategy should be considered in such patients.[26]

Another neurobiological system that may be involved in the pathogenesis of OCD is the hormonal one. Certainly, there is a frequent onset of OCD during or after pregnancy.[27] Symptoms such as thoughts of harming the baby during the peurperium may be particularly embarrassing and distressing for the patient. During pregnancy and lactation, pharmacotherapy is of course relatively contraindicated. A cognitive-behavioural psychotherapy may therefore be a good first intervention. Nevertheless, there is some evidence that certain SRIs may be acceptably safe during pregnancy, should clinical circumstances warrant this risk.

Treatment-refractory OCD

The response of drug-naive patients to an SRI may be as high as 70%. On the other hand, in large clinical trials of the SRIs, where patients who have failed other SRIs are included, the response rate may be only 50–60%.[5] Certainly, many OCD patients may respond to a trial of adequate dose (often higher in OCD than in depression) and duration (often longer in OCD than in depression).[28] A patient should certainly not be labelled as refractory to pharmacotherapy before at least one (if not more) 10–12 week trial of an SRI at high doses (e.g. fluoxetine 60 mg) has failed. Nevertheless, there remains a not insubstantial group of OCD patients who fail to respond to first-line pharmacotherapy of this disorder.

Certain patients may be particularly unlikely to respond to an SRI. These include patients with tics and perhaps with hoarding symptoms. On the other hand, it has not clearly been shown that OCD patients with poor insight (this may be particularly common in related disorders like BDD) have a worse response to pharmacotherapy. Thus every effort should be made to encourage such patients to begin these medications. The safety and possible value of medication in reducing anxious symptoms should be emphasized in order to persuade patients of the possible benefits of such treatment.

For patients who respond poorly or only partially to an SRI, a first step is to switch to another SRI. There is good evidence that this strategy is successful in some patients who have failed to respond to a first agent.[29] Meta-analyses of OCD pharmacotherapy have suggested that less-selective SRIs (such as clomipramine) may be more effective than more-selective SRIs in OCD.[30,31] On the other hand, such meta-analyses have important methodological limitations and head-to-head comparisons of different agents have not in fact confirmed this conclusion. Nevertheless, clomipramine can be recommended as a possible treatment for patients who have failed to respond to more-selective SRIs (perhaps particularly when there is comorbid severe depression[32]).

It is possible that, after failure of several different SRIs has been documented, response to other agents in this class becomes increasingly unlikely. A number of strategies have been put forward for the pharmacotherapy of such patients.

First, treatment augmentation may be attempted. Several different agents that are useful in the augmentation of serotonin reuptake inhibitors in treatment-refractory depression have been suggested, including lithium, buspirone and pindolol. More unusual strategies have also been proposed, including the benzodiazepine clonazepam, the anticonvulsants valproate and carbamazepine, the analgesic tramadol, the adrenal steroid suppressant aminoglutethimide and the antiandrogenic cyproterone acetate.[33–35] Nevertheless, those controlled trials which have taken place (e.g. of lithium, buspirone) have generally been disappointing.

The most convincing data in this area comprises those controlled trials demonstrating that dopamine blockers may be useful in augmenting SRI treatment of patients with OCD. As noted earlier, augmentation with dopamine blockers appears particularly effective in patients with comorbid tics.[26] Given their advantageous side-effect profile, use of the newer atypical neuroleptics may also be suggested in refractory OCD.[36–38] Interestingly, however, the preliminary data do not indicate that the presence of comorbid tics is necessary for an effective response to the combination of SRIs and atypical neuroleptics.

Augmentation of one SRI with a second SRI has also been suggested. Indeed, in one study the addition of sertraline to clomipramine 150 mg/d was more tolerable and more effective than further increasing the dose of clomipramine.[37] On the other hand, it is important to bear in mind the possibility of dangerous pharmacokinetic interactions between different SRIs. Certainly, patients who are being treated with a combination of such agents should be carefully monitored.[39]

A second strategy is to switch from the SRIs to an entirely different class of medication. This strategy has not, however, been well researched. Although some work has suggested that phenelzine might be useful in OCD, other studies have failed to replicate this finding. Nevertheless, in our experience and that of others, certain non-SRI agents, such as phenelzine and venlafaxine, may on occasion be effective in treatment-resistant OCD.[40] Current work using immune therapies for the treatment of OCD is particularly exciting and may ultimately lead to novel kinds of interventions for the difficult-to-treat OCD patient.[41] Once again, additional controlled trials are necessary in this area.

When OCD patients fail several different SRIs it is worthwhile to reassess the diagnosis. In addition, medical causes of OCD symptoms should be ruled out. Unfortunately, however, it is the case that some patients with clearcut OCD do not respond to several different medications. There is most certainly a need for increased research on the pharmacotherapy of this group. Current trials using high doses of SRIs, administered intravenously[42] or orally,[43] appear particularly interesting.

Perhaps the most important augmenting intervention in OCD patients who fail to respond to pharmacotherapy is, however, behavioural psychotherapy. Certainly, we now know that both pharmacotherapy and behavioural psychotherapy normalize specific brain dysfunctions on functional brain imaging.[44] There is also evidence that behavioural psychotherapy is more effective than pharmacotherapy in preventing relapse after treatment discontinuation. Nevertheless, it is also true that many patients resist behavioural therapy. Patients may argue that they have tried such strategies previously, that they will not be able to cope with increased anxiety or that the core principles of behaviour therapy – exposure and response prevention – simply cannot constitute an effective treatment.

There are several strategies for encouraging behavioural therapy. Psychoeducation is crucial – patients should be encouraged to read a good book on OCD (e.g. Baer's *Getting Control*). The effect of behaviour therapy on normalizing the brain should be emphasized.[44] Patients should also be encouraged to join a consumer support group – either in person or online – in the form of virtual internet support groups.[45] It is also important to bring in the family and educate them about OCD and its behavioural treatment. Family members should be taught how to be supportive 'coaches'. Portable computer programs may also be valuable in promoting adherence to exposure and response prevention programmes. Patients should be reassured that the process of behaviour therapy is ultimately in their hands – they have control over how quickly to work through their symptom hierarchies.

Certainly, OCD patients should as a rule be strongly encouraged to draw up a behavioural hierarchy. If the patient is unable to do this task on his or her own, it is worth spending a session with the patient in order to do so. In trying to budge the resistant patient, remember that humour may be a useful tool – most patients accept at some level that their symptoms are senseless – and with sensitivity a patient can be made to learn to laugh with the clinician at symptoms. (A well-known behaviour therapist makes a habit of touching his shoe and cajoling patients with contamination fears to shake hands before leaving the office.)

Certain symptoms may be particularly difficult to treat with behaviour therapy. Depressive symptoms may well require pharmacotherapy in addition to psychotherapy. Checkers may find it more difficult than washers to comply with exposure and response prevention techniques. Repeated seeking of reassurance from others also interferes with behavioural therapy principles. Nevertheless, in all cases, application of the general principles of behaviour therapy should be attempted. It may be particularly helpful for the therapist also to expose him or herself to the feared stimulus (participant modelling). Similarly, exposure and response prevention sessions may be needed outside the consulting office in order to obtain maximal effect. Certain symptoms of OCD may require the adaptation of general behavioural principles. For example, prompting and shaping may be needed in patients with obsessional slowness. Patients who present with obsessions and neutralizing thoughts but without overt rituals may require a variety of techniques, such as thought stopping (a distracting technique aimed at interrupting obsessions), saturation (repeating obsessions until associated distress lessens) or stimulus control (confining obsessions to a specified amount of time). More cognitively based interventions may also be useful in patients with exaggerated responsibility, unrealistic threat appraisal and other cognitive distortions.[46] When OCD symptoms remain refractory to basic exposure and response prevention techniques, referral to cognitive-behavioural therapists with a specialized knowledge of OCD may prove helpful.

Most patients with OCD are best treated as outpatients. Nevertheless, reports indicate that hospitalization or partial hospitalization with a combined programme of pharmacotherapy and behaviour therapy may be a useful step in the treatment of some resistant patients. One study showed that the majority of OCD patients admitted to a multimodal partial hospital treatment programme demonstrated improvement.[47] Another study also found that individually tailored treatments in an inpatient setting proved useful in many OCD patients with chronic symptoms.[48]

For patients who have failed multiple medication and behavioural treatments, and where the severity of the disorder is high, neurosurgery should be considered. Several uncontrolled studies have indicated that specific lesions to the cortico-striatal pathways may lead to a significant reduction in OCD symptoms.[49] Patients can be referred to specialized centres in the USA, Sweden and elsewhere for such treatments. Although electroconvulsive therapy is not thought to be particularly helpful for OCD without comorbid depression, research on transcranial magnetic stimulation in OCD may ultimately provide new methods of treatment.

Counterintuitively, some patients who do respond to treatment then begin to manifest their own particular difficulties. When symptoms that have consumed several hours a day disappear, questions arise about past wasted time, and about future plans and goals. In such cases, exploratory psychotherapy may be useful. Other successfully treated patients may unfortunately have side-effects of medication. Fortunately, the range of available SRIs often means that medication substitution is an option. There are also increasing alternatives for patients complaining of such common side-effects as decreased libido after SRI treatment. Furthermore, some (but not all) studies suggest that during maintenance pharmacotherapy of OCD it may be possible to lower the dose without loss of efficacy.[50]

Conclusion

In this chapter we have not touched on the large group of patients who are 'difficult', but not 'difficult' for the clinician. We refer to the group of patients who suffer from OCD but do not present for treatment or who decide not to embark on a recommended treatment. The size of this group may well be larger than the size of the group of patients who present with 'difficult' OCD. One of the most important issues in the future management of OCD is educating the community about OCD and encouraging people with this treatable disorder to seek ongoing help.

Indeed, OCD is one of the most rewarding psychiatric disorders to treat, precisely because patients are often relieved to receive a diagnosis and may respond well to first-line treatment. Nevertheless, as in other areas of psychiatry, there are some OCD patients who can perhaps be categorized as 'difficult'. However, with appropriate assessment and intervention, it is often possible, and indeed rewarding, to help these patients also. Further research needs to be done in order to increase the proportion of OCD patients whom clinicians are easily able to help.

Acknowledgement

Dr Stein is supported by the MRC (South Africa) Research Unit on Anxiety and Stress Disorders.

References

1. Karno M, Golding JM, Sorenson SB et al. The epidemiology of obsessive-compulsive disorder in five US communities. *Arch Gen Psychiatry* (1988) **45:** 1094–9.

2. Weissman MM, Bland RC, Canino GJ et al. The cross national epidemiology of obsessive compulsive disorder. *J Clin Psychiatry* (1994) **55S:** 5–10.

3. Zohar J, Insel TR. Obsessive-compulsive disorder: psychobiological approaches to diagnosis, treatment, and pathophysiology. *Biol Psychiatry* (1987) **22:** 667–87.

4. Insel TR. Toward a neuroanatomy of obsessive-compulsive disorder. *Arch Gen Psychiatry* (1992) **49:** 739–44.

5. Jenike MA. Pharmacologic treatment of obsessive-compulsive disorders. *Psych Clin N Am* (1992) **15:** 895–919.

6. Baer L, Minichiello WE. Behavior therapy for obsessive-compulsive disorder. In Jenike MA, Baer L, Minichiello WE (eds) *Obsessive–Compulsive Disorders: Theory and Management* (2nd edn) (Chicago, IL: Year Book Medical Publishers, 1990): 203–32.

7. American Psychiatric Association. *Diagnostic and Statistical Manual of Mental Disorders* (4th edn) (Washington, DC: American Psychiatric Press, 1994).

8. Stein DJ, Hollander E, Rowland C et al. Quality of life and pharmacoeconomic aspects of obsessive-compulsive disorder: a South African survey. *S Afr J Med* (1996) **86:** 1579–85.

9. Stein DJ, Hollander E. Serotonin reuptake blockers for the treatment of obsessional jealousy. *J Clin Psychiatry* (1994) **55:** 30–3.

10. Stein DJ, Le Roux L, Bouwer C, et al. Is olfactory reference syndrome on the obsessive-compulsive spectrum? Two cases and a discussion. *J Neuropsych Clin Neurosci* (1998) **10:** 96–9.

11. Stein DJ, Hollander E. The spectrum of obsessive-compulsive related disorders. In Hollander E (ed) *Obsessive-Compulsive Related Disorders* (Washington, DC: American Psychiatric Press, 1993): 241–72.

12. Hollander E, Liebowitz MR, Winchel R et al. Treatment of body-dysmorphic disorder with serotonin reuptake blockers. *Am J Psychiatry* (1989) **146:** 768–70.

13. Fallon BA, Javitch J, Liebowitz MR. Hypochondriasis and OCD. Overlaps in diagnosis and treatment. *J Clin Psychiatry* (1991) **52:** 457–60.

14. Pitman RK, Green RC, Jenike MA et al. Clinical comparison of Tourette's disorder and obsessive-compulsive disorder. *Am J Psychiatry* (1987) **144:** 1166–71.

15. Jenike MA, Baer L, Minichiello WE, Schwartz CE, Carey RJ. Concomitant obsessive-compulsive disorder and schizotypal personality disorder. *Am J Psychiatry* (1986) **143:** 530–2.

16. Minichiello WE, Baer L, Jenike MA. Schizotypal personality disorder: a poor prognostic indicator for behavior therapy in the treatment of obsessive–compulsive disorder. *J Anx Dis* (1987) **1:** 273–6.

17. Hermesh H, Shahar A, Munitz H. Obsessive-compulsive disorder and borderline personality disorder. *Am J Psychiatry* (1987) **144:** 120–1.

18. Baer L, Jenike MA, Black DW et al. Effects of axis II diagnoses on treatment outcome with clomipramine in 55 patients with obsessive-compulsive disorder. *Arch Gen Psychiatry* (1992) **49:** 862–6.

19. Mavissakalian M, Hamann MS, Jones B. DSM-III personality disorders in obsessive-compulsive disorder: changes with treatment. *Compr Psychiatry* (1990) **31:** 432–7.

20. Ricciardi JN, Baer L, Jenike MA, Fischer SC, Sholtz D, Buttoph ML. Changes in DSM-III-R axis II diagnoses following treatment of obsessive-compulsive disorder. *Am J Psychiatry* (1992) **149:** 829–31.

21. Hollander E, Greenwald S, Neville D et al. Uncomplicated and comorbid obsessive-compulsive disorder in an epidemiological sample. *Depression and Anxiety* (1996/1997) **4:** 111–19.

22. Stein DJ, Hollander E. Impulsive aggression and obsessive-compulsive disorder. *Psych Ann* (1993) **23:** 389–95.

23. Baker RW, Bermanzohn PC, Wirshing DA et al. Obsessions, compulsions, clozapine, and risperidone. *CNS Spectrums* (1997) **2:** 26–36.

24. Zohar J, Kaplan Z, Benjamin J. Clomipramine treatment of obsessive compulsive symptomatology in schizophrenic patients. *J Clin Psychiatry* (1993) **54:** 385–8.

25. Stein DJ. The neurobiology of obsessive-compulsive disorder. *Neuroscientist* (1996) **2:** 300–5.

26. McDougle CJ, Goodman WK, Leckman JF et al. Haloperidol addition in fluvoxamine-refractory obsessive-compulsive disorder: a double-blind placebo-controlled study in patients with and without tics. *Arch Gen Psychiatry* (1994) **51:** 302–8.

27. Neziroglu F, Anemone R, Yaryura-Tobias JA. Onset of obsessive-compulsive disorder in pregnancy. *Am J Psychiatry* (1992) **149:** 947–50.

28. Tollefson GD, Birkett M, Koran L et al. Continuation treatment of OCD: double-blind and open-label experience with fluoxetine. *J Clin Psychiatry* (1994) **55S:** 69–76.

29. Pigott TA, Pato MT, Bernstein SE et al. Controlled comparisons of clomipramine and fluoxetine in the treatment of obsessive-compulsive disorder. *Arch Gen Psychiatry* (1990) **47:** 926–32.

30. Jenike MA, Hyman S, Baer L et al. A controlled trial of fluvoxamine in obsessive–compulsive disorder: implications for a serotonergic theory. *Am J Psychiatry* (1990) **147:** 1209–15.

31. Stein DJ, Spadaccini E, Hollander E. Meta-analysis of pharmacotherapy trials for obsessive-compulsive disorder. *Int Clin Psychopharm* (1995) **10:** 11–18.

32. Hollander E, Mullen L, DeCaria CM et al. Obsessive-compulsive disorder, depression, and fluoxetine. *J Clin Psychiatry* (1991) **52:** 418–22.

33. Leonard HL, Topol D, Bukstein O et al. Clonazepam as an augmenting agent in the treatment of childhood-onset obsessive–compulsive disorder. *J Am Acad Child Adolesc Psychiatry* (1994) **33:** 792–4.

34. Chouinard G, Belanger MC, Beauclair L et al. Potentiation of fluoxetine by aminoglutethimide, an adrenal steroid suppressant, in obsessive-compulsive disorder resistant to SSRIs: a case report. *Prog Neuropsychopharmacol Biol Psychiatry* (1996) **20:** 1067–79.

35. Casas M, Alvarez E, Duro P et al. Antiandrogenic treatment of obsessive-compulsive neurosis. *Acta Psychiatr Scand* (1986) **73:** 221–2.

36. Saxena S, Wang D, Bystritsky A et al. Risperidone augmentation of SRI treatment for refractory obsessive-compulsive disorder. *J Clin Psychiatry* (1996) **57:** 303–6.

37. Ravizza L, Barzega G, Bellino S et

al. Therapeutic effect and safety of adjunctive risperidone in refractory obsessive-compulsive disorder (OCD). *Psychopharmacol Bull* (1996) **32:** 677–82.

38. Stein DJ, Bouwer C, Hawkridge S et al. Risperidone augmentation of serotonin reuptake inhibitors in obsessive-compulsive and related disorders. *J Clin Psychiatry* (1997) **58:** 119–22.

39. Szegedi A, Wetzel H, Leal M et al. Combination treatment with clomipramine and fluvoxamine: drug monitoring, safety, and tolerability data. *J Clin Psychiatry* (1996) **57:** 257–64.

40. Ananth J, Burgoyne K, Smith M et al. Venlafaxine for treatment of obsessive-compulsive disorder. *Am J Psychiatry* (1995) **152:** 1832.

41. Allen AJ, Leonard HL, Swedo SE. Case study: a new infection-triggered, autoimmune subtype of pediatric OCD and Tourette's syndrome. *J Am Acad Child Adolesc Psychiatry* (1995) **34:** 307–11.

42. Koran LM, Sallee FR, Pallanti S. Rapid benefit of intravenous pulse loading of clomipramine in obsessive-compulsive disorder. *Am J Psychiatry* (1997) **154:** 396–401.

43. Byerly MJ, Goodman WK, Christensen R. High doses of sertraline for treatment-resistant obsessive-compulsive disorder. *Am J Psychiatry* (1996) **153:** 1232–3.

44. Baxter LR, Schwartz JM, Bergman KS et al. Caudate glucose metabolic rate changes with both drug and behavior therapy for OCD. *Arch Gen Psychiatry* (1992) **49:** 681–9.

45. Stein DJ. Psychiatry on the Internet: survey of an OCD mailing list. *Psychiatric Bull* (1997) **21:** 95–8.

46. Salkovskis P. Obsessional-compulsive problems: a cognitive-behavioural analysis. *Behav Res Ther* (1985) **23:** 571–83.

47. Bystritsky A, Munford PR, Rosen RM et al. A preliminary study of partial hospital management of severe obsessive-compulsive disorder. *Psychiatr Serv* (1996) **47:** 170–4.

48. Drummond LM. The treatment of severe, chronic, resistant obsessive-compulsive disorder: an evaluation of an in-patient programme using behavioural psychotherapy in combination with other treatments. *Br J Psychiatry* (1993) **163:** 223–9.

49. Martuza RL, Chiocca EA, Jenike MA et al. Stereotactic radiofrequency thermal cingulotomy for obsessive-compulsive disorder. *J Neuropsychiatry* (1990) **2:** 331–6.

50. Mundo E, Bareggi SR, Pirola R et al. Long-term pharmacotherapy of obsessive-compulsive disorder: a double-blind controlled study. *J Clin Psychopharmacol* (1997) **17:** 4–10.

7
Anorexia nervosa

Janet Treasure

Introduction

Anorexia nervosa is renowned for being a difficult condition and yet some aspects of the disease, such as its recognition, are almost too easy to determine. Indeed, the lay public can often make the diagnosis. There has been great uncertainty across times and cultures about how the problem should be conceptualized and who is best fitted for this task. The disability caused by the illness ranges across the physical, psychological and social domains with variable levels of severity. Although it is a rare condition occurring predominantly in the teenage years, it usually persists for over 5 years and is the third commonest chronic condition of adolescence. A third fail ever to recover and the majority of these die prematurely. Treatment is the most difficult aspect. People with anorexia nervosa are at best ambivalent about help to change and at worst totally resistant. This leads to an unusual relationship between the women with anorexia nervosa and their potential helpers. Strong care-giving emotions are aroused because of the life-threatening nature of the illness and yet these drives are repulsed by the sufferer. Managing this counter-transference is very difficult, and standard practice has evolved from clinical empiricism. There are many difficulties in obtaining data upon which to mould evidence-based practices and these have not yet been overcome. In this chapter I hope to be able to shed some light on the difficulties caused by anorexia nervosa as a first step towards a solution.

History

The cultural framing of anorexia nervosa has led to wide differences in the way the condition has been managed. Bell[1] has argued that anorexia nervosa was construed as spiritual asceticism in medieval Europe. Later cases were regarded as freaks who defied the laws of science. This culminated in the unfortunate incident in which a Welsh fasting girl was subjected to the scrutiny of scientific sceptics. The claim that she did not need to eat was put to the test, which led to her rapid death.[2] In Britain, cases of anorexia nervosa were predominately managed by physicians, such as Gull[3] and Ryle.[4] Gradually over the last half of the twentieth century, especially after the recognition of bulimia nervosa by Russell in 1979,[5] psychiatrists have taken over the care. In France, on the other hand, psychiatrists such as Marce[6], Lasegue[7], Charcot (quoted in Silverman[8], and Janet[9] have been involved in the management of these cases since the middle of the nineteenth century. This wide cultural variation in the conceptualization and management of the disorder remains today. For example, in China most cases are still referred to physicians. Most Western countries now use a mixture of medical and psychological and social expertise in the management of these cases.

Diagnosis

There is usually little difficulty in diagnosing anorexia nervosa in adults in the West because the range of possible differential diagnoses is limited. In contrast, wasting conditions such as TB or AIDS will need to be considered in such countries as Africa. In children, the incidence is much lower and the presentation is often atypical because of limited cognitive development, and so the diagnosis is more difficult. Also there is a wider range of differential diagnosis in childhood, including pervasive refusal syndrome, food-avoidant emotional disorder, selective eating and functional dysphagia.

Many authorities in the field[10-12] have voiced disquiet about the diagnostic criteria regarding weight and shape concerns. They argue that because the definitions of the psychopathology are framed within contemporary Western culture they are not generalizable to other times or cultures. In Western society and particularly to women with eating disorders, the meaning of fatness encompasses negative concepts about the self, such as sloth, gluttony and selfishness. These abstract concepts about the perception of self have been operationalized into a more concrete form, such as a morbid fear of fatness or, by others, as a phobia of normal weight. However, in other cultures these concepts have different meanings. The criterion of a disturbed body image was included in classification systems in the 1980s but this was later dropped as it was not always present and was difficult to define.[13] This feature is probably a metaphor for more abstract discontent. In order to circumvent these culturally variable meanings, Russell[12] has proposed that a better definition would contain the following core features: 'that the patient avoids food and induces weight loss by virtue of a range of psychosocial conflicts whose resolution she perceives to be within her reach through the achievement of thinness and or the avoidance of fatness.' Thus aspects of the psychopathology that may be shaped by culture and education are dropped as unreliable. Nevertheless, at the moment both ICD 10 and

DSM IV continue to have criteria that relate to the perception of shape and weight.

There have been recent changes in the DSM IV criteria for anorexia nervosa, which have divided it into two subtypes.[14] The classical form is now termed anorexia nervosa restricting subtype (see Table 7.1). This is distinguished from the binge–purge subtype in which there is regular binge eating or purging behaviour (i.e. self-induced vomiting or the misuse of laxatives, diuretics or enemas). However, although these behaviours appear to be reasonable proxy measures of different subsyndromes, there are no clear-cut divisions between them. An approach that views the symptoms on dimensions may be more appropriate as patients frequently move between diagnostic categories. Over time the diagnostic criteria have also broadened. In DSM III (which drew upon Feighner's criteria) there had to be 25% weight loss. This has now decreased to a weight loss such that the weight is 15% below that of the matched population, which roughly corresponds to the ICD 10 criterion of a body mass index of less than 17.5 kg/m^2.

Comorbidity

Comorbidity with other axis I and axis II diagnoses is common in cases of anorexia nervosa presenting for treatment. In some of the atypical cases it may be difficult to decide what is the primary diagnosis. For example, there is overlap with severe obsessive-compulsive disorder, somatization and myalgic encephalitis in younger cases and with depression in older cases. Even in typical cases of anorexia nervosa additional features of depression, obsessive-compulsive disorder and social phobia are common.[15,16] Some of the comorbid conditions are a consequence of starvation, and these are ameliorated by weight gain.[17] The binge–purge subtype is associated with higher levels of depression and alcohol and substance abuse. Symptoms of post-traumatic stress disorder are also common in mixed anorexia nervosa and bulimia nervosa.[18]

A quarter of the group with restricting anorexia nervosa have avoidant, dependent or obsessive-compulsive personality types. Indeed, obsessive-compulsive personality traits are also common amongst the first-degree relatives.[19] Forty per cent of those with the binge–purge subtype have a borderline or histrionic type of personality.[20,21]

Epidemiology

Anorexia nervosa remains a rather rare condition with the incidence of new cases of 7 per 100 000 population.[18] Approximately 4000 new cases arise in the UK each year. The average duration of the disorder is 6 years.[22] The

Table 7.1   Diagnostic criteria of anorexia nervosa.

DSM-IV	ICD 10 F50
Refusal to maintain body weight over a minimal norm leading to body weight 15% below expected	Significant weight loss (Body mass index < 17.5 kg/m^2) Failure of weight gain or growth
	Weight loss self-induced by avoiding fattening foods and one or more of the following • vomiting • purging • excessive exercise • appetite suppressants • diuretics
Intense fear of gaining weight or becoming fat	A dread of fatness as an intrusive overvalued idea and the patient imposes a low weight threshold on herself
Disturbance in the way in which one's body weight, size or shape is experienced, e.g. 'feeling fat' {denial of seriousness of being underweight or undue influence of body weight and shape on self-evaluation}	
Absence of three consecutive menstrual cycles	Widespread endocrine disorder • amenorrhoea • raised growth hormone • raised cortisol • reduced T3
Restricting type binge/purging type: binge eating or vomiting/misuse of laxatives/diuretics	

prevalence in young women (the population at greatest risk) ranges from 0.1 to 1%[23–27] This puts the condition amongst the three most common chronic disorders in adolescence alongside asthma and obesity.[26] Although earlier research suggested that anorexia nervosa might have increased in frequency, the balance of evidence suggests otherwise.[28,18] However, it is possible that the binge–purge subtype of anorexia nervosa has increased.

Aetiology

Most explanations of causation are multidimensional and include genetic factors, other biological factors, psychological vulnerability, family and sociocultural setting conditions. However, one of the problems with such an all-encompassing model is that it is very difficult to prove or disprove, and it makes any attempts at prevention very difficult as vulnerabilities have to be remedied on so many fronts. One major flaw in a large proportion of the work on aetiology is that there has been a tendency to group anorexia and bulimia nervosa together or to use poorly defined subgroups, such as college girls with abnormal eating attitudes, as the basis of modelling risk factors. Given the wide difference in the history of the two conditions it would seem wise to regard them as separate entities until proved otherwise. The epidemiological data suggest that anorexia nervosa and bulimia nervosa may have different aetiological factors.

Biological factors

There are two domains of interest that are possible sites of psychopathology. One hypothesis is that there may be abnormal regulation of body composition and appetite.[29–31] Evidence to support this is the tendency for leanness to run in families and the fact that some strains of lean animals are prone to stress-related wasting. An additional variant of this model is that stress triggers the spiral of weight loss in those with a specific biological vulnerability.[32] An alternative model is that biologically determined temperamental traits, such as harm avoidance and persistence (or other components of the obsessive personality), may be either moderating or mediating factors.[33,34]

One of the key components in the control of body composition is leptin, a hormone secreted by fat cells. One hypothesis was that abnormal control of leptin regulation could underlie the weight loss in anorexia nervosa. When fat cells decrease in size the output of leptin decreases. Less leptin is transported into the brain. Low levels of leptin interfere with reproductive function and should allow the appetite system to be disinhibited, increasing food intake, with an associated decrease in metabolism and activity. The fact that reproductive function is suppressed in anorexia nervosa suggests that the abnormality of appetite and activity is downstream of leptin. Indeed, preliminary research does not suggest there is any abnormality in leptin function in anorexia nervosa.[35] The levels are low when patients are underweight, are increased with weight gain,[36] and in the normal range on recovery.[37]

An additional theory links the psychosocial aspects of anorexia nervosa with the biology of appetite. Chronic stress, for example, that is associated with submission to powerful others leads to persistent activation of the hypothalamic–pituitary–adrenal (HPA) system. In animals such a situation interferes with the normal homeostatic control of appetite.[32] This stress response disrupts the hypothalamic–pituitary axis and 5HT function.

Serotonin is of interest as a potential candidate neurotransmitter in eating disorders because of its roles in both the physiological and the psychological domains.[38,39] Serotonin is involved:

1) in eating behaviour (see Blundell and Hill[40] and Curzon[41] for reviews);
2) in animal models of anorexia nervosa[31,32] and
3) in temperamental traits, such as impulsive and emotional reactivity.[42,43]

Moreover, a fourth item could be added to this list: there is some evidence of abnormal 5HT and HPA function which persists after recovery.[44–46]

Genes as a risk factor for eating disorders

Evidence for a genetic component in the aetiology of anorexia nervosa has gradually unfolded.[33] Family studies[47,19] have found that the risk of eating disorders of the female relatives of probands with both anorexia nervosa and bulimia nervosa is increased 5–7-fold. Twenty per cent of the female relatives of anorexic probands had some form of eating disorders compared with 4% of the comparison group.[19] This has been replicated in another sample of mothers of anorexic probands (Strober, pers. comm.). In twins the concordance rates for anorexia nervosa are high, ranging from 50 to 70% depending on the phenotype.[48,49,33] Heritability is estimated to be over 50%.

Both the twin and family findings suggest that there is a specific genetic vulnerability to develop an eating disorder that does not overlap with that predisposing to other psychological disorders, such as affective disorders and alcoholism. There is also evidence of specificity between the two forms of eating disorders – that is, anorexia nervosa is more often found within the families of anorexic probands and vice versa. On the other hand, obsessive-compulsive personality disorder[50] and autistic spectrum disorder[51] are more common in the first-degree relatives of individuals with anorexia nervosa.

Association studies of candidate genes for eating disorders

Serotonin   Women with anorexia nervosa had a higher frequency of an allele of the $5HT_{2A}$ promoter region[52] than that found in a control population. This has been replicated in two other populations from the USA and Italy (Goldman and Kaye, pers. comm.) but not in two other groups[53] (Campbell and Piere, pers. comm.). A relationship between microsatellite markers in the $5HT_{2C}$ receptor and anorexia nervosa has been found (Campbell and Peire, pers. comm.) although a search for an association for alleles on this receptor was negative.[54] A linkage study of over 200 sister pairs failed to find any association with a gene on chromosome 13 in the region that codes for the 5HT receptor, but the power of this study was not great enough to detect a gene of the effect size seen in the association (Berettini, pers. comm.).

Appetite and body composition as the candidate gene No relationships was found with the β_3-adrenergic receptor gene which is associated with obesity[53] but a small relationship was found with the leptin gene (Campbell and Pieri, pers. comm.).

Social factors

Although sociocultural factors have shaped the presentation of the disorder (in that concerns about weight and fatness now predominate), it is probable that these features are not necessary (see above). For example, there is no convincing evidence that there has been an increase in the incidence of anorexia nervosa associated with the increased prevalence of dieting.[28,18] This is in contrast to bulimia nervosa. It is possible that a cultural focus on dieting serves to maintain the illness and may cause the course to be more severe, which can account for the trend for higher mortality[55] and increased readmission rates.[56] Many feminist writers have suggested that the changing roles of women and the shift in the assumptions of power and control may have lead to the emergence of eating disorders. Such arguments are made about eating disorders in general and are probably more relevant to bulimia nervosa (for a review of this area, see Fallon et al.,[57] 1994). Katzman and Lee,[58] arguing from a feminist/transcultural perspective, suggest that a phobia of control may be an appropriate definition of the psychopathology of anorexia nervosa which is free from cultural colouring.

Although there is evidence that anorexia nervosa develops in all social classes and on average in people with average intelligence, there is a tendency for women with anorexia nervosa and their families to be engaged in a struggle to attain higher ranking.[59]

Family factors

Although family factors are often included in the multidimensional aetiological model of anorexia nervosa there is little evidence to support any gross disturbance in family functioning.[60] The metaphors and explanations used in the family models are exciting and creative, which perhaps explains their widespread influence.[61,62] Minuchin[61] suggested that families of patients with anorexia nervosa showed specific traits: rigidity, lack of conflict resolution, enmeshment and over-involvement. However, some of these features appear to be a consequence of having a sick child in the family. For example, enmeshment and over-involvement are also seen in families caring for a child with cystic fibrosis.[63] In this study the main difference between anorexia nervosa families and cystic fibrosis families was that families with a child with anorexia nervosa were less adept at problem-solving. This links with the finding that patients with anorexia nervosa react to stress both in childhood and adulthood[64,65] with a helpless style of coping, with a tendency to use avoidance strategies intra- and interpersonally.

Psychological factors

The onset of anorexia nervosa usually (in 70% of cases) follows a severe life event or difficulty.[66–68] There is a tendency for these patients to have a maladaptive coping response to the triggering event, exemplified by avoidance and helplessness. This cognitive and emotional set is present from childhood.[64,65] Obsessional personality traits[69] associated with self-disgust and a sensitivity to criticism may lead to compensatory strategies, such as perfectionism and a tendency to please others and submit to their wishes.

Medical complications of anorexia nervosa

It is impossible to cover the medical complications of anorexia nervosa more than superficially. For more detailed information, the following resources are suggested: American Psychiatric Association 1992[70]; Bhanji & Mattingly, 1988[71]; Kaplan and Garfinkel, 1993[72]; Sharpe and Freeman, 1993[73]; Treasure and Szmukler, 1995.[74]

Skin and hair changes

The skin is dry, and fine downy hair, so-called lanugo hair, develops. There is often loss of head hair and this will appear thin and lifeless.

Musculoskeletal problems

Muscles   Individuals with severe anorexia nervosa have poor muscle strength and a decrease in stamina. Eventually, proximal myopathy develops with difficulty standing from a crouch or lifting the arms above the head to comb the hair. Poor muscle strength also leads to an impairment in respiratory function.[75]

Bones   Osteoporosis and pathological fractures are one of the commonest causes of pain and disability in anorexia nervosa.[74,76] The annual incidence of nonspine fractures of 0.05 per person year in anorexia nervosa is 7-fold higher than the rate reported from a community sample of women aged 15–34 years.[77] Risk factors for this complication are a long duration and an increased severity of illness.[78] Refeeding alone produces a rapid rise in bone turnover[79] and an increase in bone mineral content.[80] Insulin growth factor also increases bone turnover.[81] The value of hormone replacement therapy is uncertain. Overall it produces no effect, although it may protect against further bone loss in the subgroup who remain chronically unwell.[82] It is uncertain whether it is possible to restore bone mass to normal levels. Patients who have gained weight and have had a return of menses over many years have persistent osteopenia.[83] In the latter study duration of amenorrhoea/illness was the best predictor of osteopenia but an index of the duration of recovery was also highly correlated with outcome.

Dental changes

The commonest stigma of persistent vomiting is erosion of dental enamel, in particular from the inner surfaces of the front teeth. Eventually, dentine is exposed and the teeth become oversensitive to temperature and caries develop. Dental complications such as abnormal tooth wear are not limited to the group who vomit.[84] The other causes of poor dental health are overconsumption of acidic foods, such as fruit and carbonated drinks, and grinding and loosening of the teeth due to osteoporosis of the jaw.

Effects on the central nervous system (CNS)

Brain substance decreases in anorexia nervosa and the ventricular spaces and the sulci increase in size.[85-87] The increased resolution offered by magnetic resonance imaging (MRI) has also shown that the pituitary is smaller.[85,86] To a degree these structural abnormalities (such as loss of grey matter) despite weight recovery persist for over a year, which suggests there may be a degree of irreversible damage even in adolescents with a short history.[88] The cause of the cerebral atrophy is uncertain. It may be a general effect of starvation or may result from the high level of cortisol which is present in anorexia nervosa and which is known to be toxic to dendrites.[89,90] A post-mortem study of a 13-year-old girl who died of anorexia found that the dendrites showed evidence both of stunting of growth and of neuronal repair.[91] In addition, women with anorexia nervosa may be at greater risk for Alzheimer's disease because of their prolonged state of oestrogen deficiency. In postmenopausal women oestrogen treatment appears to delay the onset of dementia.[92] Neurophysiological abnormalities, such as vertex transients, are more common in adolescents with anorexia nervosa (56%) than in a control population (14%).[93] Also, auditory brain stem responses have been found to be abnormal.[94,95] Functional imaging – such as single photon emission computerized tomography (SPECT) studies have shown decreased flow in both the active state and after recovery.[96] Functional MRI scanning has shown an abnormal response to images of high-calorie drinks with increased activation in the insula and amygdala.[97]

Functional cognitive impairment is seen, with deficits in memory tasks, flexibility and inhibitory tasks persisting despite weight recovery.[98] On average, women who have recovered from anorexia nervosa have average IQ scores but have poorer scores on the object assembly subtest.[99]

Cardiovascular problems

The heart becomes smaller and less powerful because muscle is lost and the blood pressure and heart rate are lowered. This can lead to faints. There is poor circulation in the periphery and this leads to cold blue hands, feet and nose. At its extreme, this results in chilblains and even gangrene, in particular in children.

There have been reports of cardiac valvular problems,[100] though many of the murmurs that are heard are flow murmurs. Sudden death can occur in anorexia nervosa and may result from arrhythmias.[101] QT prolongation is common in anorexia nervosa.[102] Low potassium, which results from many of the methods of weight loss, can exacerbate this problem.

Fertility and reproductive function

Fertility is reduced in women with anorexia nervosa. In part this is due to suboptimal physical recovery. In a follow-up of 12.5 years in Denmark, the fertility rate was a third of that expected and the perinatal mortality rate was 6-fold higher.[103] The birth weight of children born to anorexic mothers is lower than average.[104] Women with anorexia nervosa may also have difficulties in feeding their children, who may become malnourished and stunted in growth.[105]

Endocrine system

The hypothalamic–pituitary–gonadal axis regresses to that of a prepubertal child. The pituitary does not secrete follicle stimulating hormone (FSH) and luteinizing hormone (LH) and the ovaries decrease in size. The ovarian follicles remain small and do not produce oestrogens or progesterone.[106] By contrast, the HPA axis is overactive, probably driven by excess corticotropin releasing factor (CRF), with high levels of cortisol that are not constrained by any feedback.[107,108]

Gastrointestinal tract

Residual gastrointestinal problems (such as irritable bowel syndrome) are common after recovery from anorexia nervosa.[81] Functional abnormalities, such as delayed gastric emptying and generalized poor motility, are related to the degree of undernutrition.[109] Anatomical abnormalities as a result of the trauma of vomiting and overeating or loss of mesenteric fat occur. Structural abnormalities such as ulcers, etc., are common.[110] It is important not to overlook the effects of the sorbitol that is present in sugar-free gums and sweets, which can cause abdominal distension, cramps and diarrhoea.[111]

Salivary glands exhibit hypertrophy and produce increased levels of amylase.[112] Pancreatitis is an extremely rare complication.[113] In cases of severe emaciation, fatty infiltration of the liver occurs and liver enzymes increase.[110]

Haematology

All components of the bone marrow are diminished but the order in which this is discernible in the peripheral blood is white cells, red cells and finally platelets. The level of marrow dysfunction relates to the total body fat mass.[114] The immune system is compromised with a decrease in CD8 T-cells.[115]

Blood chemistry

In restricting anorexia nervosa the most common abnormality is a low urea level, which is a function of a low protein intake. Low potassium levels result from vomiting or laxative and diuretic abuse. Usually, this is associated with raised levels of bicarbonate, but some laxatives can produce a metabolic acidosis. Many other salts and metabolites are reduced, for example magnesium, phosphate, calcium, sodium and glucose.

Comorbidity with physical problems

One of the most important areas of difficulties is when eating disorders develop in the context of somatic illness. This is a particular problem with diabetes mellitus: approximately a third of adolescent girls with diabetes have some form of eating disorder[116–118] and these tend to persist. It is common for these women to omit their insulin as a means of losing weight.[119] The combination of diabetes and an eating disorder leads to the development of early and severe neurovascular complications,[120–122] retinopathy (three times as prevalent in patients with highly disordered eating[117]), osteoporosis[123] and a higher mortality (5 times that of anorexia alone and 15 times that of diabetes).[124,125] Eating disorders also lead to difficulties in the management of Crohn's disease[126] and thyroid disease.[127]

Treatment of anorexia nervosa

One of the most difficult aspects of the management of anorexia nervosa is the development of a good working alliance.[128,129] Patients with anorexia nervosa are notoriously ambivalent about treatment.[130,131] Charles Lasègue in 1879[7] quoted one of his patients as saying: 'I do not suffer therefore I must be well.'

The transtheoretical model of Prochaska and DiClemente[132] is helpful in understanding these difficulties. The basic model has three dimensions, the temporal element, the processes used and the goals (see Table 7.2).[132-134]

The author has applied the transtheoretical model to women with anorexia nervosa in an inpatient unit[135] and also to people attending for out-patient care.[136] The majority of patients with anorexia nervosa are in pre-contemplation and contemplation. This has implications for the style of treatment as the processes used for each of the stages differ. If the therapist begins to talk about active change to a patient in precontemplation or contemplation, he or she will be met with resistance and hostility as there is a mismatch between the agendas of patient and therapist. It is therefore important to build a good therapeutic alliance by spending the first part of the interview eliciting the patient's readiness for change and her concerns about the illness. Motivational interviewing is helpful for people in precontemplation and contemplation[137] and has been applied in the form of motivational enhancement therapy to anorexia nervosa.[138-140] A key component of the assessment interview is to elicit the patient's concerns about her condition: physical, psychological, social, family and career and education. Patients with anorexia nervosa are usually not concerned that they have anorexia nervosa, that they are not eating and that their weight is low. They may, however, be concerned about their poor concentration that affects their ability to study, or the fact that their hair is falling out in handfuls.

An outline of the essential structure of treatment for anorexia nervosa is shown in Table 7.3.

Table 7.2   The transtheoretical approach.[133-135]

When   Five stages of change: precontemplation, contemplation, preparation/ determination, action and maintenance
How   Ten processes of change: consciousness raising, self-liberation, social liberation, counterconditioning, stimulus control, self-re-evaluation, environmental re-evaluation, contingency management, dramatic relief and helping relationships
What   Five levels of change: include symptoms/situational problems, maladaptive cognition, current interpersonal conflicts, family system conflicts and intrapersonal conflicts.

Source:
Based on Prochaska and DiClemente.

Table 7.3   Essential facets of treatment for anorexia nervosa.

- Engender motivation
- Find out what are the patients' beliefs about their illness
- Develop a good therapeutic alliance
- Formulation: links between behaviour and core schemata
- Match therapeutic processes to stage of change
- Balance move to change against degree of resistance

Current models of treatment

It is important to add a caveat to this section to warn that many of the premises of treatment are built upon clinical pragmatism rather than good evidence. There have been few randomized controlled trials, and those that have been accomplished have had very low power and have included a selected sample. General practitioners are perhaps better able to detect anorexia nervosa than many other psychiatric illnesses, and such cases are usually referred to secondary levels of care.[18,141] The standard method of treatment endorsed by the American Psychiatric Association[70] and standard psychiatric texts is inpatient treatment. Unlike most other psychiatric conditions in which the use of inpatient beds is rapidly decreasing, admission rates for anorexia nervosa in many countries are increasing.[142,143] Relapse and readmission are common.[144] Newer models of treatment are being developed which include alternative forms of management, such as day-patient and outpatient treatment[145,146] and stepped care services.[147,148]

The choice of treatment depends upon the patient's age, medical severity and the duration of the disorder. In patients under the age of 17 years, it is helpful to have the family involved in treatment.[149–151] Also, if the onset of the illness was in early adolescence – no matter what the patient's chronological age – it is usually helpful to involve the family in some capacity. Parental counselling (i.e. helping the family to understand the illness and to deal with the problems it causes) and cognitive behavioural therapy[151] are as effective and more acceptable than a traditional form of family therapy.[152]

Outpatient psychotherapy or counselling for older patients can be effective if there has not been too much weight loss (i.e. less than 25%).[153,154] A self-help book for anorexia nervosa[155] and another which combines elements of self-help with family help[138] may prove to be of benefit as adjuncts to therapy for anorexia nervosa, much as self-help books have played an important role in the management of bulimia nervosa.[156–159] Specialist psychotherapy, such as cognitive analytical therapy[139,160] or modified dynamic therapy, is more effective than supportive psychotherapy. New models of cognitive behavioural therapy have been developed[131,161] and are being tested as techniques to prevent relapse. As therapy for anorexia nervosa must be continued long term, it is important that psychological treatment is supplemented by regular medical monitoring.

Medication

One of the difficulties in the management of anorexia nervosa is that pharmacotherapy has not been found to play a major role in its management.[106,162–164] Insulin, neuroleptics, antidepressants and appetite and gastric stimulants have all been evaluated but often have a large number of side-effects to set against little benefit. A positive lead that is currently under investigation is the report by Kaye and colleagues[165] that fluoxetine may prevent relapse after inpatient treatment. This awaits confirmation, but it is possible that medications may only be effective in specific subgroups and at a certain biological stage. For example, there is the possibility that specific serotonin reuptake inhibitor (SSRI) medication requires oestrogen to be fully active.[166]

Inpatient treatment

Inpatient treatment is necessary for those with severe weight loss. This group have a poor prognosis.[167] The historical approach to the treatment of anorexia nervosa involved isolation. This was advocated in France by Charcot.[8] The use of isolation and strict behavioural regimes should now be consigned to history, as such coercive practices are deeply traumatic and reinforce the core features of the illness, which are self-disgust and ineffectiveness. Moreover, there is no evidence that strict regimes are any more effective than those that are more lenient.[168,169] Staff with expertise in the management of eating disorders can provide a judicious mixture of psychotherapy and nutritional support. This type of expertise is found in teams working in specialized units. In the UK in extreme circumstances, an anorexic patient may need to be detained under the Mental Health Act. If at all possible this should only be done within a specialized unit, where the treatment team have enough expertise to build up trust with the patient so that her extreme avoidance strategies can be left behind and the problems clearly formulated and processed.

Service acceptability

Some results suggest that as many as 50% of patients with anorexia nervosa terminate treatment prematurely.[170] Van Strein and colleagues[171] found a total drop-out rate of 38% spread over a period of years.

The factors related to compliance can be conceptualized as those that relate to the patients or family; those that relate to the therapist and therapy; and those that represent an interaction between patient and therapist variables.

Patient and family factors   Age of admission, duration of illness, educational level, social class, treatment method and engagement of the family are linked to drop-out from inpatient treatment for anorexia nervosa.[170,172,173] High levels of parentally expressed emotion, in particular, maternal criticism, are associated with poor compliance.[174,175]

Type of therapy   In a study in which patients were randomized to either inpatient or outpatient therapy, compliance with inpatient therapy was only 60%, whereas compliance with outpatient therapy, which comprised a mixture of individual and family therapy, was much higher.[176] A more lenient, flexible approach to inpatient therapy can lead to better compliance and was more acceptable to patients than traditional operant programmes.[169]

The therapeutic alliance   The interaction between doctor and patient in anorexia nervosa can have a profound effect on treatment.[128,129] Gallop and colleagues[177] measured the strength of the therapeutic alliance in patients on an eating disorder unit. Patients who remained on the unit perceived the therapeutic alliance with staff to be significantly stronger than those who left prematurely. Interestingly, there was very little correlation between the patients' and therapists' perception of the alliance.

Prognosis of anorexia nervosa

The median duration of the illness is 6 years.[22] A third of patients have a poor prognosis, even after 20 years. Mortality is 0.06% per year after onset, which means that anorexia nervosa has the highest mortality of any psychiatric illness.[55,178] Approximately one half of the deaths result from medical complications and the rest result from suicide.[21] Treatment in specialized centres probably improves the outcome, as the mortality rate in areas without a specialized service is higher.[179] Also, the outcome appears to be better in cohorts who have been recruited from clinical centres than in the one study that was able to detect cases from the school-girl population in one town.[25] Outcome is usually defined using the Morgan and Russell scales (or an equivalent) which measure outcome in terms of physical status (weight and menstruation), psychological status (specific psychopathology: attitudes to shape, weight and eating, general psychiatric comorbidity, e.g. depression and obsessive-compulsive disorder), psychosexual adjustment, socioeconomic adjustment and relationships with family. Even patients with a good outcome often have residual problems, such as abnormal attitudes to food and eating. Abnormally low serum albumin levels and a low weight (≤60% average body weight) predict a lethal course.[22]

References

1. Bell R. *Holy Anorexia* (Chicago: Chicago University Press, 1985).

2. Fowler R. *A Complete History of the Case of the Welsh Fasting Girl (Sarah Jacob) With Comments Thereon, and Observations on Death from Starvation* (London: Henry Renshaw, 1871).

3. Gull WW. The address in medicine to the annual meeting of the British Medical Association, at Oxford. *Lancet* (8 August 1869): 171–6.

4. Ryle JA. Anorexia nervosa. *Lancet* (1936) **ii:** 893–99.

5. Russell GFM. Bulimia nervosa: an ominous variant of anorexia nervosa. *Psychol Med* (1979) **9:** 429–48.

6. Marcé L-V. On a form of hypochondriacal delirium occurring during consecutive dyspepsia, and characterized by refusal of food. *J Psychol Med Men Pathology* (1860) **13:** 264–6.

7. Lasègue C. On hysterical anorexia. *Med Times Gazette* (1873) **ii:** 265–6, 367–9.

8. Silverman JA. Charcot's comments on the therapeutic role of isolation in the treatment of anorexia nervosa. *Int J Eating Dis* (1997) **21:** 295–8.

9. Janet P. *The Major Symptoms of Hysteria* (London: Macmillan, 1903).

10. Lee S. Self starvation in context: towards a culturally sensitive understanding of anorexia nervosa. *Soc Sci Med* (1995) **41:** 25–36.

11. Littlewood R. Psychopathology and personal agency: modernity, culture change and eating disorders in South Asian societies. *Br J Med Psychol* (1995) **68:** 45–63.

12. Russell GFM. Anorexia nervosa through time. In Szmukler G, Dare C, Treasure J (eds) *Handbook of Eating Disorders: Theory, Treatment, Research* (Chichester: Wiley, 1995): 5–17.

13. Hsu LKG, Sobkiewicz TA. Body image disturbance: time to abandon the concept for eating disorders. *Int J Eating Dis* (1991) **10:** 15–30.

14. American Psychiatric Association. *Diagnostic and Statistical Manual of Mental Disorders (DSM-III-R).* 4th edition revised. APA, Washington DC.

15. Laessle RG, Kittl S, Fichter MM et al. Major affective disorder in anorexia nervosa and bulimia. *Br J Psychiatry* (1987) **151:** 785–9.

16. Halmi KA, Eckert E, Marchi P et al. Comorbidity of psychiatric diagnosis in anorexia nervosa. *Arch Gen Psychiatry* (1991) **48:** 712–18.

17. Pollice C, Kaye WH, Greeno CG, Weltzin TE. Relationship of depression, anxiety and obsessionality to state of illness in anorexia nervosa. *Int J Eating Dis* (1997) **21:** 357–76.

18. Turnbull S, Ward A, Treasure J et al. The demand for eating disorder care: a study using the general practice research data base. *Br J Psychiatry* (1996) **169:** 705–12.

19. Lilenfeld LR, Kaye WH. Genetic studies of anorexia and bulimia nervosa. In Hoek WH, Treasure J, Katzman M (eds) *Neurobiology in the Treatment of Eating Disorders* (Chichester: Wiley, 1998): 169–94.

20. Braun DL, Sunday SR, Halmi KA. Psychiatric comorbidity in patients with eating disorders. *Psychol Med* (1994) **24:** 859–67.

21. Herzog DB, Keller MB, Lavori PW et al. The prevalence of personality disorders in 210 women with eating disorders. *J Clin Psychiatry* (1992) **53:** 147–52.

22. Herzog W, Schellberg D, Deter HC. First recovery in anorexia nervosa patients in the long term course: a discrete time survival analysis. *J Consult Clin Psychol* (1997) **65:** 169–77.

23. Hoek HW. The incidence and prevalence of anorexia nervosa and bulimia nervosa in primary care. *Psychol Med* (1991) **21:** 455–60.

24. Hoek HW. Review of the epidemiological studies of eating disorders. *Int Rev Psychiatry* (1993) **5:** 61–74.

25. Gillberg IC, Rastam M, Gillberg C. Anorexia nervosa outcome: six-year controlled longitudinal study of 51 cases including a population cohort. *J Am Acad Child Adolesc Psychiatry* (1994) **33:** 729–39.

26. Lucas AR, Beard CM, O'Fallon WM, Kurland LT. 50-year trends in the incidence of anorexia nervosa in Rochester, Minnesota: a population based study. *Am J Psychiatry* (1991) **148:** 917–22.

27. Rastam M, Gillberg C, Garton M. Anorexia nervosa in a Swedish urban region: a population-based study. *Br J Psychiatry* (1989) **155:** 642–6.

28. Fombonne E. Anorexia nervosa. No evidence of an increase. *Br J Psychiatry* (1995) **166:** 462–71.

29. Hebebrand J, Remschmidt H. Anorexia nervosa viewed as an extreme weight condition: genetic implications. *Hum Genetics* (1995) **95:** 1–11.

30. Treasure J, Owen JB. What can animal models tell us about the aetiology of eating disorders? *Int J Eating Dis* (1998) **21:** 307–11.

31. Treasure J, Collier D, Campbell IC. Ill fitting genes: the biology of weight and shape control in relation to body composition and eating disorders. *Psychol Med* (1997) **27:** 505–8.

32. Connan F, Treasure J. Stress, eating and neurobiology. In Hoek WH, Treasure J, Katzman M (eds) *Neurobiology in the Treatment of Eating Disorders* (Chichester: Wiley, 1998): 211–28.

33. Treasure J, Holland A. Genetic factors in eating disorders. In Szmukler G, Dare C, Treasure J (eds) *Handbook of Eating Disorders: Theory, Treatment and Research* (Chichester: Wiley, 1995): 65–82.

34. Strober M. Family-genetic perspectives on anorexia nervosa and bulimia nervosa. In Brownell K, Fairburn C (eds) *Eating Disorders: A Comprehensive Handbook* (New York: Guilford, 1995).

35. Grinspoon S, Gulick T, Askari H et al. Serum leptin levels in women with anorexia nervosa. *Clin Endocrin Metab* (1996) **81:** 3861–3.

36. Casanueva FF, Dieguez C, Popovic V et al. Serum immunoreactive leptin concentrations in patients with anorexia nervosa before and after partial recovery. *Biochem Mol Med* (1997) **60:** 116–20.

37. Brown N, Ward A, Treasure J et al. Leptin levels in anorexia nervosa (acute and long term recovered). *Int J Obesity* (1996) **20:** 37.

38. Treasure J, Campbell I. The case for biology in the aetiology of anorexia nervosa. *Psychol Med* (1994) **24:** 3–8 (editorial).

39. Study Group on Anorexia Nervosa. Anorexia nervosa – directions for future research. *Int J Eating Dis* (1995) **17:** 235–41.

40. Blundell JE, Hill AJ. Serotonin, eating disorders and the satiety cascade. In Cassano CB, Akiskal HS (eds) *Serotonin-Related Psychiatric Syndromes: Clinical Implications and Therapeutic Links. Services International Congress and Symposium Series* 165 (London: Royal Society of Medicine, 1991): 125–9.

41. Curzon G. Serotonin and appetite. *Ann NY Acad Sci* (1990) **600:** 521–31.

42. Suomi SJ. Adolescent depression and depressive symptoms: insights from longitudinal studies with rhesus monkeys. *J Youth Adolescence* (1991) **20:** 273–87.

43. Suomi SJ. Early determinants of behaviour: evidence from primate studies. *Br Med Bull* (1997) **53:** 170–84.

44. Kaye WH, Gwirstman HE, George DT et al. CSF 5-HIAA concentrations in anorexia nervosa: reduced values in underweight subjects normalise after weight gain. *Biol Psychiatry* (1988) **23:** 102–5.

45. Kaye WH, Gwirtsman HE, George DT, Ebert MH. Altered serotonin activity in anorexia nervosa after long term weight restoration: does elevated cerebrospinal fluid 5-hydroxyindoleacetic acid level correlate with rigid and obsessive behaviour? *Arch Gen Psychiatry* (1991) **48:** 556–62.

46. Ward A, Brown N, Lightman S et al. Neuroendocrine, appetitive and behavioural responses to d fenfluramine in women recovered from anorexia nervosa. *Br J Psychiatry* (1998) **172:** 351–8.

47. Strober M, Lampert C, Morrell W et al. A controlled family study of anorexia nervosa: evidence of familial aggregation and lack of shared transmission with affective disorders. *Int J Eat Disord* (1990) **9:** 239–53.

48. Holland AJ, Hall A, Murray R et al. Anorexia nervosa: a study of 34 twin pairs and one set of triplets. *Br J Psychiatry* (1984) **145:** 414–19.

49. Holland AJ, Sicotte N, Treasure J. Anorexia nervosa: evidence for a genetic basis. *J Psychosom Res* (1988) **32:** 561–71.

50. Lilenfeld LR, Kaye WH, Greeno CG et al. A controlled family study of anorexia nervosa and bulimia nervosa – psychiatric disorders in first degree relatives and effects of proband mortality. *Arch Gen Psychiatry* (1998) **55:** 603–10.

51. Wentz Nilsson E, Gillberg C, Rastam M. Familial factors in community based anorexia nervosa. A community-based study. Quoted in Gillberg C and Rastam M. The aetiology of anorexia nervosa. In Hoek WH, Treasure J, Katzman MA (eds) *Neurobiology in the treatment of eating disorders* (Chichester: Wiley, 1998): 169–94.

52. Collier DA, Arranz MJ, Li T et al. Association between 5-HT$_{2A}$ gene promoter polymorphism and anorexia nervosa. *Lancet* (1997) **350:** 412.

53. Hinney A, Lentes KU, Rosenkranz K et al. Beta 3 adrenergic receptor allele distributions in children, adolescents and young adults with obesity, underweight or anorexia nervosa. *Int J Obesity* (1997) **21:** 224–30.

54. Lentes KU, Hinney A, Zeigler A et al. Evaluation of a Cys23SER mutation within the human 5HT2C receptor gene: no evidence for an association of the mutant allele with obesity or underweight in children adolescents and young adults. *Life Sci* (1997) **61:** PL 9–16.

55. Sullivan PF. Mortality in anorexia nervosa. *Am J Psychiatry* (1995) **152:** 1073–4.

56. Nielsen S. The epidemiology of anorexia nervosa in Denmark from 1973 to 1987: a nationwide register study of psychiatric admission. *Acta Psychiatr Scand* (1990) **81:** 507–14.

57. Fallon P, Katzman MA, Wooley SC. *Feminist Perspectives on Eating Disorders* (New York: Guilford Press, 1994).

58. Katzman MA, Lee S. Beyond body image: the integration of feminist and transcultural theories in the understanding of self-starvation. *Int J Eating Dis* (1997) **22:** 385–94.

59. Gillberg C, Rastam M. The aetiology of anorexia nervosa. In Hoek WH, Treasure J, Katzman M (eds) *The Integration of Neurobiology in the Treatment of Eating Disorders* (Chichester: Wiley, 1998): 127–42.

60. Schmidt UH, Tiller JM, Treasure J. Setting the scene for eating disorders: childhood care, classification and course of illness. *Psychol Med* (1993) **23:** 663–72.

61. Minuchin S, Rosman BL, Baker L. *Psychosomatic Families: Anorexia Nervosa in Context* (Cambridge, Massachusetts: Harvard University Press, 1978).

62. Selvini-Palazzoli M. *Self-Starvation: From Individual to Family Therapy in the Treatment of Anorexia Nervosa* (London: Chaucer Human, 1974).

63. Blair C, Freeman C, Cull A. The families of anorexia nervosa and cystic fibrosis patients. *Psychol Med* (1995) **25:** 985–93.

64. Troop NA, Treasure J. Psychosocial factors in the onset of eating disorders: responses to life events and difficulties. *Br J Med Psychol* (1997) **70:** 373–85.

65. Troop NA, Treasure J. Setting the scene for eating disorders in childhood. II. Childhood helplessness and mastery. *Psychol Med* (1997) **27:** 531–8.

66. Schmidt UH, Tiller JM, Andrews B et al. Is there a specific trauma precipitating the onset of anorexia nervosa? *Psychol Med* (1997) **27:** 523–30.

67. Rastam M, Gillberg C. Background factors in anorexia nervosa. A controlled study of 51 teenage cases including a population sample. *Eur Child Adolescent Psychiatry* (1992) **1:** 54–65.

68. Gowers SG, North CD, Byram V, Weaver AB. Life event precipitants of adolescent anorexia nervosa. *J Child Psychol Psychiatry* (1996) **37:** 469–77.

69. Gillberg IC, Rastam M, Gillberg C. Anorexia nervosa 6 years after onset. Part I. Personality disorders. *Compr Psychiatry* (1995) **36:** 61–9.

70. American Psychiatric Association. Practice guidelines for eating disorders. *Am J Psychiatry* (1992) **150:** 208–28.

71. Bhanji S, Mattingly D. *Medical Aspects of Anorexia Nervosa* (London: Wright, 1988).

72. Kaplan AS, Garfinkel PE. *Medical Issues and the Eating Disorders* (New York: Brunner, Mazel, 1993).

73. Sharpe CW, Freeman CPL. The medical complications of anorexia nervosa. *Br J Psychiatry* (1993) **153:** 452–62.

74. Treasure J, Szmukler GI. Medical complications of chronic anorexia nervosa. In Szmuckler G, Dare C, Treasure J (eds) *Handbook of eating disorders: Theory, Treatment and Research* (Chichester: Wiley, 1995): 177–92.

75. Murciamo D, Rigaud D, Pinleton S et al. Diaphragmatic function in severely malnourished patients

with anorexia nervosa. Effects of renutrition. *Am J Resp Crit Care Med* (1994) **150:** 1569–74.

76. Herzog W, Deter HC, Schellberg D et al. Somatic findings at 12 year follow-up of 103 anorexia nervosa patients. In Herzog W, Deter HC, Vandereycken W (eds) *Follow-Up in the Course of Eating Disorders* (Springer Verlag: Berlin): 85–107.

77. Rigotti NA, Neer RM, Skates SJ et al. The clinical course of osteoporosis in anorexia nervosa. *JAMA* (1991) **265:** 1133–7.

78. Serpell L, Treasure J. Osteoporosis: a serious health risk in anorexia nervosa. *Eur Rev Eating Dis* (1997) **5:** 149–57.

79. Stefanis N, Mackintosh C, Abraha H et al. Dissociation of bone turnover in anorexia nervosa. *Clin Biochem* (1998) **35:** 709–16.

80. Orphanidou CI, McCarger LJ, Birmingham CL, Belzberg AS. Changes in body composition and fat distribution after short term weight gain in patients with anorexia nervosa. *Am J Clin Nutrit* (1997) **65:** 1034–41.

81. Grinspoon S, Baum H, Lee K et al. Effects of short-term recombinant human insulin-like growth-factor-I administration on bone turnover in osteopenic women with anorexia nervosa. *J Clin Endocrin Metab* (1996) **81:** 3864–70.

82. Klibanski A, Biller BMK, Schoenfeld DA et al. The effects of estrogen administration on trabecular bone loss in young women with anorexia nervosa. *J Clin Endocrin Metab* (1995) **80:** 898–904.

83. Ward A, Brown N, Treasure J. Persistent osteopenia after recovery from anorexia nervosa. *Int J Eating Dis* (1997) **22:** 71–5.

84. Robb ND, Smith BG, Geidrys-Leeper E. The distribution of erosion in the dentitions of patients with eating disorders. *Br Dental J* (1995) **178:** 171–5.

85. Dolan RJ, Mitchell J, Wakeling A. Structural brain changes in patients with anorexia nervosa. *Psychol Med* (1988) **18:** 349–53.

86. Katzman DK, Lambe EK, Mikulis DJ et al. Cerebral grey matter and white matter volume deficits in adolescent females with anorexia nervosa. *J Paediatrics* (1996) **129:** 794–803.

87. Krieg JC, Pirke KM, Lauer C, Backmund H. Endocrine, metabolic and cranial computed tomographic findings in anorexia nervosa. *Psychol Med* (1988) **18:** 349–53.

88. Lambe EK, Katzman DK, Mikulis DJ et al. Cerebral gray matter deficits after weight recovery from anorexia nervosa. *Arch Gen Psychiatry* (1997) **54:** 537–42.

89. Sapolsky RM. *Stress and the Ageing Brain and the Mechanisms of Neuron Death* (Cambridge, MA: MIT Press, 1992).

90. Sapolsky RM. Why stress is bad for your brain. *Science* (1996) **273:** 749–50.

91. Schönheit B, Meyer U, Kuchinke J et al. Morphometric investigations on lamina V pyramidal neurons in the frontal cortex of a case with anorexia nervosa. *J Brain Res* (1996) **37:** 269–80.

92. Tang MX, Jacobs D, Stern Y. Effect of oestrogen during menopause on risk and age of onset of Alzheimer's disease. *Lancet* (1996) **348:** 429–32.

93. Rothenberger A, Dumais-Huber C, Moll G, Woerner W. Psychophysiology of anorexia nervosa. In Steinhausen HC (ed) *Eating Disorders in Adolescence* (New York: Walter de Gruyter, 1995): 191–220.

94. Rothenberger A, Blanz B,

Lehmkuhl G. What happens to electrical brain activity when anorexic patients gain weight. *Eur Arch Psychiatry Clin Neurosci* (1991) **240:** 144–7.

95. Miyamoto H, Sakuma K, Kumagai K et al. Auditory brain stem response in anorexia nervosa. *Jap J Psychiatry Neurol* (1992) **46:** 673–9.

96. Gordon I, Lask B, Bryant-Waugh R et al. Childhood onset anorexia nervosa towards identifying a biological substrate. *Int J Eat Disorder* (1997) **22:** 159–65.

97. Ellison ZR, Foong J. Neuroimaging in eating disorders. In Hoek WH, Treasure J, Katzman M (eds) *Neurobiology in the Treatment of Eating Disorders* (Chichester: Wiley, 1998): 255–70.

98. Kingston K, Szmukler G, Andrews D et al. Neuropsychological and structural brain changes in anorexia nervosa before and after refeeding. *Psychol Med* (1996) **26:** 15–28.

99. Gillberg IC, Gillberg C, Rastam M, Johansson M. The cognitive profile of anorexia nervosa. A comparative study including a community based sample. *Compr Psychiatry* (1996) **37:** 23–30.

100. Johnson GL, Humphries LL, Shirley PB et al. Mitral valve prolapse in patients with anorexia nervosa and bulimia. *Arch Intern Med* (1986) **146:** 1525–9.

101. Isner JM, Roberts WC, Heymsfield SB, Yager J. Anorexia nervosa and sudden death. *Ann Intern Med* (1985) **102:** 49–52.

102. Cooke RA, Chambers JB, Singh R et al. QT interval in anorexia nervosa. *Br Heart J* (1994) **72:** 69–73.

103. Brinch M, Isager T, Tolsrup K. Anorexia nervosa and motherhood: Reproductive pattern and mothering behaviours of 50

women. *Acta Psychiatr Scand* (1988) **77:** 98–104.

104. Treasure J, Russell GFM. Intrauterine growth and neonatal weight gain in anorexia nervosa. *Br Med J* (1988) **152:** 372–6.

105. Russell GFM, Treasure J, Eisler I. Mothers with anorexia nervosa who underfeed their children: their recognition and management. *Psychol Med* (1998) **28:** 93–101.

106. Treasure J. The ultrasonographic features in anorexia nervosa and bulimia nervosa: a simplified method of measuring hormonal states during weight gain. *J Psychosom Res* (1988) **32:** 561–71.

107. Gwirtsman HE, Jaye WH, George DT et al. Central and peripheral ACTH and cortisol levels in anorexia and bulimia. *Arch Gen Psychiatry* (1989) **46:** 61–9.

108. Licinio J, Wong M, Gold PW. The hypothalamic–pituitary–adrenal axis in anorexia nervosa. *Psychiatry Res* (1996) **62:** 75–83.

109. Szmukler GI, Young GP, Lichtenstein M, Andrews D. A serial study of gastric emptying in anorexia nervosa and bulimia nervosa. *Aust NZ J Med* (1990) **20:** 220–5

110. Hall RCW, Hoffman RS, Beresford TP et al. Physical illnesses encountered in patients with eating disorders. *Psychosomatics* (1989) **30:** 174–91.

111. Ohlrich ES, Aughey DR, Dixon RM. Sorbitol abuse among eating disordered patients. *Psychosomatics* (1989) **30:** 451–3.

112. Kinzl J, Bieble W, Herold M. Significance of vomiting for hypoamylasaemia and sialadenosis in patients with eating disorders. *Int J Eating Dis* (1993) **13:** 117–24.

113. Gavish D, Eisenberg S, Berry EM et al. Bulimia: an underlying

behavioural disorder in hyperlip-idaemic pancreatitis: a prospective multidisciplinary approach. *Arch Intern Med* (1987) **147:** 705–8.

114. Lambert M, Hubert C, Depresseux G et al. Haematological changes in anorexia nervosa are correlated with total body fat mass depletion. *Int J Eating Dis* (1997) **21:** 329–34.

115. Mustafa A, Ward A, Treasure J, Peakman M. Lymphocyte subpopulations in anorexia nervosa, changes on refeeding. *Clin Immunol Immunopath* (1997) **82:** 282–9.

116. Fairburn CG, Steele JM. Anorexia nervosa in diabetes mellitus. *Br Med J* (1980) **290:** 1167–68.

117. Rydall AC, Rodin GM, Olmsted MP et al. Disordered eating behaviour and microvascular complications in young women with insulin-dependent diabetes mellitus. *New Eng J Med* (1997) **336:** 1849–54.

118. Williams G, Gill GV. Eating disorders and diabetic complications. *New Engl J Med* (1997) **336:** 1905–6.

119. Szmukler GI, Russell GFM. Diabetes mellitus, anorexia nervosa and bulimia. *Br J Psychiatry* (1983) **142:** 305–8.

120. Steele JM, Young RJ, Lloyd GG, Clarke BF. Clinical apparent eating disorders in young diabetic women: association with painful neuropathy and other complications. *Br Med J* (1987) **294:** 859–62.

121. Colas C, Mathieu P, Tchobroutsky G. Eating disorders and retinal lesions in type 1 (insulin dependent) diabetic women. *Diabetologia* (1991) **34:** 288 (letter).

122. Ward A, Troop N, Cachia M et al. Doubly disabled: diabetes in combination with an eating disorder. *Postgrad Med J* (1995) **71:** 546–50.

123. Vila G, Robert JJ, Nollet-Clemencon VL et al. Eating and emotional disorders in adolescent obese girls with insulin-dependent diabetes mellitus. *Eur Child Adolescent Psychiatry* (1995) **4:** 270–9.

124. Nielsen S, Moller-Madsen S, Isager T et al. Standardised mortality in eating disorders – a quantitative summary of previously published and new evidence. *J Psychosom Res* (1998) **44:** 413–34.

125. Nielsen S, Molbak AG. Eating disorders and type 1 diabetes: overview and summing up. *Eur Eat Dis Rev* (1998) **6:** 4–27.

126. Meadows G, Treasure J. Crohn's disease and the eating disorders. *Acta Psychiatr Scand* (1989) **9:** 413–14.

127. Tiller J, Macrae A, Schmidt U et al. The prevalence of eating disorders in thyroid disease: a pilot study. *J Psychosom Med* (1994) **38:** 609–16.

128. Vandereycken W. Naughty girls and angry doctors. *Int Rev Psychiatry* (1993) **5:** 13–18.

129. Goldner EM, Birmingham CL, Smye V. Addressing treatment refusal in anorexia nervosa: clinical, ethical and legal considerations. In Garner DM, Garfinkel PE (eds) *Handbook of Treatment of Eating Disorders* (New York: Guilford Press, 1997): 450–61.

130. Bruch H. *Eating Disorders: Obesity, Anorexia Nervosa and the Person Within* (London: Routledge & Kegan Paul, 1973).

131. Garner DM, Vitousek KM, Pike KM. Cognitive behavioural therapy for anorexia nervosa. In Garner DM, Garfinkel PE (eds) *Handbook of Treatment of Eat-*

ing Disorders (New York: Guilford Press, 1997): 94–144.

132. Prochaska JO, DiClemente CC. The transtheoretical model of change. In Norcross JC, Goldfried MR (eds) *Handbook of Psychotherapy Integration* (New York: Basic Books, 1992).

133. Prochaska JO, DiClemente CC. Transtheoretical therapy: towards a more integrative model of change. *Psychother Theory, Res Pract* (1982) **19:** 276–88.

134. Prochaska JO, DiClemente CC. Toward a comprehensive model of change. In Miller WR, Heather N (eds) *Treating Addictive Behaviors: Processes of Change* (New York: Plenum Press, 1986): 3–27.

135. Ward A, Troop N, Todd G, Treasure J. To change or not to change – How is the question. *Br J Med Psychol* (1996) **69:** 139–46.

136. Blake W, Turnbull S, Treasure J. Stages and processes of change in eating disorders. Implications for therapy. *Clin Psychol Psychother* (1997) **4:** 186–91.

137. Miller WR, Rollnick S. *Motivational Interviewing: Preparing People to Change Addictive Behavior* (New York: Guilford, 1991).

138. Treasure J. *Anorexia Nervosa. A Survival Guide for Families, Friends and Sufferers.* (Hove: Psychology Press, 1997).

139. Treasure J, Ward A. A practical guide to the use of motivational interviewing in anorexia nervosa. *Eur Eating Dis Rev* (1997) **5:** 102–114.

140. Treasure J, Ward A. Cognitive analytic therapy in the treatment of anorexia nervosa. *Clin Psychol Psychother* (1997) **4:** 62–71.

141. Van Hoeken D, Lucas AR, Hoek HW. Epidemiology. In Hoek WH, Treasure J, Katzman M (eds) *The Integration of Neurobiology in the Treatment of Eating Disorders* (Chichester: Wiley, 1998): 97–126.

142. Williams P, King M. The 'epidemic' of anorexia nervosa: another medical myth? *Lancet* (1987) **i:** 205–7.

143. Munk-Jorgensen P, Moller-Madson S, Nielsen S, Nystrup J. Incidence of eating disorders in psychiatric hospitals and wards in Denmark 1970–1993. *Acta Psychiatr Scand* (1995) **92:** 91–6.

144. McKenzie JM, Joyce PR. Hospitalisation for anorexia nervosa. *Int J Eating Dis* (1990) **11:** 235–41.

145. Kaye WH, Kaplan AS, Zucker ML. Treating eating disorder patients in a managed care environment. *Psychiatr Clin North Am* (1996) **19:** 793–810.

146. Kaplan AS, Olmsted MP. Partial hospitalisation. In Garner DM, Garfinkel PE (eds) *Handbook of Treatment of Eating Disorders* (New York: Guilford Press, 1997) (2nd edn): 354–60.

147. Royal College of Psychiatrists. *Eating Disorders. Council Report* (1992) **CR14**.

148. Treasure J. Anorexia nervosa and bulimia nervosa. In Stein G, Wilkinson G (eds) *Seminars in Adult General Psychiatry* (London: Gaskell Press, 1998).

149. Russell GF, Szmukler GI, Dare C, Eisler I. An evaluation of family therapy in anorexia nervosa and bulimia nervosa. *Arch Gen Psychiatry* (1987) **44:** 1047–56.

150. Eisler I, Dare C, Russell GFM et al. A five year follow-up of a controlled trial of family therapy in severe eating disorder: *Arch Gen Psychiatry* (1997) **54:** 1025–30.

151. Robin AL, Siegel PT, Koepke T et al. Family therapy versus individual therapy for adolescent females with anorexia nervosa. *J Dev Behav Pediatr* (1994) **15:** 111–16.

152. Le Grange D, Eisler I, Dare C, Russell GFM. Evaluation of family therapy in anorexia nervosa: a pilot study. *Int Eating Dis* (1992) **12:** 347–57.

153. Channon S, De Silva P, Hemsley D, Perkins R. A controlled trial of cognitive behavioural and behavioural treatment of anorexia nervosa. *Behav Res Ther* (1989) **27:** 529–35.

154. Crisp AH, Norton K, Gowers S et al. A controlled study of the effect of therapies aimed at adolescent and family psychopathology in anorexia nervosa. *Br J Psychiatry* (1991) **159:** 325–33.

155. Crisp AH, Joughin N, Halek C, Bowyer C. *Anorexia Nervosa. The Wish to Change* (Hove: Psychology Press, 1996).

156. Treasure J, Schmidt U, Troop N et al. First step in managing bulimia nervosa: a controlled trial of a therapeutic manual. *Br Med J* (1994) **308:** 686–9.

157. Treasure J, Schmidt U, Troop N et al. Sequential treatment for bulimia nervosa incorporating a self care manual. *Br J Psychiatry* (1996) **168:** 94–8.

158. Cooper PJ, Coker S, Fleming C. An evaluation of the efficacy of supervised cognitive behavioral self-help for bulimia nervosa. *Psychosom Res* (1996) **140:** 281–7.

159. Waller D, Fairburn CG, McPherson A et al. Treating bulimia nervosa in primary care – a pilot study. *Int J Eating Dis* (1996) **19:** 99–103.

160. Treasure J, Todd G, Brolley M et al. A pilot study of a randomised trial of cognitive analytic therapy vs educational behavioural therapy for adult anorexia nervosa. *Behav Res Ther* (1995) **33:** 363–7.

161. Wolff G, Serpell L. Finding an appetite for life: a cognitive model of anorexia nervosa. In Hoek H, Treasure J, Katzman M (eds) *The Integration of Neurobiology in the Treatment of Eating Disorders* (Chichester: Wiley, 1998): 407–30.

162. Martinez-Raga J, Treasure J. Pharmacological Treatment for Eating Disorders. In Kerwin R (ed) *Drug treatment in Psychiatry* (in preparation).

163. Mayer LES, Walsh BT. The treatment of eating disorders. In Hoek H, Treasure J, Katzman M (eds) *Neurobiology in the Treatment of Eating Disorders* (Chichester: Wiley, 1998): 395–7.

164. Jimerson DC, Wolfe BE, Brotman AW, Metzger ED. Medications in the treatment of eating disorders. *Psych Clin N Am* (1996) **19:** 739–54.

165. Kaye WH, Weltzin TE, Hsu G et al. Relapse prevention with fluoxetine in anorexia nervosa: a double blind placebo controlled study. 150th APA meeting 178 (May 17th 1997).

166. Schneider LS, Small GW, Hamilton SH et al. Estrogen replacement and response to fluoxetine in a multicenter geriatric depression trial. Fluoxetine Collaborative Study Group. *Am Geriatric Psychiatry* (1997) **5:** 97–106.

167. Hebebrand J, Himmelmann GW, Herzog W et al. Prediction of low body weight at long term follow-up in acute anorexia nervosa by low body weight at referral. *Am J Psychiatry* (1997) **154:** 566–9.

168. Touyz SW, Beaumont PJV, Glaun D et al. A comparison of lenient and strict operant condi-

tioning programmes in refeeding patients with anorexia nervosa. *Br J Psychiatry* (1984) **144:** 517–20.

169. Touyz SW, Beaumont PJ, Dunn SM. Behaviour therapy in the management of patients with anorexia nervosa. A lenient, flexible approach. *Psychother Psychosom* (1987) **48:** 151–6.

170. Vandereycken W, Peirloot R. Drop out during inpatient treatment of anorexia nervosa: A clinical study of 133 patients. *Brit J Med Psychol* (1983) **56:** 145–56.

171. Van Stein DC, van der Ham DC, van Engeland H. Drop out characteristics in a follow-up study of 90 eating disorder patients. *Int J Eating Dis* (1992) **12:** 341–3.

172. Silverman JA. Anorexia nervosa: clinical observation in a successful treatment plan. *J Pediatr* (1974) **84:** 68–73.

173. Warren W. A study of anorexia nervosa in young girls. *J Child Psychol Psychiatry* (1968) **9:** 27–40.

174. Szmukler GI, Eisler I, Russell GFM, Dare C. Anorexia nervosa, parental expressed emotion and dropping out of treatment. *Br J Psychiatry* (1985) **147:** 265–71.

175. Van Furth EF, van Strein DC, Martina LML et al. Expressed emotion and the prediction of outcome in adolescent eating disorders. *Int J Eating Dis* (1996) **20:** 19–32.

176. Gowers S, Norton K, Halek C, Crisp AH. Outcome of outpatient psychotherapy in a random allocation treatment study of anorexia nervosa. *Int J Eat Disord* (1994) **15:** 165–77.

177. Gallop R, Kennedy SH, Stern D. Therapeutic alliance on an inpatient unit for eating disorder. *Int J Eat Disord* (1994) **16:** 405–10.

178. Patton, GC. Mortality and eating disorders. *Psychol Med* (1988) **18:** 947–51.

179. Crisp AH, Callender JS, Halek C, Hsu LKG. Long term mortality in anorexia nervosa. A 20-year follow-up of the St George's and Aberdeen cohorts. *Br J Psychiatry* (1992) **161:** 104–7.

8
Treatment of chronic fatigue syndrome

Trudie Chalder, Alicia Deale and Simon Wessely

Introduction

Although it is not a new disease[1] there is no doubt that in the last 10 years there has been a dramatic rise in the number of patients thought to be suffering from chronic fatigue syndrome (CFS). Such patients are now frequently referred to general medical clinics. Many are referred to psychiatrists, either because the general practitioner thinks that the problem may be psychological, or because patients who are perceived as difficult to help often end up in the psychiatric clinic. More charitably, we hope, this referral is because of a growing acceptance of the positive role psychological medicine can play in the management of this otherwise debilitating and intractable condition.[2]

Between half and three-quarters of patients with CFS meet criteria for an identifiable psychiatric diagnosis. Some will believe, rightly or wrongly, that they have a physical illness called myalgic encephalomyelitis (ME) and may be reluctant to see the psychiatrist. The patient may be desirous of an organic diagnosis or may request sophisticated investigations which have thus far not been carried out. Consultations can leave both patient and doctor feeling dissatisfied. Given that the morbidity of CFS is not a matter for dispute,[3,4] this is an unsatisfactory situation.

This chapter will consider the different aetiological factors that have been associated with CFS and will go on to describe a multifactorial model of CFS that will focus on making a distinction between precipitating and perpetuating factors. Rehabilitation based on this model will be outlined and difficulties encountered in the delivery of this approach addressed. The evidence for such an approach will be presented.

Epidemiology

It is helpful to view fatigue on a continuum, with fatigue as a symptom at one end of the spectrum and CFS with all its associated disability at the other. Prevalence rates vary, but, in the UK, approximately 10% of general practice attenders have chronic fatigue,[5] while approximately 1%

have CFS, exact proportions depending on the diagnostic criteria used.[6] This chapter is concerned primarily with the group of patients who fall into the latter category. By the time they reach secondary care the majority of patients will have been investigated by their GP and any physical causes will have been diagnosed. For the majority of patients investigations will be normal.[7,8] However, recent longitudinal studies, conducted on hospital populations, show that left untreated the majority of people affected by this condition remain functionally impaired for several years.[2]

Operational criteria

Patients with CFS have been referred to by a variety of labels: ME and postviral fatigue syndrome are commonly used, but the broader and aetiologically neutral term CFS is preferred.[9] Operational criteria from the UK, USA and Australia all require a main complaint of disabling fatigue, as well as other symptoms such as sleep disturbance, mood disorder and muscle pain, with no identifiable organic disease and marked disability.[10-13] The UK criteria are the only criteria that include mental as well as physical fatigue.[12] The symptoms should be present for 6 months and patients suffering from physical diseases, known to produce fatigue, should be excluded. Patients with depression and anxiety are not excluded, but the presence of a major mental illness such as schizophrenia would be considered an exclusion criterion.

Clinical description

Patients complain of exhaustion. They say that this subjective state is unfamiliar and unlike the sort of tiredness they used to feel when well. The fatigue is usually exacerbated by activity and even minor exertions can leave the patient feeling unwell for days. Many patients complain of additional symptoms such as headache, pain and flu-like symptoms. Disability varies considerably. At the more severe end of the spectrum an inability to work is common, with some confined to a wheelchair or bed bound. Most patients will complain of abnormal sleep patterns, particularly onset or sleep maintenance insomnia, hypersomnia and daytime sleepiness. Of particular interest is patients' beliefs about the cause of their problem. Many hold strong physical illness attributions. Some worry they have a chronic viral infection while others believe they have some sort of immune dysfunction.

From the doctor's perspective, views tend to be divided. Some believe the problem to be psychiatric, i.e. a form of depression or anxiety, while others view it as an organic disease of uncertain aetiology. This mind–body split, which prevails in our society, can be unhelpful at the best of times but is particularly so when considering a heterogeneous condition such as CFS.

Prognosis

The prognosis in CFS is poor, particularly for adult patients seen in specialist settings.[2] Fewer than 10% of CFS patients referred to specialist settings make a full recovery, and about 10–20% appear to worsen over time.[14–16] Some patients improve over time, but the rates of improvement range from 8%[17] to 63%.[16] Most improved patients remain functionally impaired, unable to work or undertake any significant social or physical activity.[16]

Aetiology

CFS and muscle dysfunction

Many patients with CFS complain of weakness and postexertional fatigue. This led researchers to consider the possibility of a neuromuscular cause. However, studies of dynamic muscle function have demonstrated that muscle strength, endurance and fatiguability are normal in most patients.[18–21] Examination of muscle tissue showed some evidence of a persistent virus[22] but these findings are difficult to replicate and it seems unlikely that a factor such as this would be solely responsible for the degree of disability seen in these patients. Furthermore, the mental fatigue which is so common in CFS cannot be associated with neuromuscular dysfunction. It seems far more plausible that central mechanisms underlie the experience of physical and mental fatigability, confirmed by evidence of dysfunction in the hypothalamic–pituitary–adrenal axis and possible central neurotransmitter dysregulation.[23,24]

The role of viruses

Most patients will describe having experienced a viral infection at the onset of their fatigue.[14,25] There are many reasons why attributing the cause of fatigue to a virus is appealing, not least because viruses are extremely common. Making an external attribution for symptoms protects the person from blame and feelings of guilt. Self-esteem remains intact and the stigma of a psychiatric diagnosis is avoided.[26–29] However, there is no evidence that common viruses cause chronic fatigue[30] and, although delayed recovery occurs in a small percentage of patients after more serious infections such as glandular fever,[31] hepatitis[32] and meningitis,[33] it seems unlikely that a virus alone could be responsible for causing such profound disability as is witnessed in patients with CFS.

An immune dysfunction?

A number of abnormalities have been shown in the immune system of patients with CFS,[34] but these are both inconsistent and insubstantial. The findings are difficult to interpret and, at present, add little to the understanding of CFS or its treatment.

The overlap between psychiatric disorder and CFS

There are a number of studies that show an overlap between CFS and psychiatric disorders such as depression, anxiety and somatization disorder.[35–38] There are a number of possible reasons for this. It has been suggested that depression is an understandable consequence of a physical illness. However, some studies show clearly that the rate of psychiatric disorder is higher in CFS than in other medical conditions with a similar degree of associated disability.[25,39,40] The idea that CFS is a form of depression has also been suggested. However, despite the clear overlap in symptoms and diagnostic criteria, not everyone fulfils criteria for depression (even when using the Centers for Disease Control criteria), which requires multiple symptoms, resulting in patients with psychiatric disorder being actively selected.[39] At least a quarter have no psychiatric disorder at all. Depression with profound fatigue has been termed atypical depression, but only 14% of these patients fulfil criteria for CFS.[41]

It does seem plausible that CFS, in some, is a stress response that differs from depression. There is now convincing evidence that, in contrast to depressed patients, those with CFS show increased activity at sites of 5-HT neurotransmission.[24,42,43] Similarly, while patients with depression show high levels of the stress hormone cortisol, representing a state of heightened arousal, CFS patients have reduced levels of cortisol.[23,24] The most robust way of determining the relationship between psychiatric disorder and CFS is to take a prospective longitudinal view. There is now evidence of an association between previous psychiatric disorder and CFS.[6]

Neuropsychiatry

There is no doubt that patients experience substantial complaints of cognitive dysfunction. With regards to global intellectual functioning, research to date is unequivocal. There is no decline or primary deficit in intellectual functioning.[44–48] Similarly, there is no evidence of sensory or perceptual impairments in CFS.[49,50] What seems to be emerging is a picture of a mismatch between the subject's own perception of cognitive disturbance, and the level of actual decrements in performance determined on testing.[51] Although selective attention may be impaired,[52] formal deficits in memory seem unlikely. Patients with CFS may have a bias for processing somatic or fatigue-related information, and increased attention to bodily sensations may well affect attentional processes. However, higher cognitive functioning such as planning, organizing, problem-solving and conceptualization do not appear to be affected.

Perhaps the best publicized, but the least researched, area is that of neuroimaging. Studies using magnetic resonance techniques have concentrated on the appearance of punctate foci of high signal intensity (so-called 'unexplained bright objects' – UBOs). These have either been substantially increased, moderately increased or not increased at all compared with controls.[53]

It is also too early to judge the results of functional neuroimaging studies. There are several studies using functional neuroimaging techniques such as single photon emission tomography (SPET) in CFS. None are without problems.[53] In one study[54] a substantially increased number of defects was seen in CFS subjects compared with normal controls, while there was no difference in the number or situation of defects between CFS and depressed controls. There were, however, differences in the patterns of radionucleotide uptake between depression and CFS. Another study found that brainstem perfusion was significantly reduced in CFS subjects compared with controls, with depressed patients showing intermediate values.[55] Other groups do not report brainstem perfusion values because of the technical difficulties of imaging this small structure. Any interpretation of this finding must await its independent replication. It is, however, most unlikely that this will be a test for ME, as frequently claimed by the media.

A multifactorial model of CFS

A host of specific physical and psychological causes has been implicated in CFS. However, because of the subjective, heterogeneous nature of the condition it is likely that a complex interaction of physiological, cognitive, behavioural and affective factors is responsible for both its development and maintenance. A cognitive behavioural model takes into account such factors (Table 8.1).

Predisposing and precipitating factors

Examining the role of predisposing and precipitating factors in the development of CFS is complicated and costly: consequently, research in this area is preliminary. Some studies suggest that the premorbid personalities of patients with CFS are characterized by a marked hyperactivity or workaholism and achievement orientation, perfectionism and high standards for work performance.[56–58] However, although there is evidence of

Table 8.1   Factors which contribute to the development and maintenance of CFS.

Predisposing factors
- Family history of illness during childhood
- Unhelpful core beliefs about the meaning of symptoms, e.g. physical symptoms are dangerous

Precipitating factors
- Negative life events/chronic stress
- Illness/disease, i.e. infection
- Psychiatric disorder
- Lack of social support

Perpetuating factors

Behavioural
- Reduction of activities
- Frequent visits to the doctor/hospital
- Poor sleep routine
- Avoidance of tasks/specific places

Cognitive
- Fear of making symptoms worse
- Physical illness attributions
- Symptom focusing
- Influenced by memory of past aversive experiences
- Feeling out of control

Affective
- Demoralization
- Low mood
- Frustration

Social and cultural
- Mind–body dualism
- Misinformation in the media
- Unhelpful advice
- Being disbelieved
- Role of family and friends

Physiological
- Deconditioning
- Loss of morbidity
- Lack of fitness
- Weakness and wasting

an association between negative components of perfectionism and fatigue in female nurses, this has not been shown in CFS patients.[59]

In a primary care study, an increased number of negative life events, lack of social support, prior psychological distress and the presence of infection were all independently associated with fatigue.[30,60] This result concurs with one of the cross-sectional studies. Retrospectively, patients with CFS report infection and life stress as being associated with the onset of their illness.[61,62]

Conflicting results have also been obtained. Although Bruce-Jones et al. found an association between social adversity and depression this did not apply to postviral fatigue syndrome.[63] Another study[64] compared CFS and irritable bowel syndrome patients with normal controls in terms of the number of life events and social support experienced prior to the onset of their illness. The CFS group did not experience more life events than the other two groups but they perceived less overall support both pre- and post-onset of their illness.

The prevailing culture has also to be taken into account. As CFS (referred to in the media as ME) is being promoted as a disease with an as yet undiscovered physical cause, it is likely that this will influence individuals' beliefs about symptoms and illness.

Perpetuating factors

Once fatigue has been triggered, the problem is both maintained and made worse by cognitive and behavioural factors, such as fear and avoidance.

Illness attributions and cognitions

Most patients with somatic complaints, regardless of the type, have a tendency to misinterpret innocuous physical symptoms persistently as evidence of something more serious. In CFS, specific attributions and beliefs are likely to influence fear and avoidance behaviour.[57,65] These include beliefs about the nature of the illness, beliefs about the meaning of symptoms, fears about the consequences of activity and fear that activity or exercise will make symptoms worse.[29,66] In chronic illness generally, such beliefs are associated with a perpetuation of disability and symptoms.[67] Longitudinal studies have demonstrated that making physical illness attributions for fatigue predicts the degree of disability in patients with CFS.[16,29,62] In an effort to control and reduce symptoms, patients become hypervigilant and oversensitized to bodily sensations. This symptom focusing may serve to exacerbate unpleasant sensations and has been shown to be associated with fatigue in patients with CFS.[68]

Behaviour

Prolonged rest and avoidance of activity are central in sustaining the cycle of symptoms and disability in CFS.[69,70] Sharpe et al.[62] found that avoiding exercise predicted disability, while Ray et al.[68] found an association between functional impairment and accommodating to the illness in patients with CFS. The long-term physiological consequences of inactivity are deleterious.

Summary

Symptoms of fatigue can therefore be precipitated by a stressor, such as an infection, a negative life event or chronic stress, and are perpetuated by physical illness attributions, fearful cognitions and avoidance coping strategies. The model described here was adapted from other models which have achieved acceptance in understanding and treating chronic pain[69] and lead on to a number of possible interventions. In accordance with the model, success should result from reducing avoidance behaviour and addressing unhelpful thoughts and fears about the effects of activity and exercise.

A rehabilitation programme based on cognitive behaviour therapy (CBT)

The main aim of treatment is to enable patients to carry out their own rehabilitation with some support and guidance from their therapist. Treatment will involve the introduction of a consistent, graded approach to activity, establishing a sleep routine and using cognitive strategies to help combat unhelpful thoughts that are interfering with the rehabilitative process. Success, however, depends on several things. A thorough assessment should be carried out that will form the basis of a formulation of the patient's problem. This formulation will be shared with the patient before treatment starts. It should help the process of engagement and will form part of the rationale for treatment. Throughout treatment, progress is reviewed constantly and goals adjusted in collaboration with the patient.[71]

Who should treat

Outpatient treatment can be conducted by a competent psychiatrist who has had some training and experience of cognitive behaviour therapy (CBT). Alternatively, nurse behavioural therapists, psychologists, occupational therapists or physiotherapists may be competent in this field. Whatever the discipline, it is necessary that they possess specific skills in delivering psychological treatment.

Assessment

The assessment should include not only a detailed description of symptoms but also, more importantly, a detailed behavioural analysis of what the patient is able to do in relation to the work, home, private and social aspects of his or her life.[72] The quality and quantity of sleep should be inquired about. A detailed account of activity, rest and sleep patterns should be obtained by asking the patient to keep a diary for 2 weeks.[73] This will be used as a guide for setting the initial behavioural goals and can be used throughout treatment to monitor progress. Specific fears about the consequences of activity and exercise should be elicited, as should more general ideas about the nature of the illness. Circumstances surrounding the onset should be discussed, as this information may be useful when giving the patient a rationale for treatment: lifestyle factors may need to be addressed during treatment. It is important at this stage to inquire about the presence of depression and/or anxiety.[72] If severe, such disorders may require treatment in their own right, either before CBT or concurrently.

Engagement

Engaging the patient and forming a therapeutic alliance are part of a continuing process. While the therapist is carrying out the assessment, the patient, who may be sensitive to being disbelieved, may be on the lookout for evidence that the therapist thinks the problem is 'all in the mind'. During this early stage of treatment, the therapist should be explicit in conveying belief in the reality of the symptoms and should pay careful attention to the language used. The term 'psychological' should be avoided: this is a broad term that means different things to different people and it may also set the scene for disagreement between the patient and therapist. The patient's symptoms are real, and it helps to state and restate this. Rather than debating whether the problem is physical or psychological (a mind–body split is unhelpful in any illness), it is far more useful to direct the discussion towards how the problem can best be managed, taking into account physiological, behavioural and cognitive factors.

Rationale for treatment

Offering the patient a rationale for treatment should be a prerequisite of any intervention. It stands to reason that having an understanding of how and why treatment works will aid compliance. It can be helpful to offer the patient a formulation of his or her problems, using a cognitive behavioural framework. Information gathered during the assessment will be utilized during this process. A distinction is made between precipitating and perpetuating factors.

The rationale will obviously vary depending on the individual's circumstances but, essentially, the patient should be told that the emphasis will be on establishing a consistent level of activity every day – regardless of symptoms. The amount of activity is then gradually increased and rest decreased as the patient becomes more confident. It can be helpful to point out that rest is useful in an acute illness but is rarely restorative in the longer term. A sleep routine should also be established as quickly as possible.

The rationale should be repeated several times throughout treatment. It is useful to ask the patient to explain the rationale to the therapist to determine whether this has been clearly understood, and also to discuss any concerns. Before commencing treatment, it is important that the patient is clear about what the treatment entails and that the patient agrees to at least try what is being offered. The aims of treatment should be explicitly negotiated and agreed. These aims are best defined in terms of specific and realistic achievements, such as returning to work or swimming a certain number of lengths every day.

It may be important to address the role of continuing investigations and other treatments, as these may detract from the rehabilitation process. It is better, therefore, to call a halt to further investigations and treatments and to give the patient a positive diagnosis of CFS before commencing CBT.

Structure

Patients are usually seen fortnightly for up to 15 sessions of face-to-face treatment. Follow-ups are carried out at 3 and 6 months and then at 1 year to monitor progress and to tackle any residual problems. Questionnaires are given to assess fatigue, disability and psychological distress before and after treatment and at follow-up. At the beginning of treatment, long-term targets are negotiated with the patient just to ensure that both the therapist and patient are working towards similar goals. At every subsequent session, short-term goals are agreed upon. Patients should keep hourly records of their activity and rest throughout treatment so that progress can be monitored and problems discussed. Problems should be anticipated, and problem-solving strategies used to elicit effective coping. Discussion during sessions often revolves around exploring issues that may be preventing the patient from making changes.

Active scheduling

Goals are negotiated initially using the baseline diaries and typically involve a variety of specific tasks; usually these include a mixture of social, work and leisure-related activities. Short walks or tasks carried out in even chunks throughout the day are ideal, and these should be interspersed with rests. The emphasis is on consistency and breaking the association between experiencing symptoms and stopping activity. The goals (e.g. walking for 10 minutes three times daily) are gradually built up as tolerance to symptoms increases, until the longer-term targets are reached. This usually takes several months. Fatigue levels do not decrease very much initially but, between discharge and follow-up, marked reductions in fatigue should be expected. Tasks such as reading (which require concentration) can be included, but mental functioning does seem to improve in synchrony with physical functioning.

Establishing a sleep routine

Early on in treatment, patients should be asked to keep a diary of bedtime, sleep time, wake-up time and get-up time. The total number of hours spent asleep is calculated and a variety of strategies should then be used to improve both the quality and quantity of sleep. A routine of going to bed and getting up at a pre-planned time, whilst simultaneously cutting out daytime catnaps, helps to prevent insomnia. Change in sleep routine can be made slowly depending on the severity of the problem. For those who sleep too much, the amount of time spent asleep can be reduced gradually (for a detailed description of sleep management, see Morin[74]).

Modifying negative and unhelpful thinking

The main aim of this component of CBT is to prevent unhelpful thoughts from blocking progressive increases in activity. Information about the nature of CFS and the process of rehabilitation should be shared with the patient throughout treatment, as many patients will have been given incorrect or misleading information about their illness. Explanations regarding the physiological effects of inactivity can help patients comply with activity scheduling. The patient should be reassured about the safety of exercise, and written self-help information that reinforces these messages can be helpful. In reality, unhelpful beliefs about the harmful effects of exercise will diminish as the patient becomes more active and confident. However, some will need more structured cognitive therapy using traditional methods (see Beck et al.[75]). Specific negative thoughts, such as 'My muscles will be damaged by exercising too much', should be recorded in a diary. Patients should be encouraged to elicit alternative, less-catastrophic interpretations of events. These too should be recorded in a diary and discussed during consultations. In some patients core beliefs and dysfunctional assumptions relating to perfectionism or self-worth can be addressed in the conventional way.

Tackling psychosocial problems

Related social or psychological difficulties will often emerge during treatment. It is important these are tackled in a problem-solving way; otherwise they may prevent further progress.[76] It is important, however, to keep the focus on rehabilitation: being distracted from the main task in hand may lead to treatment failure. Improvements in one particular area of a patient's life will usually generalize to other areas.

Treatment: traditional approaches

Acyclovir (an antiviral drug[77]) and immunoglobulins[78] have been evaluated for use in CFS. Neither were found to be efficacious. Although both evening primrose oil and magnesium achieve better results, it is difficult to know how these impact on levels of disability.

One would have imagined, given the overlap between depression and CFS, that antidepressants would be helpful in the treatment of CFS. However, despite promising beginnings,[79,80] a recent randomized controlled trial of antidepressants found no effect in CFS with or without depression.[81] The lack of a placebo response is difficult to explain and future trials are awaited before passing a final judgement on this issue. Undoubtedly, it is the authors' experience that some patients with an obvious mood disorder improve on antidepressants.

Evidence for the efficacy of CBT

An uncontrolled pilot study carried out at the National Hospital for Neurology in London[82] resulted in a 70% improvement rate in those who commenced treatment. A 4-year follow-up reassuringly confirmed that patients who had initially improved retained their gains.[83] Since then, two randomized controlled trials have demonstrated that the 70% improvement rate in the pilot study was a robust finding. The first trial carried out in Oxford randomized 60 patients to either CBT or treatment as usual. Seventy-three per cent of the patients in the CBT group improved in terms of fatigue disability and illness beliefs.[84] The second trial, carried out by the authors at King's College Hospital, controlled for nonspecific treatment factors by comparing CBT with a relaxation control. At 6-months' follow-up, 70% of the CBT group and 19% of the control group had improved.[85]

An exercise trial carried out by Fulcher et al. at St Bartholomew's Hospital, London, in which 66 CFS patients (with no psychiatric disorder or sleep disturbance) were randomized to either aerobic exercise or flexibility exercises, demonstrated about a 55% improvement rate in the exercise group, compared with 26% in the control group.[86] This provides evidence for using exercise as part of the rehabilitation programme, although some patients may be fearful of attempting aerobic exercise at the beginning of treatment. Given that walking is an important component of CBT, it appears that the two approaches have much in common.

Predictors of outcome

Various studies have shown that poor outcome, in untreated groups, is associated with older age, greater functional impairment, multiple somatic complaints, comorbid psychiatric disorder and holding a belief that the illness is due solely to physical causes.[15,16,62,87] Little is known about outcome predictors in patients treated with CBT. Physical illness attributions do not appear to be associated with poor outcome in patients who have received CBT.[83,85] In one randomized controlled trial, poor outcome appeared to be related to patients negotiating medical retirement.[85] In the authors' experience, severe depression can also lead to treatment failure.

Special issues

The angry patient

Many patients are initially ambivalent towards the idea of seeing a psychiatrist. It is better to address such feelings immediately on seeing the patient, and to sympathize openly with their plight. 'Did you think that seeing me meant your symptoms were not being taken seriously?' can lead to direct questions about the experience of disconfirmation and the perceived stigmatization implicit in referral to a psychiatric service. The value of simple compassion should never be underestimated.

The insurance assessment

The issue of benefits and insurance payments is exceptionally difficult in this area, and can lead to misunderstandings unless carefully handled. Disability systems and insurance agencies are sceptical about CFS – the combination of a disorder based entirely on self-report (without any agreed diagnostic test) and sometimes profound disability understandably causes some concern.[88] Much of the self-help literature concerns the iniquities of the various benefits systems and both the personal and political strategies to overcome them.

It is helpful to adopt a pragmatic approach to this problem. When asked to comment on benefits or insurance claims, the authors support the patient as much as is possible but, rarely, support claims for permanent disability or medical retirement until all reasonable methods of rehabilitation have been tried. Difficulties for the therapist arise when there are clear conflicts of interest – for example, when stress at work contributed to the development of CFS and a return to work would exacerbate the symptoms. In some cases a gradual return to work can be helpful.

Role of the spouse/parent

A poor marital relationship can be a relevant component in a range of social stressors. However, researchers have recently reported an apparently paradoxical result in the context of CFS. Greater marital satisfaction was associated with more fatigue – the presumed link being via overprotective and oversolicitous behaviours.[89] Hence, if it is felt that either partners or parents are encouraging disability – albeit inadvertently – then it is just as important to engage them in the treatment as the individual patient.[90,91] Relatives or friends often act as co-therapists in CBT. This role can be especially helpful in the management of CFS, as significant others may otherwise unwittingly reinforce illness beliefs and avoidance behaviour.

Conclusions

There is now substantial evidence that graded activity (which includes some form of exercise, such as walking) decreases levels of fatigue and reduces disability in patients with CFS. Psychiatrists will reduce the likelihood of alienating the patient by paying careful attention to engagement. Future research should focus on training a variety of health professionals in this approach, particularly in the primary care setting.

References

1. Wessely S. Old wine in new bottles: neurasthenia and 'ME'. *Psychol Med* (1990) **20:** 35–53.

2. Joyce J, Hotopf M, Wessely S. The prognosis of chronic fatigue and chronic fatigue syndrome: a systematic review. *Q J Med* (1997) **90:** 223–33.

3. Komaroff A, Fagioli L, Doolittle T et al. Health status in patients with chronic fatigue syndrome and in general population and disease comparison groups. *Am Med* (1996) **101:** 281–90.

4. Buchwald D, Pearlman T, Umali J, Schmaling K, Katon W. Functional status in patients with chronic fatigue syndrome, other fatiguing illnesses, and healthy controls. *Am J Med* (1996) **171:** 364–70.

5. David A, Pelosi A, McDonald E et al. Tired, weak or in need of rest: fatigue among general practice attenders. *Br Med J* (1990) **301:** 1199–22.

6. Wessely S, Chalder T, Hirsch S, Wallace P, Wright D. Psychological symptoms, somatic symptoms and

psychiatric disorder in chronic fatigue and chronic fatigue syndrome: a prospective study in the primary care setting. *Am J Psychiatry* (1996) **153:** 1050–9.

7. Valdini A, Steinhardt S, Feldman E. Usefulness of a standard battery of laboratory tests in investigating chronic fatigue in adults. *Family Practice* (1989) **6:** 286–91.

8. Lane T, Matthews D, Manu P. The low yield of physical examinations and laboratory investigations of patients with chronic fatigue. *Am J Med Sci* (1990) **299:** 313–18.

9. Report of the Royal College. *Chronic Fatigue Syndrome: Report of a Joint Working Group of the Royal Colleges of Physicians, Psychiatrists and General Practitioners* (London, 1996).

10. Holmes G, Kaplan J, Gantz N et al. Chronic fatigue syndrome: a working case definition. *Ann Intern Med* (1988) **108:** 387–9.

11. Lloyd A, Hickie I, Boughton R, Spencer O, Wakefield D. Prevalence of chronic fatigue syndrome in an Australian population. *Med J Aust* (1990) **153:** 522–8.

12. Sharpe M, Archard L, Banatvala J et al. Chronic fatigue syndrome: guidelines for research. *J Royal Soc Med* (1991) **84:** 118–21.

13. Fukuda K, Straus S, Hickie I, Sharpe M, Dobbins J, Komaroff A. The chronic fatigue syndrome: a comprehensive approach to its definition and study. *Ann Intern Med* (1994) **121:** 953–9.

14. Petersen P, Schenck C, Sherman R. Chronic fatigue syndrome in Minnesota. *Minnesota Med* (1991) **74:** 21–6.

15. Vercoulen J, Swanink C, Fennis J, Galama J, van der Meer J, Bleijenberg G. Prognosis in chronic fatigue syndrome: a prospective study on the natural course. *J Neurol Neurosurg Psychiatry* (1996) **60:** 489–94.

16. Wilson A, Hickie I, Lloyd A et al. Longitudinal study of the outcome of chronic fatigue syndrome. *Br Med J* (1994) **308:** 756–60.

17. Tirelli U, Marotta G, Improta S, Pinto A. Immunological abnormalities in patients with chronic fatigue syndrome. *Scand J Immunol* (1994) **40:** 601–8.

18. Lloyd A, Hales J, Gandevia S. Muscle strength, endurance and recovery in the postinfection fatigue syndrome. *J Neurol Neurosurg Psychiatry* (1988) **51:** 1316–22.

19. Stokes M, Cooper R, Edwards R. Normal strength and fatigability in patients with effort syndrome. *Br Med J* (1988) **297:** 1014–18.

20. Riley M, O'Brien C, McCluskey D, Bell N, Nicholls D. Aerobic work capacity in patients with chronic fatigue syndrome. *Br Med J* (1990) **301:** 953–6.

21. Rutherford O, White P. Human quadriceps strength and fatigability in patients with post-viral fatigue. *J Neurol Neurosurg Psychiatry* (1991) **54:** 961–4.

22. Wessely S, Thomas PK. The chronic fatigue syndrome ('myalgic encephalomyelitis' or 'postviral fatigue'). In Kennard C (ed) *Recent Advances in Neurology* (Edinburgh: Churchill Livingstone, 1990): 85–132.

23. Demitrack M, Dale J, Straus S et al. Evidence for impaired activation of the hypothalamic–pituitary–adrenal axis in patients with chronic fatigue syndrome. *J Clin Endocrinol Metab* (1991) **73:** 1224–34.

24. Cleare A, Bearn J, Allain T et al. Contrasting neuroendocrine responses in depression and chronic fatigue syndrome. *J Affect Disorders* (1995) **35:** 283–9.

25. Wessely S, Powell R. Fatigue syndromes: a comparison of chronic 'postviral' fatigue with neuromus-

cular and affective disorder. *J Neurol Neurosurg Psychiatry* (1989) **52:** 940–8.

26. Helman C. Feed a cold and starve a fever. *Culture, Med, Psychiatry* (1978) **7:** 107–37.

27. Katz B, Andiman W. Chronic fatigue syndrome. *J Paediatrics* (1988) **113:** 944–7.

28. Greenberg D. Neurasthenia in the 1980s: chronic mononucleosis, chronic fatigue syndrome, and anxiety and depressive disorders. *Psychosomatics* (1990) **31:** 129–37.

29. Chalder T, Power M, Wessely S. Chronic fatigue in the community: 'a question of attribution'. *Psychol Med* (1996) **26:** 791–800.

30. Wessely S, Chalder T, Hirsch S, Pawlikowska T, Wallace P, Wright D. Post infectious fatigue: a prospective study in primary care. *Lancet* (1995) **345:** 1333–8.

31. White P, Thomas J, Amess J, Grover S, Kangro H, Clare A. The existence of a fatigue syndrome after glandular fever. *Psychol Med* (1995) **25:** 907–16.

32. Berelowitz G, Burgess A, Thanabalasingham T, Murray-Lyon I, Wright D. Post-hepatitis syndrome revisited. *J Viral Hepatitis* (1995) **2:** 133–8.

33. Hotopf M, Noah N, Wessely S. Chronic fatigue and minor psychiatric morbidity after viral meningitis: a controlled study. *J Neurol Neurosurg Psychiatry* (1996) **60:** 504–9.

34. Strober W. Immunological function in chronic fatigue syndrome. In Straus S (ed) *Chronic Fatigue Syndrome* (New York: Mark Dekker, 1994): 207–40.

35. Abbey S, Garfinkel P. Chronic fatigue syndrome and the psychiatrist. *Can J Psychiatry* (1990) **35:** 625–33.

36. Kendell R. Chronic fatigue, viruses and depression. *Lancet* (1991) **337:** 160–2.

37. David AS. Postviral fatigue syndrome and psychiatry. *Br Med Bull* (1991) **47:** 966–88.

38. Fischler B, Cluydts R, De Gucht V, Kaufman L, DeMeirleir K. Generalised anxiety disorders in chronic fatigue syndrome. *Acta Psychiatr Scand* 1996 (in press).

39. Katon W, Buchwald D, Simon G, Russo J, Mease P. Psychiatric illness in patients with chronic fatigue and rheumatoid arthritis. *J Gen Intern Med* (1991) **6:** 277–85.

40. Wood G, Bentall R, Gopfert M, Edwards R. A comparative psychiatric assessment of patients with chronic fatigue syndrome and muscle disease. *Psychol Med* (1991) **21:** 619–28.

41. Zubieta J, Engleberg N, Yargic L, Pande A, Demitrack M. Seasonal variation in patients with chronic fatigue; comparison with major mood disorders. *J Psychiatr Res* (1994) **28:** 13–22.

42. Bakheit A, Behan P, Dinan T, Gray C, O'Keane V. Possible upregulation of hypothalamic 5-hydroxytryptamine receptors in patients with postviral fatigue syndrome. *Br Med J* (1992) **304:** 1010–12.

43. Sharpe M, Clements A, Hawton K, Young A, Sargent P, Cowen P. Increased prolactin response to buspirone in chronic fatigue syndrome. *J Affect Disorders* (1996) **41:** 71–6.

44. Altay H, Abbey S, Toner B, Salit I, Brooker H, Garfinkel P. The neuropsychological dimensions of post infectious neuromyasthenia (chronic fatigue syndrome): a preliminary report. *Inter J Psychiatry Med* (1990) **20:** 141–9.

45. Cope H, Pernet A, Kendall B, David A. Cognitive functioning and magnetic resonance imaging in chronic fatigue. *Br J Psychiatry* (1995) **167:** 86–94.

46. Grafman J, Schwartz V, Scheffers M, Houser C, Straus S. Analysis of neuropsychological functioning in

patients with chronic fatigue syndrome. *J Neurol Neurosurg Psychiatry* (1993) **56:** 684–9.

47. Riccio M, Thompson C, Wilson B, Morgan R, Lant A. Neuropsychological and psychiatric abnormalities in myalgic encephalomyelitis: a preliminary report. *Br J Med Psychol* (1992) **31:** 111–20.

48. Scheffers M, Johnson R, Grafman J, Dale J, Straus S. Attention and short-term memory in chronic fatigue syndrome patients: an event-related potential analysis. *Neurology* (1992) **42:** 1667–75.

49. Prasher P, Smith A, Findley L. Sensory and cognitive event-related potentials in myalgic encephalomyelitis. *J Neurol Neurosurg Psychiatry* (1990) **53:** 247–53.

50. Sandman C, Barron J, Nackoul K, Goldstein J, Fidler F. Memory deficits associated with chronic fatigue immune dysfunction syndrome. *Biol Psychiatry* (1993) **33:** 618–23.

51. Schmaling K, DiClementi J, Cullum M, Jones J. Cognitive functioning in chronic fatigue syndrome and depression: a preliminary comparison. *Psychosom Med* (1994) **56:** 383–8.

52. Joyce E, Blumenthal S, Wessely S. Memory, attention and executive function in chronic fatigue syndrome. *J Neurol Neurosurg Psychiatry* (1996) **60:** 495–503.

53. Cope H, David A. Neuroimaging in chronic fatigue syndrome. *J Neurol Neurosurg Psychiatry* (1996) **60:** 471–3.

54. Schwartz RB, Komaroff AL, Garada BM et al. SPECT imaging of the brain: comparison of findings in patients with chronic fatigue syndrome, AIDS dementia complex and major unipolar depression. *AJR Am J Roentgenol* (1994) **162:** 943–51.

55. Costa D, Tannock C, Brostoff J. Brainstem perfusion is impaired in patients with myalgic encephalomyelitis/chronic fatigue syndrome. *Q J Med* (1995) **88:** 767–73.

56. Salit I. Sporadic post-infectious neuromyasthenia. *Can Med Assoc J* (1985) **133:** 659–63.

57. Surawy C, Hackmann A, Hawton K, Sharpe M. Chronic fatigue syndrome: a cognitive approach. *Behav Res Ther* (1995) **33:** 535–44.

58. Ware N, Kleinman A. Culture and somatic experience – the social course of illness in neurasthenia and chronic fatigue syndrome. *Psychosom Med* (1992) **54:** 546–60.

59. Magnusson A, Nias D, White P. Is perfectionism associated with fatigue? *Psychosom Res* (1996) **41:** 377–84.

60. Chalder T, Neeleman J, Power M, Wessely S. Factors contributing to the development and maintenance of fatigue in primary care. (London: Institute of Psychiatry, PhD Thesis, 1998).

61. Komaroff A, Buchwald D. Symptoms and signs in chronic fatigue syndrome. *Rev Infect Dis* (1991) **13:** S8–S11.

62. Sharpe M, Hawton K, Seagroatt V, Pasvol G. Follow up of patients with fatigue presenting to an infectious diseases clinic. *Br Med J* (1992) **302:** 347–52.

63. Bruce-Jones W, White P, Thomas J, Clare A. The effect of social adversity on the fatigue syndrome, psychiatric disorders and physical recovery, following glandular fever. *Psychol Med* (1994) **24:** 651–9.

64. Lewis S, Cooper C, Bennett D. Psychosocial factors and chronic fatigue syndrome. *Psychol Med* (1994) **24:** 661–71.

65. Wessely S, Butler S, Chalder T, David A. The cognitive behavioural management of the post-

viral fatigue syndrome. In Jenkins R, Mowbray J (eds) *Postviral Fatigue Syndrome* (Chichester: Wiley, 1991): 305–34.

66. Deale A, Chalder T, Wessely S. Illness beliefs and outcome in chronic fatigue syndrome: do patients need to change their beliefs in order to get better? *J Psychosom Res* (1998) **45:** 77–83.

67. Sensky T. Patients' reaction to illness. *Br Med J* (1990) **300:** 622–3.

68. Ray C, Jeffries S, Weir W. Coping with chronic fatigue syndrome: illness responses and their relationship with fatigue, functional impairment and emotional status. *Psychol Med* (1995) **25:** 937–45.

69. Philips C. Avoidance behaviour and its role in sustaining chronic pain. *Behav Res Ther* (1987) **25:** 273–9.

70. Chalder T, Butler S, Wessely S. In patient treatment of chronic fatigue syndrome. *Behav Psychother* (1996) **24:** 351–65.

71. Deale A, Wessely S. A cognitive behavioural approach to chronic fatigue syndrome. *Therapist* (1994) **2:** 11–14.

72. Sharpe M, Chalder T, Palmer I, Wessely S. Chronic fatigue syndrome: a practical guide to assessment and management. *Gen Hosp Psychiatry* (1997) **19:** 185–99.

73. Chalder T. *Coping with Chronic Fatigue* (London: Sheldon Press, 1995).

74. Morin CM. *Insomnia. Psychological Assessment and Management* (New York: Guilford, 1993).

75. Beck A, Rush A, Shaw B, Emery G. *Cognitive Therapy of Depression* (New York: Guilford Press, 1979).

76. Hawton K, Salkowskis P, Kirk J, Clark D. *Cognitive Behaviour Therapy for Psychiatric Problems* (Oxford: Oxford Medical Publications, 1990).

77. Straus S, Dale J, Tobi M et al. Acyclovir treatment of the chronic fatigue syndrome: lack of efficacy in a placebo-controlled trial. *N Engl J Med* (1988) **319:** 1692–8.

78. Anon. Pseudo-outbreak of infectious mononucleosis – Puerto Rico, 1990. *Morbid Mortal Weekly* (1991) **40:** 552–55.

79. Lynch S, Seth R, Montgomery S. Antidepressant therapy in the chronic fatigue syndrome. *Br J Gen Pract* (1991) **41:** 339–42.

80. Goodnick P, Sandoval R. Psychotropic treatment of chronic fatigue syndrome and related disorders. *J Clin Psychiatry* (1993) **54:** 13–20.

81. Vercoulen J, Swanink C, Zitman F et al. Fluoxetine in chronic fatigue syndrome; a randomized, double-blind, placebo-controlled study. *Lancet* (1996) **347:** 858–61.

82. Butler S, Chalder T, Ron M, Wessely S. Cognitive behaviour therapy in chronic fatigue syndrome. *J Neurol Neurosurg Psychiatry* (1991) **54:** 153–8.

83. Bonner D, Butler S, Chalder T, Ron M, Wessely S. A follow up study of chronic fatigue syndrome. *J Neurol Neurosurg Psychiatry* (1994) **57:** 617–21.

84. Sharpe M, Hawton K, Simkin S et al. Cognitive behaviour therapy for chronic fatigue syndrome; a randomized controlled trial. *Br Med J* (1996) **312:** 22–6.

85. Deale A, Chalder T, Marks I, Wessely S. A randomised controlled trial of cognitive behaviour versus relaxation therapy for chronic fatigue syndrome. *Am J Psychiatry* (1997) **154:** 408–14.

86. Fulcher K, White P. Randomised controlled trial of graded exercise in patients with the chronic fatigue syndrome. *Br Med J* (1997) **314:** 1647–52.

87. Clark M, Katon W, Russo J, Kith P, Sintay M, Buchwald D. Chronic fatigue; risk factors for symptom persistence in a 2.5-year follow up study. *Am J Med* (1995) **98:** 187–95.

88. Lechky O. Life insurance MDs sceptical when chronic fatigue syndrome diagnosed. *Can Med Assoc J* (1990) **143:** 413–15.

89. Schmaling K, diClementi J. Interpersonal stressors in chronic fatigue syndrome: a pilot study. *J Chron Fatigue Synd* (1995) **1:** 153–8.

90. Vereker M. Chronic fatigue syndrome: a joint paediatric-psychiatric approach. *Arch Dis Childhood* (1992) **67:** 550–5.

91. Feder H, Dworkin P, Orkin C. Outcome of 48 pediatric patients with chronic fatigue; a clinical experience. *Arch Fam Med* (1994) **3:** 1049–55.

9
The psychopharmacological treatment of substance abuse (including alcoholism)

Michael Soyka

Introduction

Our understanding of the biological basis of addiction has increased significantly over the past decade. The biological mechanisms underlying clinical phenomena such as relapse and craving have been studied in great depth in animal studies at the neurochemical level (for a review, see Koob and LeMoal[1]) and at the molecular level (for a review, see Nestler and Aghajanian[2]). Although more clinical studies are necessary to explore the psychological and biological mechanisms of addiction further, a range of research-based pharmacotherapies for addiction has been established (for a review, see O'Brien[3] and Soyka[4]). The pharmacological treatment of substance abuse disorders has a number of different aspects. Some drugs are used for the treatment of withdrawal symptoms (i.e. for detoxification), others are used for the treatment of neuropsychiatric complications of substance use (e.g. delirium, hallucinations) or comorbid psychiatric disorder (e.g. depression, schizophrenia), and some are used for maintenance therapy or relapse prevention. This chapter deals mainly with the latter, although some drugs (e.g. antidepressants) may also be used for the treatment of detoxification or comorbid psychiatric disorder. There are some substance use disorders in which a number of pharmacological agents have been examined or introduced into clinical practice, such as alcoholism or opioid dependence, while in others (such as hallucinogens), little advice about such agents can be given. As some drugs discussed might be applied to the treatment of different substance use disorders, the major clinical guidelines for their pharmacological use are presented. Since there is no pharmacological basis for the prevention of relapse in the use of volatile substances, hallucinogens and cannabis, this chapter concentrates on the treatment of opioid dependence, cocaine use disorders, other stimulant abuse and alcoholism.

General aspects

A number of clinical and epidemiological studies suggest that substance abuse, especially alcoholism, is among the most prevalent psychiatric disorders in most Western countries. In the US Epidemiological Catchment Area study (ECA), 6 month prevalence estimates for alcoholism were found to be 2.9% (males 6.5%, females 0.3%), while in the Upper Bavarian Study prevalence estimates for severe alcoholism were found to be 3.1% (males 10.4%, females 0.8%; for a review, see Fichter et al.[5]). Lifetime prevalence for alcoholism in different regions of the USA was found to be 8–12%, while in the Munich region the prevalence rate was estimated to be 13% for males.[6] Per capita consumptions of pure alcohol in Germany and France (11.5 l/year) are somewhat higher than in Great Britain (7.3 l), Italy (8.6 l) or the USA (6.81 l). Six-month prevalence rates for drug abuse were higher in the USA compared with most European countries, such as Germany (0.9% vs. 0.3%), but it seems noteworthy that all the more recent statistics and findings suggest that use of illicit drugs has been increasing over the last decade. The drugs of preference change over time, with opioids and cannabis being most frequently used. While hallucinogens were popular in the 1960s and consumption decreased over time, the intake of hallucinogens and so-called designer drugs has again increased in recent years. Psychostimulant abuse (cocaine, 'crack' and others) is also very prevalent in the USA and Europe. Unfortunately, many drug users consume a large number of different drugs so that a definitive therapeutic strategy is often difficult to propose. Nevertheless, the principles of pharmacological treatment are discussed for the different groups of drugs.

Opioid dependence

Narcotics such as heroin are widely used in Western countries. In the USA, recent general population surveys suggest that 1.3% of the population may have used heroin at least some times in their lives.[7] In Europe, lifetime prevalence estimates for heroin consumption are considerably lower. In Western countries heroin is by far the most commonly abused opioid. It is usually injected, but can also be smoked and inhaled.

The abstinence-orientated treatment of heroin users has proved effective, but only a minority of patients remain abstinent. Both mortality and delinquency are high in heroin users. A long-term (24-year) follow-up study of heroin users showed that 28% of the patients had died, 29% were abstinent, 23% had positive urine tests for opioids and 18% were in prison.[8] Psychosocial treatment approaches in opioid addiction have been studied in great detail in a number of studies, including the Drug Abuse Reporting Program ($n = 44\,000$), the Treatment Outcome

Table 9.1   Possible pharmacological agents for use in opioid dependence.

Agent	Dose	Comments
Opiate agonists		
Methadone	50 mg or more	• Widely accepted • Can be given orally (daily) • Long half-life • Severe withdrawal symptoms
LAAM	70–100 mg	Three-times weekly administration possible
Heroin		Few studies conducted so far (e.g. Switzerland); highly controversial issue
Mixed agonists/antagonists		
Buprenorphine	4–12 mg (or more)	A number of studies conducted; possibly effective in detoxification and maintenance
Antagonists		
Naltrexone	50 mg daily or 100–100–150 three-times weekly	Predominantly effective in highly motivated opiate addicts

Prospective Study ($n = 11\,000$) and the ongoing Drug Abuse Treatment Outcome Study (for a review, see Simpson and Sells[9] and Hubbard et al.[10]), among others. Abstinence rates of opioid addicts in many follow-up studies range only between 10 and 20% (for a review, see Maddux and Desmond[11]).

Pharmacological treatment

For the treatment of opioid addicts a number of possible pharmacological agents can be used (see Table 9.1). Both opioid agonists and antagonists can be given. To date, methadone maintenance therapy is by far the most widely accepted treatment approach but some other alternative pharmacological strategies could be tried.

Opioid agonists

Methadone maintenance
Following the introduction of methadone maintenance in the USA by Dole and Nyswander,[12] the low abstinence rates in follow-up studies of heroin

addicts, high mortality rates and the severe medical and psychosocial consequences of heroin consumption found to exist in other countries led to the introduction of further methadone maintenance programmes. Methadone is an opioid agonist with a clear analgesic effect, a substantial abuse potential and cross-tolerance to heroin. Its long half-life (>24 hours) permits once-daily dosage. The clinical settings in which methadone is delivered to the patient vary significantly between countries. In some countries methadone is delivered by clinics or physicians, who give methadone directly to the patient (the USA, Germany). In other countries the drug is available by prescription through pharmacies (the UK, Austria) or via GPs (the UK). Most studies suggest that methadone maintenance may reduce heroin consumption, mortality, risk of HIV infection and crime in opioid addicts.[13,14] Few patients participating in methadone maintenance therapy appear to return to continuous drug-free abstinence,[15] although in follow-up studies Maddux and Desmond found that 9–21% of patients on methadone treatment were drug-free. For methadone maintenance, a daily dosage of 50 mg or more is usually recommended, but tolerance of methadone varies widely between patients and lower dosages might be sufficient in some, higher doses in others. McGlothin and Anglin reported higher abstinence rates in patients with high dosages of methadone (82–92 mg) compared with low dosages (43 mg on average).[16] Plasma levels of methadone are only infrequently measured during treatment, although a significant number of pharmacological interactions between methadone and other drugs are known (see Tables 9.2–5). Clinical guidelines for methadone treatment programmes have been proposed by a number of expert groups.[17–20] Inclusion and exclusion criteria for opioid addicts to be entered into methadone programmes vary considerably among different countries. Initially in the USA only addicts between the ages of 21 and 40 who were addicted to heroin for at least 4 years and who had relapsed repeatedly after several detoxifications were included in treatment programmes. Today the FDA/NIDA regulations allow heroin addicts with a 1 year addiction history (including physical dependence) to enter treatment programmes. Repeated urine toxicology is necessary to exclude/verify substance abuse.

Among the positive predictors of treatment outcome is client engagement in programme counselling. In general, the efficacy of methadone treatment programmes varies considerably, depending on the different treatment settings and patient and staff characteristics.[21] In many countries, methadone treatment programmes are receiving intensive public and scientific attention.[22,23] Methadone can also be used for opioid detoxification.

Some of the problems frequently encountered in methadone treatment programmes should be mentioned. First, dosage is important. As mentioned above, a minimum dose of 50 mg is often recommended although

Table 9.2   Drugs which are contraindicated (may precipitate withdrawal).

Generic name	Action use	Brands/examples
Naltrexone	Opioid antagonist used for treatment of alcoholism and/or blockade of opioid effects	ReVia™
Buprenorphine, butorphanol, dezocine, nalbuphine, pentazocine	Pain relievers with opioid-antagonist activity	Buprenex®, Stado®, Dalganr®, Nubain®, Talwin®
Tramadol	Synthetic analgesic (not considered opioid antagonist, but does decrease levels of opiates)	Ultram®
Nalmefene, naloxone	Reversal of opioid effects	Revex™, Narcan®

Adapted from *Addiction Treatment Forum Newsletter* (1997), Soyka[17] and Gross.[18]

Table 9.3   Drugs which may lower plasma levels of methadone or decrease methadone effects.

Generic name	Action/use	Brands/examples
Butabarbitone sodium, mephobarbitone, phenobarbitone, pentobarbitone, secobarbitone	Barbiturate sedatives and/or hypnotics	Bitosol Sodium®, Mebaral®, Nembutal®, phenobarbital, Seconal®
Carbamazepine	Anticonvulsant for epilepsy and trigeminal neuralgia	Aretol®, Tegretol®
Ethanol	Chronic use	wine, beer, whisky, etc.
Phenytoin	Control of seizures	Dilantin®
Rifampicin	Treatment of pulmonary tuberculosis	Rifadin®, Rifamate®, Rifater®, Rimactane®
Urinary acidifiers, ascorbic acid	Keeps calcium soluble, controls urine-induced skin irritations, vitamin C	K-Phos®, vitamin C (large doses)

Adapted from *Addiction Treatment Forum Newsletter* (1997), Soyka[17] and Gross.[18]

Table 9.4   Drugs which may increase plasma levels of methadone or increase methadone effects.

Generic name	Action/use	Brands/examples
Amitriptyline	Treatment of depression and anxiety	Elavil®, Endep®, Etrafon®, Limbitrol®, Triavil®
Cimetidine	H_2 receptor antagonist for the treatment of gastric and duodenal ulcers, and gastric reflux disease	Tagamet®
Diazepam	Control of anxiety and stress	Dizac™, Vairelease®, valium
Ethanol	Acute use	wine, beer, whisky, etc.
Fluvoxamine maleate	Serotonin reuptake inhibitor for treatment of depression and compulsive disorders	Luvox™
Ketoconazole	Antifungal agent	Nizoral® tablets
Urinary alkalinizers	Treatment of kidney stones, gout therapy	Bicitra®, Polycitra®

Adapted from *Addiction Treatment Forum Newsletter* (1997), Soyka[17] and Gross.[18]

Table 9.5   Drugs whose pharmacokinetics may be altered by methadone.

Generic name	Action/use	Brands/examples
Desipramine	Tricyclic antidepressant	Norpramin®
Zidovudine	Initial treatment of HIV	Retrovir®, AZT combinations

Adapted from *Addiction Treatment Forum Newsletter* (1997), Soyka[17] and Gross.[18]

some patients obviously need more, others less. Many expert groups recommend a dose range of up to 80–120 mg/day. Since many patients entering methadone treatment programmes receive psychotropic or other pharmacological agents, possible pharmacological interactions have to be considered carefully. Secondly, many patients in methadone treatment programmes suffer from mild to severe psychiatric symptoms, especially depression or insomnia. In these cases additional psychotropic medication has to be evaluated carefully. Thirdly, the possible side-effects of methadone have to be considered. These include sedation, vegetative dysregulation, sweating, sleep disorders, impaired libido, affective symptomatology, depression, constipation, impaired concentra-

Table 9.6   Pharmacological agents used in cocaine use disorders.

Substance	Author	Comments
Antidepressants		
Desipramine	Gawin et al.[97]	Significant effect
	Fischman et al.[99]	Weak effect
	Arndt et al.[24]	
Fluoxetine	Batki et al.[100]	Weak effect
Dopamine agonists		
Amantadine	Tennant and Sagherian[101]	Hardly any effect
Bromocriptine		
Dopamine antagonists		
Flupenthixol	Gawin et al.[98]	No effect
		Positive preliminary data
Carbamazepine	Halikas et al.[102]	Effect not yet proven
Methylphenidate	Gawin and Kleber[103]	Effect not yet proven

tion or cognitive function and loss of appetite or weight loss, among others. Psychomotor performance and driving ability might also be impaired. Fourthly, besides the intake of other substances, alcohol abuse is frequently overlooked in methadone patients. Alcohol may both potentiate and antagonize methadone's effect by interaction with the microsomal ethanol oxidising system (MEOS) in the liver.

LAAM

Laevo-alpha-acetylmethadol (LAAM) was introduced into clinical practice in the USA in 1993. LAAM is a pro-drug that is metabolized into nor-LAAM and dinor-LAAM, two potent opioid agonists that, compared with methadone, have a slower onset of action and a longer duration of action (up to 72 hours). The drug can be administered orally, intravenously or subcutaneously. LAAM basically acts at the mu-opioid receptor. LAAM can be given 3 times a week (70–100 mg, maximum 120 mg). An initial dose of 30 mg is recommended, with an increase of 5–10 mg every second day. If the dose is increased too quickly, side-effects such as sedation or hypotonia may occur. Possible advantages of LAAM compared with methadone are its long half-life and action, its comparatively slow onset of action and the 3 times a week regimen. Although LAAM has been studied for over two decades,[25–31] its possible clinical benefit in certain subgroups of opioid addicts is not entirely clear. The drug is hardly used outside the USA.

Buprenorphine

Buprenorphine is a potent opioid analgesic that might be an alternative to other opioid agonists.[32] Pharmacologically, buprenorphine is a partial mu- and kappa-agonist with an antagonistic effect on delta-opioid receptors. Buprenorphine 0.5 mg is equivalent to morphine 10 mg. The drug can be given intravenously, intramuscularly or sublingually. The dose required for the treatment of opioid addicts ranges between 4–8 (12) and 16 (32) mg/day. Although a number of clinical studies have been conducted, buprenorphine's place in the treatment of opioid dependence has yet to be determined. Some recent studies suggest that buprenorphine might be as effective as methadone in the treatment of opioid dependence.[33,34] Higher dosages of buprenorphine (12 mg) were found to be more effective than lower dosages (4 mg) in reducing illicit opioid (but not cocaine) use.[35] The drug has recently been introduced into clinical practice in France (Subutex) and is apparently widely used there. In the USA, the Food and Drug Administration is currently evaluating buprenorphine as a drug for the treatment of opioid dependence. It is also currently under investigation in a number of European countries. Since the withdrawal syndrome after buprenorphine treatment is comparatively mild, a possible role for buprenorphine might be found in the treatment of pregnant heroin addicts.

Morphine sulphate

Morphine sulphate is a very potent analgesic used predominantly to relieve pain in patients with carcinoma. It can be taken orally, with maximum plasma concentrations 4–7 hours after intake. The drug is used only in Austria for the treatment of opioid-dependent patients.[36]

Heroin

The use of heroin in the treatment of opioid-dependent patients is an extremely controversial issue that cannot be discussed in detail here. Some authors claim a reduced mortality rate in severely dependent opioid addicts under heroin maintenance.[37] The clinical data to support this finding are very inconclusive at present. Few heroin maintenance programmes have as yet been conducted. In Switzerland a heroin programme has been initiated that is currently being evaluated; another is to be launched in Austria and other countries will probably follow. The risks (i.e. overdose) of heroin treatment are obvious.

Opioid antagonists

Naltrexone

Treating opioid-dependent patients with opioid antagonists such as naltrexone is a different approach from the maintenance strategies discussed above. Naltrexone is used as an adjunct to ensure abstinence, and it can be recommended for highly motivated or short-term dependent opioid users. Naltrexone 50 mg can block the opioid receptor for at least 24 hours. It can be given orally daily (50 mg) or 3 times a week (100–100–150 mg). A number of clinical trials have been published which show some efficacy of naltrexone in the treatment of opioid dependence, but they also suggest a low retention rate. Important side-effects are nausea, vomiting and elevation of liver enzymes in some cases. The drug is also used for the treatment of alcoholism (see below).

Cocaine use disorders

Cocaine is a substance produced by the coca plant. It is used in very different preparations including coca paste (cocaine hydrochloride that can be insufflated or dissolved and injected – sometimes being mixed with heroin e.g. 'speedball' and 'crack'). Crack 'rocks' can be inhaled after placing them in a small pipe and heating them. This kind of preparation is characterized by its rapid onset of physiological action.

The pharmacological basis of cocaine's action is well understood. Cocaine blocks the dopamine reuptake transporter and causes an increase of dopamine at postsynaptic receptors.[38] Cocaine may also affect serotonergic neurotransmission.[39] Typical effects of cocaine or crack are mood elevation, euphoria, hypervigilance, restlessness, grandiosity, talkativeness and interpersonal sensitivity (for a review, see Woody et al.[40]). Acute intoxication is associated with impaired impulse control and judgement, paranoid reactions and ideation, and tactile and auditory hallucinations, among others. Aggression and violence are a frequent complication, especially in 'crack' consumption. Chronic consumption is associated with mood disorders, especially depression, irritability, anhedonia and anergia, emotional lability and impaired social functioning. Cognitive deficits, and disturbances of attention and concentration are also frequent. More severe complications are organic mental disorders with delusions and hallucinations closely resembling paranoid schizophrenia. There is no clear-cut withdrawal syndrome in cocaine users, but dysphoric mood, agitation, depression, insomnia or hypersomnia and psychomotor retardation are frequent.

Treatment

For cocaine abusers a number of therapeutic settings have been established including both inpatient and outpatient rehabilitation, family assessment and involvement, addiction counselling, behavioural approaches and self-help programmes. Few of these psychosocial approaches have been scientifically evaluated (for a review, see Woody et al.[40]), but most studies published so far and clinical experience suggest that relapses in cocaine abusers are frequent. A number of different pharmacological agents have been suggested in cocaine users, including tricyclic antidepressants (TCAs), specific serotonin reuptake inhibitors (SSRIs) (such as fluoxetine), dopamine antagonists (such as bromocriptine and amantadine), dopamine antagonists (such as flupenthixol) and a number of other drugs, including carbamazepine. The major studies and findings published so far are summarized in Table 9.6.

Since none of the medications tested has proved to be effective overall, the possible beneficial effects of medication given to cocaine users remain a matter of debate. From a clinical point of view it makes sense to focus on the treatment of psychopathological symptoms in cocaine users, especially depression (which may lead to relapse). Desipramine has been shown to have some effect in facilitating cocaine abstinence in at least some studies,[40] and might be the antidepressant to be tried first. Alternatively, SSRIs might be given. SSRIs such as sertraline or other antidepressants such as bupropion have been shown as to be effective in reducing cocaine abuse in open clinical trials.[41,42] The other possible treatment approach is blocking the dopamine receptor to prevent cocaine's action at the receptor. Flupenthixol, a 'classic' neuroleptic with both D1 and D2 antagonism that is widely used as an antipsychotic in Europe (but not the USA), can be given by intramuscular injection and might be a possible alternative to TCAs or SSRIs. Unfortunately the empirical basis for administering this drug to cocaine users is limited. It is currently under investigation for the treatment of alcohol abuse in Germany (see below).

Other psychostimulants

A wide range of stimulants is available, with amphetamines being the most important group. Amphetamines may be subdivided into stimulating N-substituted amphetamines, hallucinogenic methoxyphenethylamines and entactogenic methylenedioxyamphetamines/butamines. These can cause a wide range of psychiatric complications including increased violence, paranoid reactions and psychosis, confusional states, emotional lability syndromes, bizarre sexual behaviour and depression, among others.[43,44]

The pharmacological treatment of stimulant abuse has not been studied in great detail. For the treatment of depressive syndromes, TCAs such as imipramine and desipramine have been advocated. The issue remains controversial.[44] Alternatively, SSRIs may be used, but no controlled trials are available.

Pharmacotherapy of alcoholism

The efficacy of both inpatient and, to a lesser extent, the outpatient treatment of alcoholism has been demonstrated in a large number of experimental and prospective studies.[45,46] Relapse prevention, however, still remains a major challenge in alcohol therapy. Even after mid-term or even long-term inpatient treatment, abstinence rates in alcoholics hardly exceed 30–40% in all major prospective studies. Both self-help groups and psychotherapeutic approaches (such as coping skills, supportive or family therapy) have their place in the prevention of relapse in alcoholism.

A number of psychotropic agents have been used in alcohol treatment. Apart from disulfiram treatment,[47] TCAs and lithium, various other substances have been tested in an attempt to increase abstinence rates in alcoholics, most with little or no success. In recent years some more promising anti-craving drugs have been introduced into clinical practice.

New agents

Although the pathophysiological and neurochemical basis of alcohol dependence, craving and relapse is not yet fully understood, there is increasing evidence that a number of neurotransmitters and receptors are involved in the development of alcohol tolerance and dependence and in mediating the psychotropic effects of alcohol. Both the dopaminergic and serotonergic system,[48,49] the opioid/endorphin system and, more recently, the glutamate system[50,51] have been found to be influenced by alcohol. Alcohol's effect on these neurotransmitters and receptors is very complex and conflicting results and findings have been published.

For some time, the acute and chronic biological effects of alcohol on neuronal structures and cells, neurotransmitters and receptors have been studied in various species, but only recently have these findings led to new and challenging treatment approaches in the management of alcoholism. A variety of substances have been examined as adjuncts in the prevention of relapse in alcoholism, including serotonergic substances, especially SSRIs, buspirone, dopaminergic drugs and opiate antagonists (such as naltrexone or nalmefene) or the glutamate modulator acamprosate. Some of these have found general acceptance as anti-craving drugs.

Acamprosate
The use of N-methyl-D-aspartate (NMDA) antagonists for the treatment of alcohol-related disorders has been advocated repeatedly, but most non-competitive NMDA antagonists have proved too toxic for clinical use in humans.

The only glutaminergic drug used clinically for the treatment of

alcoholism so far is the homotaurinate derivate, calcium acetylhomotauri-
nate (acamprosate). The pharmacological profile of acamprosate has
been studied in detail: the drug is hydrophilic and poorly absorbed in the
gastrointestinal tract. It has a half-life of about 3.2 hours, has no pharmacologically active metabolite and is eliminated by renal excretion. Animal
studies have shown that the drug crosses the blood–brain barrier.[52]
Acamprosate was found to reduce CA^{2+} fluxes and the postsynaptic efficacy of excitatory amino acid neurotransmitters such as L-glutamate
(especially NMDA subtype), thus lowering the neuronal excitability.[53]
There is no evidence of a withdrawal syndrome or abuse potential from
acamprosate either in animals or humans. In the animal model, acamprosate was also found not to generalize for the alcohol cue, suggesting
that it is not a substitution drug. Acamprosate is a potent antagonist of
the excitatory amino acids' stimulatory effect. It seems to lower neuronal
excitability due to a reduction of CA^{2+} fluxes and it blunts the action of
excitatory amino acids (for a review, see Littleton[54]).

Acamprosate proved to be efficient in the reduction of alcohol intake
in animal models without changing ethanol toxicity.[55] Acamprosate is
usually well tolerated with few side-effects (see below). Its major disad-
vantage is the comparatively high dosage needed (1.3–2 g = 4–6
tablets/day).

The efficacy of acamprosate was evident in all but one of the studies
conducted so far (Figure 9.1). In the German Study, a total of 272 alcoholic patients recruited in 14 collaborating centres took part in a randomized, double-blind placebo-controlled study (phase III study) that
comprised a 48-week treatment phase and a 48-week drug-free follow-
up.[4,56] Some 134 (49.3%) of the patients completed the study after 1 year.
Patients on acamprosate showed significantly higher abstinence rates
within the first 60 days of treatment (67% vs. 50%) and throughout the
further study (45% vs. 25%).[57] Very few side-effects were recorded,
mainly diarrhoea and headache. No significant differences could be
demonstrated with respect to serious adverse reactions.

In most studies reviewed, patients with a body weight of more than
60 kg received 2 g acamprosate/day; below this weight, they received
1.3 g/day. A significant effect of acamprosate on the relapse rates in
alcoholics has been demonstrated in large studies in Austria conducted
by Whitworth et al.[58] and in France by Paille et al.[59] Other studies have
also proved acamprosate's effect on relapse prevention.[60,61]

Few side-effects and adverse reactions were observed during the
studies, with diarrhoea and nausea being the most frequent complications. Tolerance was usually good. The toxicity of the drug is mainly
related to the calcium part of the molecule; thus patients with hyper-
parathyroidism should not be treated with acamprosate. There is no evidence of any psychotropic effect or potential abuse for acamprosate
that could account for its observed effect on alcohol intake, and

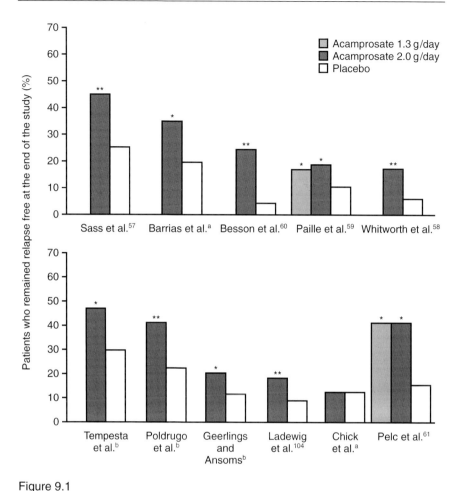

Figure 9.1

Survival analysis of acamprosate and placebo in alcohol-dependent patients. (Top) Studies with a 12-month (48-week) treatment phase; (bottom) studies with a 3 to 6-month treatment phase.
[a] These studies are unpublished, but were reported in the review of Soyka[4]; [b] these studies are unpublished; * indicates 0.05 vs. placebo; ** indicates 0.01 vs. placebo.

apparently there is no potential abuse[55] or interaction with ethanol toxicity. Acamprosate has gained approval for the treatment of alcoholism in most European Community countries, while it is still currently being studied in the USA.

Opioid antagonists (naltrexone and nalmefene)

Some of the major psychotropic and reinforcing effects of alcohol are believed to be mediated via the opioid endorphin system. There is substantial evidence from numerous animal studies and from some clinical studies that suggests acute alcohol intake stimulates opioid receptors (especially delta-subtype), while in chronic exposure an opioid receptor dysfunction may be part of the biological basis of alcohol craving and relapse. Animal data are consistent with the hypothesis that alcohol drinking is reinforced, in part, by enhanced opioid receptor activity. Most animal studies show that opioid antagonists reduce excessive alcohol intake without reducing the ingestion of other biologically important reinforcers.[62,63] Opioid receptor antagonists may help to reduce craving and relapse rates in alcoholics. A further theory suggests that cues associated with drinking may act like a 'priming dose' of alcohol and elicit an appetitive motivational response, possibly through endogenous opioid release. Volpicelli et al. reported that the major effect of opioid antagonists (such as naltrexone) may be a reduced feeling of being 'high' after alcohol consumption in chronic alcoholics.[64]

Naltrexone   In recent years two opioid receptor antagonists, naltrexone and, to a lesser extent, nalmefene, have been examined as possible anti-craving drugs. For naltrexone (a nonselective long-acting opioid receptor antagonist), the two major placebo-controlled double-blind studies so far have been conducted by Volpicelli et al.[65] and O'Malley et al.[66,67] In a 3-month double-blind study (naltrexone 50 mg vs. placebo) of 70 alcohol-dependent outpatients at a veterans hospital, Volpicelli et al. were unable to demonstrate a significant effect of naltrexone on abstinence rates (57% of the patients drinking in this group, 46% in the placebo group): only 23% of the patients in the naltrexone group (but 54% in the placebo group) relapsed.[65] 'Relapse', as in the O'Malley et al. study,[66] was defined as a substantial alcohol intake: self-reporting of five or more drinks during one or more drinking session, self-report of drinking five or more days within 1 week or coming to a treatment appointment with a blood alcohol concentration of more than 100 mg/dl. A similar effect was found by O'Malley et al., who also examined the efficacy of two different psychotherapeutic approaches for relapse prevention, coping skills therapy and supportive therapy in 97 alcohol-dependent individuals.[66] The major findings were that naltrexone treatment reduced the number of days in which alcohol was consumed and increased the time of relapse to heavy drinking. The highest overall rates of continuous abstinence were found in the group of patients who received naltrexone plus supportive therapy. Among those subjects who started to drink alcohol again, those on naltrexone plus coping skills therapy had the lowest rate of relapse. In the 6-month off-treatment phase, O'Malley et al. showed that the effect of naltrexone therapy on abstinence rates persisted only through the first month of follow-up, and that the effect of medication condition diminished over time.[66] Although naltrexone was usually well tolerated in the two studies mentioned, there is some concern about its side-effects. Obviously, nausea is a frequent problem in naltrexone treatment. The question whether naltrexone causes elevation of liver enzymes in alcoholics cannot be finally answered as yet but, if so, it seems to be a rare phenomenon. The side-effect profile of naltrexone has been examined in detail in an open-label treatment study of 500 alcoholics by Croop et al.[68] The most frequent side-effects were nausea (10%), headache (7%), dizziness, nervousness and fatigue (4% each), insomnia and vomiting (3%).

The results of a double-blind placebo-controlled 3-month trial followed by a 3-month open label phase with naltrexone conducted in the UK (79 patients on placebo, 85 on naltrexone) were less favourable.[69] This was basically due to an extremely high drop-out rate. Although there was no effect of naltrexone on abstinence rates, according to intention-to-treat analysis there was an advantage in the active drug on subjects who complied to treatment. McCaul reported the results of a study into alcoholics with and without comorbid opiate or cocaine dependence with three treatment groups (placebo vs. 50 mg vs. 100 mg naltrexone).[70] This study also failed to show any significant effect on alcohol intake. More long-term (6 or 12-month) studies are needed for naltrexone to explore its beneficial effects. A 3-month, placebo-controlled double-blind study with naltrexone 50 mg/day has recently been completed in Germany and another 6-month study is currently being undertaken in Sweden. In the USA studies have been funded by the National Institute of Alcoholism and Alcohol Abuse. It seems likely that naltrexone will find approval for the treatment of alcoholism in most European Community Countries in the near future.

Nalmefene   A possible alternative to naltrexone is the opiate antagonist, nalmefene, a drug with a similar pharmacological profile. A pilot study conducted by Mason et al. has suggested that it may reduce alcohol intake in alcoholics.[71] Nalmefene is not available in Europe.

Dopaminergic drugs

The mesolimbic-mesohippocampal dopaminergic system, and especially the nucleus accumbens, are believed to be major sites of action of most drugs with abuse potential, such as cocaine, psychostimulants and probably alcohol. These were found to increase dopamine release in the nucleus accumbens.[48] There also is a close functional relationship between the dopaminergic and the opiate/endorphin system. In animals, chronic alcohol consumption results in a dysfunction in dopaminergic neurotransmission, a decreased dopamine release and a probable supersensitivity of dopamine receptors, which might form the basis of alcohol dependence or craving.

Several dopaminergic drugs have been tested as possible anti-craving medications. Despite numerous preclinical studies that suggest that the dopaminergic system may be involved in mediating the reinforcing effects of alcohol, the clinical studies conducted so far have not provided a realistic therapeutic perspective. To date, the most promising results in animals have been reported with bromocriptine, a long-acting nonselective dopaminergic agonist. A small 6-month, double-blind placebo-controlled study of bromocriptine in 50 alcoholics showed reduced ethanol craving and drinking behaviour as well as a reduction of depressive symptoms and improved social function.[72] However, no quantifiable drinking data are given in the report. A more recent study by Dongier et al. has failed to show any significant effect of bromocriptine on alcohol consumption.[73] Lawford et al. conducted a 6-week trial in 83 detoxified patients which, they claimed, showed a selective effect of bromocriptine in patients with the A1 dopamine receptor D2 gene allele.[74] To date, bromocriptine cannot be recommended for the treatment of alcoholism.

A number of preclinical and clinical findings have also suggested a possible anti-craving effect for tiapride, a dopamine antagonist benzamide (for a review, see Peters and Faulds[75]). However, this drug failed to show any significant effect in a large, 6-month, placebo-controlled double-blind trial conducted in Germany in 1994 (unpublished data). Another dopaminergic drug is flupenthixol, a neuroleptic drug with a D1/D2-antagonistic profile that is currently under investigation in a double-blind placebo-controlled trial in Germany.[4] This drug has also been examined as an anti-craving drug in cocaine abusers. Flupenthixol is the only anti-craving drug so far to be administered intramuscularly (10 mg/every 2 weeks).

Drugs for the treatment of comorbid psychiatric disorder

Serotonergic drugs

A significant number of studies point at a dysfunction in the serotonergic neurotransmission, at least in a subtype of alcoholics. Alcoholics were found to have low cerebrospinal fluid (CSF) levels of 5-HT metabolites, and there is an inverse relationship between 5-HIAA levels in the CSF and time elapsed since last alcohol intake. An attractive hypothesis suggests that, since alcohol enhances 5-HT release, alcohol consumption could normalize low levels of 5-HT in the brain. A dysfunction in the serotonergic neurotransmission may predispose to alcohol consumption and relapse, and has thus to be considered as one of the major targets for treatment with anti-craving drugs (for a review, see Soyka[4]).

SSRIs

A number of animal studies have shown that SSRIs such as zimeldine, citalopram, viqualine, fluoxetine and others decrease alcohol consumption. A modest effect (9–17% reduction of alcohol consumption) has also been shown in some short-term, placebo-controlled double-blind studies in nondepressed heavy drinkers with zimeldine, citalopram, viqualine and fluoxetine.[76,77] Moncrieff and Drummond[78] pointed at the selection procedures in most of these studies: patients had been recruited from the general population through advertisements, and several hundred applicants had been excluded before the commencement of the trial. They also argued that noncompleters were excluded from the analysis and, hence, questioned the findings of these studies. Unfortunately, the major studies conducted with SSRIs in recent years have predominantly shown unfavourable results.[76] Tiihonen et al. showed more favourable results for citalopram.[79]

It has been shown that the SSRIs (such as fluoxetine) are able to reduce depressive symptomatology as well as postdischarge alcohol consumption in depressed alcoholics, as demonstrated by Cornelius et al.[80,81] At present, the SSRIs may have their place in alcoholic patients with comorbid affective disorder but cannot be recommended for relapse prevention in nondepressed alcoholics.

Serotonergic agonists
In open trials in alcoholics with symptoms of anxiety, buspirone was found to reduce both anxiety and the desire to drink.[82] In placebo-controlled trials, buspirone reduced alcohol craving, anxiety and depression, while the decrease in alcohol consumption in their study was equal to that in the placebo group.[83] Similar results were shown by Tollefson et al.,[84] who did not measure alcohol consumption in their study, while Malcolm et al.[85] failed to demonstrate any effect of buspirone on measures either of anxiety or alcohol intake. The most promising results have been demonstrated in a study by Kranzler et al., who studied 61 patients in a 12-week placebo-controlled trial and who found reduced anxiety and a slower return to heavy alcohol consumption in the buspirone group as well as fewer drinking days during the follow-up period.[86] A more recent study by Malec et al. failed to show a clear effect of buspirone on drinking behaviour in nonanxious alcoholics.[87] At present, buspirone seems to be an interesting drug in the prevention of relapse in alcoholics with comorbid anxiety disorder.

TCAs
Earlier studies failed to show any effect of TCAs on alcohol consumption.[88] For depressed alcoholics, TCAs such as desipramine were found to decrease depressive symptomatology but not alcohol intake.[89] A similar effect was reported for imipramine by McGrath et al. who, in a 12-week, randomized placebo-controlled trial, demonstrated that imipramine treatment was effective for the treatment of primary depression among actively drinking alcoholics while there was no overall effect on drinking outcome – although patients whose mood improved showed decreased alcohol consumption that was more marked in those treated with imipramine.[90] Nunes et al. conducted an open trial in 60 depressed alcoholics and found imipramine to have some impact on the relapse rate

in patients with dysthymia.[91] Of 60 depressed alcoholic patients who completed an open trial with imipramine, 27 (45%) responded with improvement in both mood and drinking behaviour, and 8 (13%) responded after further dosage increases or treatment with disulfiram. In a subsequent 6-month, randomized discontinuation trial, 4 of 23 subjects relapsed during imipramine treatment and 7 of 10 relapsed while taking placebo. Mason et al. also reported positive effects of desipramine on affective symptomatology in alcoholics.[92] Apart from the usual side-effects, TCAs were found to prolong the PR interval in the ECG of alcoholics[93] and to induce the hepatic microsomal system which might result in reduced plasma levels of various substances including TCAs[94], although the latter phenomenon is not specific for alcoholics. Taking the studies so far published and the potential risks of using TCAs for alcoholism into account, there is little reason why TCAs should not be used in nondepressed alcoholics for the prevention of relapse.

Table 9.7   Clinical guidelines for pharmacotherapy in the prevention of relapse in alcoholics.[4]

Drugs of first choice	Recommendations/comments
Acamprosate (1.3–2 g/day)	Few side-effects, mainly diarrhoea No psychotropic effects Clear increase in abstinence rates Approval for treatment of alcoholics in most EC countries, not the USA
Naltrexone (50 mg/day)	Decrease in alcohol consumption Should not be given to patients taking opiates Beware of hepatotoxicity Nausea quite frequent Approval for treatment of alcoholics in the USA, Canada and Austria
Drugs in patients with comorbid psychiatric disorder	
Buspirone	Probable effect in comorbid anxiety disorder
SSRIs	Patients with affective disorder may benefit Possible effect of fluvoxamine in alcoholic amnestic disorder
Valproate	Patients with bipolar disorder may benefit Beware of hepatotoxicity
Lithium	Patients with bipolar disorder may benefit Beware of intoxication
Flupenthixol	Patients with schizophrenia may benefit Typical side-effects of neuroleptics

Other possible alternatives

A number of other pharmacological agents have been examined as possible anti-craving drugs, but most have not yet been shown to be effective (for a review, see Soyka[4]). The possible use of mood stabilizers for relapse prevention in alcoholism has not been studied in much detail. Carbamazepine is possibly effective as an anti-craving drug.[95] Due to its liver toxicity, the use of valproate in alcoholic patients may be limited, but in patients with acute bipolar affective episodes valproate may be effective in decreasing the intake of abusive substances as shown in an open pilot study by Brady et al.[96]

Few anti-craving drugs have been registered: acamprosate in most EC countries and naltrexone in the USA, Canada and Austria (and in the near future possibly in more EC countries). Other possible anti-craving drugs (such as buspirone) have been approved for the treatment of other psychiatric disorders but may be used in alcoholism. A list of available anti-craving drugs is given in Table 9.7.

References

1. Koob GF, Le Moal M. Drug abuse: hedonic homeostatic dysregulation. *Science* (1997) **278:** 52–8.

2. Nestler EJ, Aghajanian GK. Molecular and cellular basis of addiction. *Science* (1997) **278:** 58–63.

3. O'Brien CP. A range of research-based pharmacotherapies for addiction. *Science* (1997) **278:** 66–70.

4. Soyka M. Relapse prevention in alcoholism – recent advances and future possibilities. *CNS Drugs* (1997) **4:** 313–27.

5. Fichter MM, Narrow NE, Roper MT et al. Prevalence of mental illness in Germany and the United States. Comparison of the Upper Bavarian study and the Epidemiological catchment area program. *J Nerv Ment Dis* (1996) **184:** 598–606.

6. Bronisch T, Wittchen HV. Lifetime and 6-month prevalence of abuse and dependence of alcohol in the Munich follow-up study. *Eur Arch Psychiatry Clin Neurosci* (1992) **241:** 273–82.

7. National Institute on Drug Abuse. *National Household Survey on Drug Abuse: Population Estimates, 1991.* DHHS Publication (ADM) 92-1887 (Washington, DC: US Government Printing Office, 1992).

8. Hser Y, Anglin MD, Powers K. A 24 year follow-up of California narcotic addicts. *Arch Gen Psychiatry* (1993) **50:** 577–84.

9. Simpson DD, Sells SB (eds) *Opioid Addiction and Treatment: A 12-Year Follow-up* (Malabar, FL: Keiger, 1990).

10. Hubbard RL, Marsden ME, Rachal JV et al. *Drug Abuse Treatment: A National Study of Effectiveness* (Chapel Hill, NC: University of North Carolina Press, 1989).

11. Maddux JF, Desmond DP. Methadone maintenance and recovery from opioid dependence. *Am J Drug Alcohol Abuse* (1992) **18:** 63–74.

12. Dole VP, Nyswander ME. A medical treatment for diacetylmorphine (heroine) addition. *JAMA* (1965) **193:** 646–50.

13. Ward J, Mattik RP, Hall W. *Key Issues in Methadone Maintenance Treatment* (Sydney: New South Wales University Press, 1992).

14. Des Jarlais DC, Friedman SR, Woods J, Milliken J. HIV infection among intravenous drug users: epidemiology and emerging public health perspectives. In Lowinson JH, Ruiz P (eds) *Substance Abuse: A Comprehensive Textbook* (Baltimore, MD: Williams & Wilkins, 1992): 734–43.

15. Soyka M, Banzer K, Buchberger R, Völkl M, Naber D. Methadon-Substitution Opioidabhängiger. *Nervenheilkunde* (1997) **16:** 347–52.

16. McGlothin WH, Anglin MD. Long-term follow-up of clients of high- and low-dose methadone programs. *Arch Gen Psychiatry* (1981) **38:** 1055–63.

17. Soyka M. *Drogen- und Medikamentenabhaengigkeit* (Stuttgart: Wissenschaftliche Verlagsgesellschaft, 1998).

18. Gross A, Soyka M. Pharmakotherapie bei Methadonsubstituierten Opiatabhängigen-Interaktionen mit anderen Pharmaka. *Psychopharmakotherapie* (1997) **4:** 101–4.

19. Center for Substance Abuse Treatment. *State Methadone Treatment Guidelines. Treatment Improvement Protocol Series* 1 (Rockville, MD: US Department of Health and Human Services, 1993).

20. Buehringer G, Gastpar M, Heinz U et al. *Methadon Standards* (Stuttgart: Enke, 1995).

21. Ball JC, Ross A. *The Effectiveness of Methadone Maintenance Treatment: Patients, Programs, Services and Outcomes* (New York: Springer-Verlag, 1993).

22. Advisory Council on the Misuse of Drugs. *AIDS and Drug Misuse Update* (London: HMSO, 1993).

23. Institute of Medicine. *Federal Regulation of Methadone Treatment* (Washington, DC: National Academy Press, 1995).

24. Arndt IO, Dorozynski L, McLellan AT et al. Desipramine treatment of cocaine dependence in the methadone-maintained patient. *Arch Gen Psychiatry* (1992) **49:** 888–93.

25. Blaine JD, Renault PF (eds). *Rx: 3x/week LAAM Alternative to Methadone. National Institute on Drug Abuse Research Monograph* 8. *DHEW Publication (ADM)* 76-347 (Washington, DC: US GPO, 1976).

26. Blaine JD, Renault PF. Clinical use of LAAM. *Ann Acad* (1978) **31:** 214–31.

27. Freedman RR, Czertko G. A comparison of three weekly LAAM and daily methadone in employed heroine addicts. *Drug Alcohol Depend* (1981) **8:** 215–22.

28. Marcovici M, O'Brien C, McLellan T, Kacian J. A clinical controlled study of 1-alpha-acetylmethadol in the treatment of narcotic addiction. *Am J Psychiatry* (1981) **138:** 234–6.

29. Savage C, Karp EG, Curran SF, Hanlon TE, McCabe OL. Methadone/LAAM maintenance: a comparison study. *Compr Psychiatry* (1976) **17:** 415–24.

30. Tennant SF, Rawson RA, Pumphrey E, Scecof R. Clinical experience with 959 opioid-dependent patients with levo-alpha-acetylmethadol (LAAM). *J Subs Abuse Treat* (1986) **3:** 195–202.

31. Trueblood B, Judson BA, Gold-

stein A. Acceptability of methadyl acetate (LAAM) as compared with methadone in a treatment program of heroin addicts. *Drug Alcohol Depend* (1978) **3:** 125–32.

32. Johnson RE, Cone EJ, Henningfield JE, Fudala PJ. Use of buprenorphine in the treatment of opiate addiction. I. Physiologic and behavioural effects during a rapid dose induction. *Clin Pharmacol Ther* (1989) **46:** 3–9.

33. Johnson RE, Jaffe JH, Fudala PJ. A controlled trial of buprenorphine treatment for opioid dependence. *JAMA* (1992) **267:** 20.

34. Strain EC, Stitzer ML, Liebsohn IA, Bigelow GA. Comparison of buprenorphine and methadone in the treatment of opioid dependence. *Am J Psychiatry* (1994) **151:** 1025–30.

35. Schottenfeld RS, Pakes JR, Oliveto A, Ziedonis D, Kosten TR. Buprenorphine vs methadone maintenance treatment for concurrent opioid dependence and cocaine abuse. *Arch Gen Psychiatry* (1997) **54:** 713–20.

36. Fischer G, Presslich O, Diamant K, Schneider C, Pezavas L, Kasper S. Oral morphine-sulphate in the treatment of opiate dependent patients. *Alcoholism* (1996) **32:** 35–43.

37. Bammer G. Should the controlled provision of heroin be a treatment option? Australian feasibility considerations. *Addiction* (1993) **88:** 467–75.

38. Gawin FH, Ellinwood EH. Cocaine and other stimulants. *New Engl J Med* (1988) **318:** 1173–82.

39. Nestler EJ. Molecular neurobiology of drug addiction. *Neuropsychopharmacology* (1994) **11:** 77–87.

40. Woody GE, Mercer DE, Auriacombe M. Cocaine use disorders: diagnosis and treatment. In Rommelspacher H, Schuckit MA (eds) *Baillière's Clinical Psychiatry. Vol. 2. Drugs of Abuse* (London and Philadelphia, PA: Baillière Tindall, 1996): 461–77.

41. Margolin A, Kosten T, Petrakis I et al. Bupropion reduces cocaine abuse in methadone-maintained patients. *Arch Gen Psychiatry* (1991) **48:** 87 (letter).

42. Kosten TR, McCane-Katz E. Substance abuse: new pharmacotherapies. In Oldham J, Riba M (eds) *Review of Psychiatry* (Washington, DC: American Psychiatric Press, 1995): 105–26.

43. Angrist B. Amphetamine psychosis: clinical variations of the syndrome. In Cho AK, Segal DS (eds) *Amphetamine and its Analogs* (San Diego, CA: Academic Press, 1994): 387–414.

44. Ellinwood EH, Lee TH. Psychopathology and treatment of amphetamine abuse. In Rommelspacher H, Schuckit MA (eds) *Baillière's Clinical Psychiatry. Vol. 2. Drugs of Abuse* (London and Philadelphia, PA: Baillière Tindall, 1996): 487–500.

45. Soyka M. *Die Alkoholkrankheit* (Weinheim and London: Chapman & Hall, 1995).

46. Hester RK, Miller WR. *Handbook of Alcoholism Treatment* (New York: Pergamon Press, 1989).

47. Fuller RK, Branchey L, Brightwell DR et al. Disulfiram treatment of alcholism: a Veterans Administration cooperative study. *JAMA* (1986) **256:** 1449–55.

48. DiChiara G, Imperato A. Drugs abused by humans preferentially increase synaptic dopamine concentrations in the mesolimbic system of freely moving rats. *Proc Nat Acad Sci USA* (1988) **85:** 5274–8.

49. Sellers EM, Higgins GA, Sobell MB. 5-HT and alcohol abuse. *Trends Pharmacol Sci* (1992) **13:** 69–75.

50. Lovinger DM, White G, Weight FF. Ethanol inhibits NMDA-activated ion current in hippocampal neurons. *Science* (1989) **243:** 1721.

51. Tsai G, Gastfriend DR, Coyle JT. The glutamatergic basis of human alcoholism. *Am J Psychiatry* (1995) **152:** 332–40.

52. Durbin P, Hulot T, Chabac S. Pharmacodynamics and pharmacokinetics of acamprosate: an overview. In Soyka M (ed) *Acamprosate in Relapse Prevention of Alcoholism* (Berlin, Heidelberg and New York: Springer, 1996): 47–64.

53. Zieglgänsberger W, Hauser C, Wetzel C et al. Actions of acamprosate on neurons of the central nervous system. In Soyka M (ed) *Acamprosate in Relapse Prevention of Alcoholism* (Berlin, Heidelberg and New York: Springer, 1996): 65–70.

54. Littleton J. Acamprosate – how does it work? *Addiction* (1995) **90:** 1179–88.

55. Grant KA, Woolverton WL. Reinforcing and discriminative stimulus effects of Ca-acetyl homotaurine in animals. *Pharmacol Biochem Behav* (1989) **32:** 607–11.

56. Soyka M. Clinical efficacy of acamprosate in the treatment of alcoholism. In Soyka M (ed) *Acamprosate in Relapse Prevention of Alcoholism* (Berlin, Heidelberg and New York: Springer, 1996): 155–71.

57. Sass H, Soyka M, Maa K, Zieglgänsberger W. Relapse prevention by acamprosate: results from a placebo controlled study in alcohol dependence. *Arch Gen Psychiatry* (1996): 673–80.

58. Whitworth AB, Fischer F, Lesch OM et al. Comparison of acamprosate and placebo in long-term treatment of alcohol dependence. *Lancet* (1996) **347:** 1438–42.

59. Paille FM, Guelfi JD, Perkins AC et al. Double-blind randomized multicentre trial of acamprosate in maintaining abstinence from alcohol. *Alcohol Alcohol* (1995) **30:** 239–47.

60. Besson J, Aeby F, Kasas A et al. Combined efficacy of acamprosate and disulfiram for enhancing abstinence of chronic alcoholic patients during a one year post detoxification period. *Neuropsychopharmacology* (1994) **10(Suppl 2):** 74S.

61. Pelc I, LeBon O, Verbanck P. Acamprosate in the treatment of alcohol dependence: a six month post-detoxification study. *Alcohol Clin Exp Res* (1994) 38A (abstract).

62. Hoffman PL, Urwyler S, Tabakoff B. Alterations in opiate receptor function after chronic ethanol exposure. *J Pharmacol Ther* (1982) **222:** 182–9.

63. Ulm RR, Volpicelli JR, Volpicelli LA. Opiates and alcohol self-administration in animals. *J Clin Psychiatry* (1996) **56(Suppl 7):** 5–14.

64. Volpicelli JR, Alterman AI, Hayashida M, O'Brien CP. Naltrexone in the treatment of alcohol dependence. *Arch Gen Psychiatry* (1992) **49:** 876–80.

65. Volpicelli JR, Watson NT, King AC et al. Effect of naltrexone on alcohol 'high' in alcoholics. *Am J Psychiatry* (1995) **152:** 613–15.

66. O'Malley SS, Jaffe AJ, Chang G et al. Naltrexone and coping skills therapy for alcohol dependence. A controlled study. *Arch Gen Psychiatry* (1992) **49:** 881–7.

67. O'Malley SS, Jaffe AJ, Chang G

et al. Six-month follow-up of naltrexone and psychotherapy for alcohol dependence. *Arch Gen Psychiatry* (1996) **53:** 217–74.

68. Croop RS, Labriola DF, Wroblewski JM, Nibbelink DW. A multicenter safety study of naltrexone as adjunctive pharmacotherapy for individuals with alcoholism. *Alcohol Clin Exp Res* (1995) **19:** 16A.

69. Croop RS, Chick J. American and European trials of naltrexone. Paper presented at the symposium, 'International Update: New Findings on Promising Medications'. Joint Scientific Meeting, 8th ISBRA congress and RSA meeting, Washington, DC, 1996.

70. McCaul ME. Efficacy of naltrexone for alcoholics with and without comorbid opiate or cocaine dependence. Paper presented at the symposium 'International Update: New Findings on Promising Medications', Joint Scientific Meeting 8th ISBRA congress and RSA meeting, Washington, DC, 1996.

71. Mason BJ, Ritvo EC, Morgan RO et al. A double-blind, placebo-controlled pilot study to evaluate the efficacy and safety of oral nalmefene HCL for alcohol dependence. *Alcohol Clin Exp Res* (1994) **18:** 1162–7.

72. Borg V. Bromocriptine in the prevention of alcohol abuse. *Acta Psychiatr Scand* (1983) **68:** 100–10.

73. Dongier M, Vachon L, Schwartz G. Bromocriptine in the treatment of alcohol dependence. *Alcohol Clin Exp Res* (1991) **15:** 970–7.

74. Lawford BR, Young RM, Rowell JA et al. Bromocriptine in the treatment of alcoholics with the D2 dopamine receptor allele. *Nat Med* (1995) **1:** 337–41.

75. Peters DH, Faulds D. Tiapride. A review of its pharmacology and therapeutic potential in the management of alcohol dependence syndrome. *Drugs* (1994) **47:** 1010–32.

76. Balldin J, Berggren U, Bokström K et al. Six-month open trial with Zimeldine in alcohol-dependent patients: reduction in days of alcohol intake. *Drug Alcohol Depend* (1994) **35:** 245–8.

77. Naranjo CA, Poulos CX, Bremner KE, Lanctôt KL. Citalopram decreases desirability, liking, and consumption of alcohol in alcohol-dependent drinkers. *Clin Pharmacol Ther* (1992) **51:** 729–39.

78. Moncrieff J, Drummond DC. New Drug Treatments for Alcohol Problems: A Critical Appraisal. *Addiction* (1997) **92:** 939–47.

79. Tiihonen J, Ryynänen O-P, Kauhanen J et al. Citalopram in the treatment of alcoholism: a double-blind placebo-controlled study. *Pharmacopsychiatry* (1996) **29:** 27–9.

80. Cornelius JR, Fisher BW, Salloum IM et al. Fluoxetine trial in depressed alcoholics. *Alcohol Clin Exp Res* (1992) **16:** 362.

81. Cornelius J, Salloum IM, Cornelius MD et al. Fluoxetine trial in suicidal depressed alcoholics. *Psychopharmacol Bull* (1993) **29:** 195–9.

82. Kranzler HR, Myers RE. An open trial of buspirone in alcoholics. *J Clin Psychopharmacol* (1989) **9:** 379–80.

83. Bruno F. Buspirone in the treatment of alcoholic patients. *Psychopathology* (1989) **22(Suppl 1):** 49–59.

84. Tollefson GD, Montague-Clouse J, Tollefson SL. Treatment of comorbid generalized anxiety in a recently detoxified alcohol population with a selective serotonergic drug (buspirone). *J Clin*

Psychopharmacol (1992) **12:** 19–26.

85. Malcolm R, Anton RF, Randall CL et al. A placebo-controlled trial of buspirone in anxious impatient alcoholics. Alcohol Clin Exp Res (1992) **16:** 1007–13.

86. Kranzler HR, Burleson JA, Del Boca FK et al. Buspirone treatment of anxious alcoholics. A placebo-controlled trial. Arch Gen Psychiatry (1994) **51:** 720–31.

87. Malec E, Malec T, Gagné MA, Dongier M. Buspirone in the treatment of alcohol dependence: a placebo-controlled trial. Alcohol Clinical Exp Res (1996) **20:** 307–12.

88. Ciraulo DA, Jaffe JH. Tricyclic antidepressants in the treatment of depression associated with alcoholism. J Clin Psychopharmacol (1981) **1:** 146–50.

89. Mason BJ, Kocsis JH. Desipramine treatment of alcoholism. Psychopharmacol Bull (1991) **27:** 155–61.

90. McGrath PJ, Nunes EV, Stewart JW et al. Imipramine treatment of alcoholics with primary depression. A placebo-controlled clinical trial. Arch Gen Psychiatry (1996) **53:** 232–40.

91. Nunes EV, McGrath PJ, Quitkin FM et al. Imipramine treatment of alcoholism with comorbid depression. Am J Psychiatry (1993) **150:** 963–5.

92. Mason BJ, Kocsis JH, Ritvo EC et al. A double-blind, placebo-controlled trial of desipramine for primary alcohol dependence stratified on the presence or absence of major depression. JAMA (1996) **275:** 761–7.

93. Ciraulo DA, Barnhill JG, Jaffe JH et al. Intravenous pharmacokinetics of 2-hydroxyimipramine in alcoholics and normal controls. J Stud Alcohol (1990) **1:** 366–72.

94. Ciraulo DA, Barnhill JG, Jaffe JH. Clinical pharmacokinetics of imipramine and desipramine in alcoholics and normal volunteers. Clin Pharmacol Ther (1988) **43:** 509–18.

95. Mueller TI, Rudden S, Stout R et al. Carbamazepine for alcohol dependence – a pilot study. Alcohol Clin Exp Res (1995) **19(Suppl):** 17A (abstract).

96. Brady KT, Sonne SC, Anton R, Ballenger JC. Valproate in the treatment of acute bipolar episodes complicated by substance abuse: a pilot study. J Clin Psychiatry (1995) **56:** 118–21.

97. Gawin FH, Kleber HD, Byck R et al. Desipramine facilitation of initial cocaine abstinence. Arch Gen Psychiatry (1989) **46:** 117–21.

98. Gawin FH, Allen D, Humblestone B. Outpatient treatment of 'crack' cocaine smoking with flupenthixol decanoate: a preliminary report. Arch Gen Psychiatry (1989) **46:** 322–5.

99. Fischman MW, Foltin RW, Nestadt G et al. Effects of desipramine maintenance on cocaine selfadministration by humans. J Pharmacol Exp Ther (1990) **253:** 760–70.

100. Batki SL, Manfredi LB, Jacob P et al. Fluoxetine for cocaine dependence in methadone maintenance: quantitative plasma and urine cocaine/benzoylecgonine concentrations. J Clin Psychopharmacol (1993) **13:** 242–50.

101. Tennant FS, Sagherian AA, Double-blind comparison of amantadine and bromocriptine for ambulatory withdrawal from cocaine dependence. Arch Int Med (1987) **147:** 109–12.

102. Halikas J, Kemp K, Kuhn K et al. Carbamazepine for cocaine

addiction? *Lancet* (1989) **1:** 623–4.

103. Gawin GH, Kleber HD. Methylphenidate treatment of cocaine abusers without attention deficit disorder: a negative report. *Am J Drug Alcohol Abuse* (1985) **11:** 193–7.

104. Ladewig D, Knecht T, Lehert P et al. Acamprosat – Ein Stabilisierungsfaktor in der Langzeitentwöhnung von Alkoholabhängigen. *Ther Umschau* (1993) **59:** 182–8.

10
Behavioural disturbances in old age

Franz Müller-Spahn and Cristoph Hock

Depression and dementia are the most common psychiatric disorders in the elderly. In the past 10 years, a large number of epidemiological studies in the community have been conducted to detect the prevalence of mental disorders in the elderly.[1–4]

Twenty-four per cent of the elderly above the age of 70 manifested clearly defined psychiatric disorders, whereas approximately half of the elderly were free of symptoms.[4] This indicates that overall psychiatric morbidity appears not to be increased in the elderly compared with the younger population. Of the elderly people in society, many demonstrate that a satisfactory and happy life is possible despite medical illness, disabilities or social and economic problems. This chapter reviews diagnostic and current treatment strategies of mental disorders in the elderly.

Depression in the elderly

Depression is not a normal feature of ageing, and it occurs in about 10–15% of the elderly above the age of 65. Among community-dwelling residents over the age of 65, approximately 15% manifest depressive symptoms, 1–2% meet criteria for a major depression and 2% for dysthymia.[5] Substantially higher rates are reported for subsyndromal depression in the same population.[6] Subsyndromal depression does not meet ICD-10 or DSM-IV criteria for major depression or dysthymia; however, it is associated with an increased risk of major depression.[7] In the Berlin Ageing Study of the elderly[4] (70 to >100 years of age), prevalence rates were 4.8% for major depression, 9.1% for all DSM-III-R specified disorders and 26.9% for subthreshold depression.[4] Although the Epidemiological Catchment Area Study (ECA)[2] showed an age-associated decline in the prevalence rates of major depression, there is evidence that masked depression, minor depression, depression secondary to medical conditions and organic depression have higher prevalence rates in the elderly than in younger subjects.[8] Table 10.1 summarizes the characteristic features of depression in the elderly.

Table 10.1   Characteristics of depression in the elderly.

- Decline in the prevalence rates of major depression with advancing age and increase in minor depression, in depression secondary to medical illness and in organic depression.
- Increase in subsyndromal depression.
- Marked fluctuations in symptoms.
- Depression may be masked by somatic complaints.
- Concomitant presence of dementia may impair the reporting and recognition of depressive symptoms.

Recognition of depression in the elderly seems to be more difficult than in younger patients. The classic clinical features of a depressive episode decrease and become masked with advancing age. It is estimated that depression is undiagnosed in up to 40% of the elderly population. This may be attributed to a number of factors. First, although the ICD-10 and DSM-IV criteria for major depressive episodes can be applied to depression in the elderly, the overall clinical picture may differ considerably from that in younger patients. Major depressive episodes in the elderly are primarily characterized by diffuse and changing somatic complaints, increased neurasthenic syndromes, psychomotor restlessness and agitation, anxiety syndromes, increased delusions and hypochondriac syndromes, as well as increased feelings of guilt and insufficiency. In the elderly, these syndromes are often triggered by psychosocial or physical problems. Secondly, doctors as well as patients and their relatives frequently assume that depressive symptoms in the elderly are normal psychological consequences of the ageing process itself. This may be due to the fact that patients are more willing to report somatic problems and frequently forget previous depressive symptoms, especially if these are mild. On the other hand, clinicians may be more concerned about medical illness and may therefore fail to recognize depressive symptoms.

Late-onset depression seems to be associated with a lower frequency of family history of depression and a higher frequency of cognitive impairment, deep white matter changes, cerebral atrophy, medical comorbidity and mortality. Depressive symptoms in the elderly may frequently be associated with a number of organic factors. Further conditions that contribute to depression in the elderly include cerebrovascular and cardiovascular diseases, sensory loss, osteoarthritis, neoplasms, dementia and infections. Approximately 50–60% of acute stroke patients, especially with left-sided lesions of the frontal region and the basal ganglia, manifest a clinically significant depression. The frequency of depression secondary to medical conditions ranges from 20 to 80% and seems to depend on the extent of impairment of social mobility. The question of whether duration of phases is prolonged and the tendency to chronicity is increased remains a matter of debate. The severity of concomitant medical disorders and the degree of social support are among the major factors influencing the course of illness. Thirdly, polypharmacy and the presence of dementia may also impair the recognition of depression.

A large number of social and demographic risk factors have been analysed in recent years. Severe life events, lack of supportive social network and physical illness (in particular multimorbidity) appear to increase greatly the risk of depression.

Suicides are more frequent in elderly than in younger depressed patients and appear to be more spontaneous and of greater violence. The highest rate of suicide for any age group occurs in the elderly.[9] Elderly men who have been recently widowed, who suffer from insomnia or chronic physical illness and feelings of worthlessness and hopelessness, and who have no (or weak) social support systems, are at highest risk.

The consequences of unrecognized depression in the elderly are dramatic. They include loss of quality of life, social isolation, increased mortality (suicide), enhanced vulnerability to certain physical illnesses, premature admission to nursing homes and large financial burden. The prognosis of depression in late life is generally similar to that in younger subjects, and therefore previously held notions of an unfavourable response to treatment in the elderly need to be revised.

A number of studies indicate that depression in the elderly is often insufficiently treated with antidepressants. In the Berlin Ageing Study,[4] undertreatment was observed in 44% of depressed patients. Only 6% of patients were treated with antidepressants, and 40% with benzodiazepines. Pharmacological treatment with traditional antidepressants in aged patients may bring about complex clinical situations. Altered pharmacokinetics and pharmacodynamics associated with ageing, accompanying physical disorders such as cardiovascular disease or prostate hypertrophy, as well as common polypharmacy in the elderly, have to be taken into account. The recommendation 'start low, go slow' should be strictly followed. Most of the classical antidepressants available today are of comparable clinical efficacy but may differ in terms of tolerability. Comparative analyses on atypical antidepressants (e.g. mianserin), reversible inhibitors of monoamine oxidase-A inhibitors, selective serotonin reuptake inhibitors (SSRIs) and tricyclics (TCAs) revealed no statistical difference between outcome measures.[10] TCAs are characterized by a high potential for anticholinergic side-effects, including memory impairment, delirium, behavioural toxicity and cardiovascular dysfunctions, in particular orthostatic hypotension. Elderly patients appear particularly susceptible to these side-effects, probably due to diminished capacities in central regulatory systems. The sedative and anticholinergic properties of TCAs may substantially impair psychomotor performance and cognition and the abilities of daily living. Nevertheless, the effectiveness of TCAs in the elderly seems to be similar to that in young patients. Secondary amines (such as nortriptyline) that have a smaller effect on orthostatic hypotension are generally better tolerated. In the quest for new antidepressants with fewer adverse effects, a large number of new compounds have been developed recently and introduced into the market. SSRIs and moclobemide – a reversible monoamine oxidase A inhibitor (MAOAI) – venlafaxine (a selective serotonin and noradrenaline reuptake inhibitor) and mirtazapine (a noradrenergic and specific serotonergic antidepressant) have been demonstrated to be as efficacious as traditional TCAs in the treatment of depression. Currently, five different SSRIs are available in Europe: citalopram, fluoxetine, fluvoxamine, paroxetine and sertraline. Their clinical efficacy and tolerability have been demonstrated in a large number of placebo-controlled, double-blind studies. The antidepressant, anxiolytic and antiaggressive effects, the lack of sedative and anticholinergic properties, and the wide therapeutic window suggest that these drugs may be useful in the treatment of depressed patients with concomitant medical illnesses. (Table 10.2 summarizes current treatment strategies with second or third-generation antidepressants.)

Table 10.2   Examples of antidepressants used in the treatment of the elderly.

Type	Compound	Starting dose (mg/day)	Average dose (mg/day)
TCAs	Nortriptyline	10	60–150
SSRIs	Citalopram	10	20–40
	Fluoxetine	10	20–40
	Fluvoxamine	50	100–200
	Paroxetine	10	20–40
	Sertraline	25	50–150
MAOI	Moclobemide	75	300–450
SNRI	Venlafaxine	37.5	75–150
NASSA	Mirtazapine	15	15–45

Notes:
TCAs = tricyclic antidepressants; SSRIs = selective serotonin reuptake inhibitors; MAOI = monoamine oxidase inhibitor; SNRI = selective serotonin and noradrenaline reuptake inhibitors;
NASSA = noradrenergic and specific serotonergic antidepressant.

Behavioural disturbances in dementia

Behavioural disturbances are common and important features of dementia (Table 10.3). However, in the past, research into Alzheimer's disease (AD) focused primarily on the detection and management of cognitive dysfunctions, whereas behavioural disturbances were neglected.[11] The relationship between cognitive and behavioural disturbances has not been clearly elucidated. Behavioural disturbances, such as aggressiveness, cause considerable problems for the demented patient's caregivers, and are one of the major factors precipitating institutionalization.[12]

There is some evidence that behavioural disturbances correlate with the different stages and the cognitive deterioration associated with AD. Behavioural symptoms seem to become more frequent during moderate stages. In severe stages, significant cognitive impairment becomes predominant and behavioural disturbances gradually less problematic.[12]

There are many methodological problems in the detection and assessment of behavioural dysfunction in patients with AD. For instance, the prevalence rates of depression range between 10 and 80%. This might be due to several factors. First, prevalence rates for depression are higher in studies of inpatients in psychiatric wards. Secondly, caregivers generally rated AD patients as more depressive than did the patients themselves.[13] Thirdly, varying definitions of depression have been applied. Fourthly, the assessment of depression in demented patients may be difficult because many symptoms (such as weight loss, apathy and insomnia) may be common features in dementia as well as in depression. Finally, because of cognitive impairment, it is often difficult to obtain information from patients with moderate and severe dementia.

The behavioural disturbances observed in dementia are not the result of uniform aetiology. They represent a broad category of disturbances that are often multifactorial, multiform and dynamic. In addition to the basic neurobiological changes in the degenerating brain, other factors such as primary personality, social environment and the behaviour of the

Table 10.3   The frequency of behavioural disturbances of dementia.

Depression	up to 60%
Anxiety	up to 80%
Delusions and hallucinations	up to 40%
Aggression	up to 60%
Agitation, wandering	up to 70%
Sleep disturbances	up to 70%
Sexual disinhibition	up to 10%

caregiver contribute greatly to the clinical picture of behavioural disturbances. Loss of neurons has been considered a major pathophysiological event in AD. Certain populations of neurons tend to be lost
selectively. These include large neurons of association cortices and certain nuclei, including the cholinergic cells of the basal nuclear complex
and the serotonergic cells of the dorsal raphe. In addition to the loss of
acetylcholine and serotonin, alterations in noradrenergic systems occur.
This is, for example, reflected by decreases in noradrenaline levels and
increases in levels of the metabolite 3-methoxy-4-hydroxyphenylglycol
(MHPG).[14] Thus, as the extent of alterations in cholinergic, serotonergic
and noradrenergic neurotransmission may vary during the disease
process, several combinations of neurotransmitter imbalances may
occur. While major depression in primary dementia was associated with
increased degeneration of the brainstem aminergic nuclei (especially the
locus coeruleus) and relative preservation of the cholinergic nucleus
basalis Meynert, psychosis in primary dementia was associated with
increased neurodegenerative changes in the cortex, but not with
increased degeneration of the aminergic nuclei.[15] Neurochemically, both
depression and psychosis in dementia have been associated with modest decreases in the levels of serotonin in the brain.[15] In conclusion, alterations in serotonergic neurotransmission may be associated with either
depression or psychosis depending on the functional integrity of other
neurotransmitter systems in the neuronal environment and association
networks.

In late stages of dementia, physical disability, apathy and communication failure have been associated with more severe tangle pathology in
the parahippocampal gyrus, frontal and parietal neocortex, as well as
with lower neuron counts in the hippocampus and basal nucleus of
Meynert.[16] Features of the Kluver–Bucy syndrome have been associated
with lower counts of large neurons in the parahippocampal gyrus and
parietal neocortex, but not with plaques or tangle formations or with neuronal loss in subcortical nuclei. Neurodegenerative processes in various
brain regions, including neurotransmitter imbalances, constitute the
physiological substrate, where personality and social and psychological
factors play a modifying role. Personality changes are most common in
AD and affect approximately 70% of patients.[17] These include a lack of
interest in the environment (disengagement) or inappropriate social
behaviour (disinhibition). Depending on the patient's primary personality,
different poles of personality traits may become more predominant. In
addition, environmental factors may exert a certain influence on the progression of AD. Unfamiliar surroundings, for instance, may worsen the
patient's difficulties. A low level of competence or excessive external
demands have been found to be predictive of maladaptive behaviour. On
the other hand, the environment may also have a therapeutic influence. A
supportive and positive atmosphere may affect the course of dementia,

at least as regards the patient's physical, social and psychological well-being.[18] Changes in personality are a major burden for relatives and caregivers, who often have difficulties in accepting the patient's loss of established roles and function in families or partnerships. The presence and competence of the social networkers, as well as the compliance and skills of the caregivers, largely decide whether a demented patient with severe behavioural disturbances can live in the community or needs to be institutionalized.

The symptoms of dementia can be conceptualized in several ways. The most common concepts broadly distinguish cognitive and noncognitive domains.[19] Other dichotic concepts have been proposed (e.g. cognitive vs. behavioural or cognitive vs. psychiatric disturbances). All these concepts have limitations, considering the complex interaction between cognitive and noncognitive symptoms. However, the assessment of behavioural disturbances in dementia is important. The symptoms are major sources of the caregiver's burden and of premature institutionalization. The disturbances are likely to be responsive to pharmacological or nonpharmacological treatments.[20] Two major means to assess noncognitive behavioural disturbances in dementia have been proposed: the BEHAVE-AD Scale[21] and the BRSD (Behaviour Rating Scale for Dementia) of the CERAD (Consortium to Establish a Registry for Alzheimer's Disease) programme.[22] Reisberg and colleagues[21] identified seven major categories of behavioural domain symptoms in AD (the BEHAVE-AD Scale):

1. Paranoid and delusional symptoms.
2. Hallucinatory disturbances.
3. Activity disturbances.
4. Aggressiveness.
5. Diurnal rhythm disturbances.
6. Affective disturbances.
7. Anxieties and phobias.

Behavioural domain symptoms are characteristic in AD, but none of these symptoms occurs in all patients. Most of the behavioural domain symptoms of AD frequently occur at later stages of the disease. The BRSD of the CERAD considers a wide variety of symptoms in eight areas: depressive features, psychotic features, defective self-regulation, irritability and agitation, vegetative features, apathy, aggression and affective lability.[22] Other scales include the ADAS non-cog[23] (Alzheimer's Disease Assessment Scale, noncognitive part), the NBRS[24] (Neurobehavioral Rating Scale), the NPI[25] (Neuropsychiatric Inventory) and the CMAI[26] (Cohen–Mansfield Agitation Inventory), as well as the PAS[27] (Pittsburgh Agitation Scale). The comprehensive assessment of the effects of pharmacological interventions on behaviour should include not only those instruments designed to measure behaviours in dementia *per se* but also instruments that measure cognitive changes and health-related quality of life.[12] For example, the use of high doses of antipsychotics may completely abolish an undesirable behaviour (as shown by an improvement on behavioural scales) but may cause sedation and may impair cognitive performance. Such negative consequences could be detected by measuring changes in the severity of dementia and changes in the ability to perform the basic functions of daily living. Therefore, a proper assessment should include behavioural, cognitive and quality-of-life domains.[12] In clinical practice, these scales may be useful for the documentation of changes that occur during pharmacological or behavioural therapies or to evaluate the effect of substances during clinical trials.

Depression

Differential diagnosis between a primary depression with cognitive disturbances and neurodegenerative dementia associated with depression (30–40% of cases) can be clinically difficult or sometimes impossible. This is particularly true in the early stages of dementia. Patients with AD exhibit depressive symptoms (such as lowered mood in 20–60% of cases), and 10–30% meet the criteria for a major depressive episode.[28] The presence of dementia symptoms may impair the reporting and recognition of depressive symptoms. Depression in dementia has psychological and neurobiological causes. It may result from the patient's recognition of the severity of his or her cognitive impairment or from neurotransmitter dysfunctions associated with the underlying disease process.[29] Major depression tends to manifest first in patients with mild to moderate cognitive decline, whereas in the advanced stages of dementia there might be insufficient brain tissue to maintain any depressive affect.[30]

When depressive symptoms combined with severe cognitive disturbances occur, a careful review of the psychiatric and medical history should be undertaken. Further, assessment of neuropsychological deficits, psychopathological state, concomitant neurological signs, and time of onset of illness and the time course of the disease will help in finding the appropriate diagnosis (Table 10.4). However, it is currently unclear whether depressed mood in the elderly is an early sign or a risk factor for dementia. Transmitter deficiencies are not restricted to cholinergic pathways but include a variety of other neurotransmitters, such as serotonin and noradrenaline. Serotonergic dysfunctions have been associated with a variety of psychopathological symptoms, including irritability, suicidality, insomnia, aggressive behaviour and anxiety. There is some evidence that the new generation of antidepressants, in particular the SSRIs and moclobemide, may exert beneficial effects on cognition and behavioural disturbances in addition to their well-known antidepressant properties.

Table 10.4 Differentiating depression from dementia.

Clinical features	Depression	Dementia
Psychopathology		
Orientation	Adequate	Impaired
Thinking, memory and reasoning	Temporarily diminished ability to think or concentrate Fluctuate with mood	Progressive memory decline (short term, later long term) Difficulties in learning new things Substantial deficits in thinking and reasoning
	More 'I don't know' answers	More 'near miss' answers Deficits are more pronounced at night
	Tend to emphasize disabilities	Tend to conceal disabilities
Language dysfunctions	Absent	Presence of anomic aphasia in early AD
Apraxia	Absent	Frequent
Agnosia	Absent	Frequent
Mood	Persistent, moderate to severe symptoms of depression Higher scores of feelings of helplessness, worthlessness or excessive or inappropriate guilt, loss of libido True suicidal ideation	Frequently single depressive symptoms Only 10–30% meet criteria for major depression
Sleep disturbance	Difficulties in falling asleep Shallow sleep More severe early morning awakening	Breakdown of the sleep–wake cycle Nocturnal wandering Daytime sleepiness, naps
Executive functions		
Judgement and insight	Specifically disturbed (fluctuate with mood)	Generally impaired
Verbal fluency	Not affected	Affected early
Planning, sequential organization	Not generally affected	Generally impaired
Treatment outcome with antidepressants	Improvement of depressive symptoms and cognitive dysfunctions	Improvement of depressive symptoms
History of psychiatric disorder		
Past history of affective disorders	Frequent (depressive episodes)	Rare
Family history of affective disorders	Frequent	Rare
Family history of dementia	Rare	Frequent
Onset of illness	Usually acute	Insidious
Duration and course of illness	Usually less than 6 months	More than 6 months' progressive deterioration

Anxiety

Anxiety occurs in 50–80% of patients with AD.[28] However, in contrast to depression and agitation, anxiety has been less well studied in patients with dementia. This may be due to the fact that anxiety may at least in part overlap with such symptoms as agitation and depression. Anxiety and depression often coexist in the elderly, and these conditions may be difficult to disentangle. Feelings of loss and hopelessness, and increased feelings of worthlessness combined with sleep, appetite and cognitive disturbances, may be associated with anxiety as well as with depression. Antidepressant medication, in particular the SSRIs, may improve both syndromes.[31] Benzodiazepines should be used with caution in demented patients with anxiety, because of the risk of worsening cognitive function, of daytime sleepiness, delirium and of gait disturbances. Benzodiazepines may lead to disinhibition. Elderly patients taking long-acting benzodiazepines are more likely to fall than those taking short-acting agents[32] without such active metabolites as lorazepam (e.g. 0.5–1 mg every 4–6 hours) and oxazepam. Compared with classical benzodiazepines, alprazolam has been suggested by some authors to be characterized by a considerable anxiolytic potential, with lower risk of dependency. However, these studies have been subjected to critical discussions and debates. Antidepressant drugs of several classes have been shown to exert positive effects on anxiety syndromes. SSRIs and reversible MAOIs (moclobemide) may be beneficial in the elderly because of their low anticholinergic potency. Buspirone, a generally well tolerated nonbenzodiazepine anxiolytic and 5-HT_{1A} agonist, may be added to the pharmacological repertoire for anxiety disorders in the elderly (e.g. 5 mg every 4–5 hours).

Delusions and hallucinations

Psychotic symptoms (delusions and hallucinations) are frequent and prominent manifestations of dementia. They most often manifest for the first time in patients with moderate to severe cognitive decline. It has to be emphasized, however, that the first symptom in A Alzheimer's original case report was characterized by a paranoid ideation.[33] Some 40–80% of AD patients show psychotic symptoms[34] – on average about 30%. The occurrence of psychotic symptoms in AD patients seems to be independent of psychiatric history, and delusions appear to be more frequent than hallucinations (10–70% vs. 3–33%).[35] Some studies propose a more rapid progression of disease when the dementia syndrome is associated with psychotic symptoms. Lopez et al.[36] reported a more rapid rate of decline, as measured by the Mini-Mental State Examination[37] (MMSE), and a specific deficiency in receptive language, as well as a greater frequency of aggression and hostility, in AD patients with delusions and hallucinations than in patients without such symptoms. Electro-encephalogram (EEG) analysis showed a significantly greater proportion of moderately abnormal EEGs, and spectral analysis confirmed the increased amount of delta and theta activity. These authors concluded that AD patients with delusions and hallucinations have a greater degree of cerebral dysfunction and more focal neuropsychological defects, which may indicate an additional localized (e.g. vascular) brain pathology. Cummings proposed that lesions in the right temporal cortex might cause abnormal perceptual input to the limbic system and, consequently, the development of hallucinations and delusions.[38] Schneider and Sobin performed a meta-analysis of controlled trials of neuroleptic treatments in dementia.[39] They showed that neuroleptic treatment moderately accelerated the improvement rate in agitated demented patients. The use of new antipsychotics with a significantly lower potential for extrapyramidal side-effects (e.g. clozapine, risperidone, sertindole, olanzapine, quetiapine, etc.) might be advantageous (Table 10.5). Preliminary experience suggests a possible indication of clozapine for dementia with Lewy bodies (DLB). However, so far, clinical experiences with these new substances in dementia are limited. Low starting doses are recommended (e.g. 0.5 mg/day of haloperidol, 10–25 mg/day of thioridazine, 0.5 mg/day of risperidone and 12.5 mg/day of clozapine).

Aggression

Aggressiveness is one of the most challenging behavioural disturbances in dementia. It upsets the patient's family members and the staff, and cannot be tolerated because of the risk of injury. It is probably the main reason why physicians are called in to assess and treat patients.[17] Burns et al.[28] assessed behavioural abnormalities and psychiatric symptoms in 187 diagnosed as having probable AD by the NINCDS-ADRDA criteria,[40] and found that 20% of patients showed signs of aggressiveness. Interestingly, several studies suggested a relationship between anxiety, impulsivity, mood and aggression.[41] At the neurochemical level, most of these signs may be linked to a serotonergic deficit in the brain. Because

Table 10.5   The dosing of representative neuroleptics for elderly patients.

Generic name	Brand name	Dosage (mg/day)
Haloperidol	Haldol	0.25–3
Thioridazine	Melleril	25–150
Clozapine	Leponex	12.5–75
Risperidone	Risperdal	0.5–2
Olanzapine	Zyprexa	5–10

aggressive patients do not always respond to medication, one-to-one nursing in a quiet room is sometimes indicated. Occasionally, mechanical restraints are inevitable.[17] In addition, low-potency neuroleptics with a low anticholinergic potential may be helpful (e.g. pipamperone 20–120 mg/day, melperone 10–150 mg/day).

Agitation and wandering

Nineteen of the 107 patients with AD studied by Burns et al. exhibited excessive walking behaviour.[28] These signs can be observed in the setting of a hospital ward or in a patient at home. This finding is in agreement with Teri et al.,[42] who reported a prevalence of wandering of 21%.[42] This disturbance appears to be associated significantly with the severity of dementia. Schneider and Sobin reviewed the benefit of neuroleptic treatment in agitated patients with dementia and showed that the therapeutic effects were only modest.[39] Alternatively, non-neuroleptic medications (including lithium, propanolol, pindolol, trazodone, carbamazepine, buspirone, L-deprenyl and citalopram) have been investigated, most of them in anecdotal case vignettes or case series.[39] Most of these patients had been nonresponders or intolerant to neuroleptics. Schneider and Sobin conclude that there is little, if any, evidence to suggest that non-neuroleptic medication is more effective than neuroleptics in treating agitated behaviour in dementia patients.[39] Wandering and agitation in dementia appeared to increase with the duration of the illness.

Numerous nonpharmacological treatment approaches have been described, including behavioural management, environmental modifications, interventions using sound and light, and social interaction groups.[12]

Sleep disturbances

Sleep disturbances tend to occur in both AD and depressive disorder. However, in AD, the sleep disturbances are characterized by fragmented sleep or an interruption of the day–night sleep cycling.[17] Sleep disturbances in AD patients appear to become progressively worse as the disease progresses, although the severity of this problem varies considerably among individual patients. Disrupted sleep may not always be related to the dementia itself. Often, the problem is secondary to other medical or environmental conditions.[43] Thus, many patients with sleep disturbances receive pharmacological treatment (particularly benzodiazepines and sedative hypnotics) that may be inappropriate or excessive. If benzodiazepines are used, the application of substances with a short half-life is recommended (e.g. oxazepam). In some cases, paradoxical effects have been reported. Alternatively, low-potency neuroleptics with low anticholinergic effects (e.g. pipamperone 10–60 mg) or atypical neuroleptics (melperone 10–100 mg) may be helpful. New nonbenzodiazepine hypnotics, such as zolpidem (10 mg) – an imidazopyridine derivative – and zopiclone (3.75–7.5 mg) – a cyclopyrrolone derivative – may be included in the psychopharmalogical repertoire. Both show a favourable side-effect profile when compared with the classical benzodiazepines, and may have a lower potential for dependency.

Sexual disinhibition

Of the 178 patients investigated by Burns et al., 7% showed signs of sexual disinhibition.[28] There is a tendency for sexual disinhibition in severe dementia. Sexual behaviour is generally not well tolerated in clinical settings and is often annoying to the staff.[17] Although major tranquillizers are frequently used, there seems to be no specific treatment for sexual behavioural disturbances. Nonpharmacological treatments are often recommended, including pleasant environments, music therapy and adequate social activities (such as doing the laundry and setting the table). These treatments – along with good medical and nursing practices – should provide a convenient atmosphere and appear to be reasonable, although they have never been evaluated in controlled studies.

Anxiety disorder

The frequency of anxiety seems to increase with advancing age.[44] Between 10 and 20% of the elderly residing in the community show symptoms of anxiety for which medical attention is sought.[45] Phobic disorders are among the most common psychiatric diagnoses in the elderly.[29] Overall, the prevalence of anxiety disorders is greater in women than in men and remains high throughout life, peaking at about the age of 55 and diminishing slightly thereafter. Factors associated with ageing (such as social isolation, decreased autonomy, financial insecurity, poor health and impending debts) may be expected to increase the prevalence of anxiety in later life. Nevertheless, it is possible that elderly people with anxiety do not present themselves to the health services or are not recognized by them, which could lead to hidden morbidity.[46] Flint reviewed the epidemiology and comorbidity of anxiety disorders in the elderly (>65 years).[47] Total anxiety rates in studies that examined the elderly alone varied considerably, from 0.7% in the New York study by Copeland et al.[48] to 18.6% in the study of Bergmann.[49] Copeland et al.[48,50] and the 'national survey of psychotherapeutic drug use'[51] studied generalized anxiety disorder in addition to phobias and found that, even when a hierarchical approach to the diagnosis of anxiety disorders was used, phobias were less common than generalized anxiety disorder.[47] In fact, Copeland and co-workers reported that only 0.7% of their subjects in Liverpool reach the criteria for phobia.[48] The case rate in London and

New York, on the other hand, was 0.0%.[50] According to the Epidemiologic Catchment Area data, panic disorder was the least common among the anxiety disorders.[2] In the elderly, there was a 0.2% prevalence in females and 0.0% prevalence in males. Frequent comorbid conditions in late life were depression, dementia, alcohol abuse and dependence, and medical illnesses. Anxiety, like depression, is sometimes difficult to diagnose because it ranges along a continuum from a normal state to distress, to a disabling, to a fully developed disorder.[31] Sudden onset of anxiety in the elderly should alert the clinician to possible organic aetiologies. The core symptoms of anxiety (autonomic hyperactivity, moderate restlessness and sleep disturbances) may be prodromal symptoms of delirium or dementia. As with depression, a thorough mental status and physical examination is required to search for relevant cognitive deficits associated with these as well as other neurobehavioural disorders.[31] Anxiety and depression may also coexist in the elderly, and it may be difficult to distinguish between them.

Benzodiazepines are the most frequently prescribed anxiolytics.[52] Because of pharmacokinetic and pharmacodynamic changes in the elderly, benzodiazepines with shorter half-lives that are eliminated by conjugation (e.g. oxazepam, lorazepam), as opposed to hepatic oxidation (diazepam), are preferred in this population. As a result of the risk of side-effects (such as cognitive deficits, cerebellar dysfunction and abuse or dependency), benzodiazepine prescription should be restricted to a short time period. Alternatives include nonbenzodiazepine anxiolytics such as the 5-HT_{1A} agonist buspirone. In addition, low-potency neuroleptics (such as prothipendyl) or atypical neuroleptics (such as melperone) have been used with some positive effects. Among the antidepressants, reversible MAOIs as well as the SSRIs are essentially equivalent in their effectiveness for reducing anxiety, whether or not there is accompanying major depressive disorder.[29] The excellent clinical efficacy of cognitive behavioural therapy in young patients has been confirmed in many studies. However, there are only a very few reports on cognitive behavioural treatment for geriatric patients with anxiety disorders.[53] This treatment strategy should be part of the overall management concepts for elderly patients.

Late-life psychosis and paranoid syndromes in the elderly

Late-life psychosis includes psychoses secondary to general medical conditions (e.g. metabolic and encephalopathies), dementia with psychosis, mood disorders with psychotic features, schizophrenia, delusional disorders and other disorders with psychotic symptoms.[54] In general, late-life schizophrenia can be considered as a prototypical chronic psychosis. Late-life schizophrenia is defined by manifestation after the age of 45 years. Some studies suggest that approximately 10% of all patients with schizophrenia may have onset of symptoms after the age of 45.[55] Late-life schizophrenia is more common in women than in men and shows fewer negative symptoms (such as social withdrawal or emotional blunting) than schizophrenia that comes on in earlier life. Pearlson et al. demonstrated some psychopathological differences between early and late-onset schizophrenia.[56] Those patients with a later age of onset were more likely to have persecutory delusions and visual, olfactory and auditory hallucinations, and were less likely to have thought disorder and affective flattening.

The effective doses of antipsychotic drugs for late-life schizophrenia are as low as one-third of those required for patients of younger ages. Some authors separate late-life paraphrenia from late-life schizophrenia, although the former concept has not been supported by the DSM-IV. Approximately 10% of all patients admitted to psychiatric hospitals have late paraphrenia.[57] The disorder is characterized by a well-organized system of delusions, with or without auditory hallucinations, and with preservation of intellectual abilities, affect and personality. Paranoid and schizoid traits are frequently reported, but personality disorders occur in only 50% of patients. Prognosis is poor. The majority of patients show little or no response to neuroleptic treatment. A number of special considerations are necessary when managing elderly patients.[53] Approximately 80% of the elderly have at least one chronic serious physical illness and may be receiving multiple drug therapies (polypharmacy). In addition, elderly patients frequently have sensory defects, such as visual or auditory impairments. Further, age-associated cognitive impairments may result in poor or noncompliance. Finally, pharmacokinetic and pharmacodynamic changes in the elderly may render them at greater risk of serious adverse affects, such as tardive dyskinesia (TD). Jeste et al. reported a 1-year incidence of TD of 26.1% and a 3-year incidence of 59.8% among neuropsychiatric patients over the age of 45 years.[58] On the other hand, the frequency of relapses is clearly increased in patients who do not receive maintenance therapy. Therefore, the flexible use of conventional antipsychotic drugs at their lowest effective dosages is generally recommended in patients with late-life schizophrenia. As the use of haloperidol is associated with an increased risk for TD, the use of atypical neuroleptics (such as clozapine or risperidone) or the use of new antipsychotics (such as olanzapine, sertindole or quetiapine) may be considered. When using clozapine, its high anticholinergic potential and the necessity for blood monitoring have to be taken into account. In general, a flexible dose regimen, and the use of substances with a low anticholinergic potential and without cardiovascular side-effects, may be of benefit for late-life schizophrenic patients.

References

1. Meller I, Fichter M, Schröppel H, Beck-Eichinger N. Mental and somatic health and need for care in octo- and nonagenarians. *Eur Arch Psychiatry Clin Neurosci* (1993) **242:** 286–92.

2. Regier DA, Boyd JH, Burke JD Jr et al. One-month prevalence of mental disorders in the United States: based on five Epidemiologic Catchment Area sites. *Arch Gen Psychiatry* (1988) **45:** 977–86.

3. Baltes P, Meyer K, Helmchen H, Steinhagen-Thiessen E. The Berlin Aging Study (BASE): overview and design. *Ageing and Society* (1993) **13:** 483–515.

4. Linden M, Kurtz G, Baltes M et al. Depression bei Hochbetagten. Ergebnisse der Berliner Altersstudie. *Nervenarzt* (1998) **69:** 27–37.

5. Johnson J, Weissman M, Klerman G. Service utilization and social morbidity associated with depressive symptoms in the community. *JAMA* (1992) **267:** 1478–83.

6. Judd L, Rapaport M, Paulus M et al. Subsyndromal symptomatic depression: a new mood disorder. *J Clin Psychiatry* (1994) **55(Suppl 4):** 18–28.

7. Salzman C. Depressive disorders and other emotional issues in the elderly: current issues. *Int Clin Psychopharmacol* (1997) **12(Suppl):** 37–42.

8. Müller-Spahn F, Hock C. Clinical presentation of depression in the elderly. *Gerontology* (1994) **40(Suppl):** 10–14.

9. Valente S. Recognizing depression in elderly patients. *Am J Nurs* (1994) **94:** 19–24.

10. Mittmann N, Herrmann N, Einarson T et al. The efficacy, safety and tolerability of antidepressants in late life depression: a meta-analysis. *J Affect Disorders* (1997) **46:** 191–217.

11. Zaudig M. Assessing behavioural symptoms of dementia of the Alzheimer type: categorical and quantitative approaches. *Int Psychogeriatrics* (1996) **8(Suppl 2):** 183–200.

12. Herrmann N, Lanctôt KL, Naranjo CA. Behavioural disorders in demented elderly patients. Current issues in pharmacotherapy. *CNS Drugs* (1996) **6:** 280–300.

13. Weiner M, Svetlik D, Risser R. What depressive symptoms are reported in Alzheimer's patients. *Int J Geriat Psychiatry* (1997) **12:** 648–52.

14. Raskind MA, Peskind ER. Neurobiologic bases of noncognitive behavioral problems in Alzheimer disease. *Alz Dis Assoc Disorders* (1994) **8(Suppl 3):** 54–60.

15. Zubenko GS. Etiology, clinicopathologic and neurochemical correlates of major depression and psychosis in primary dementia. *Int Psychogeriatrics* (1996) **8(Suppl 3):** 219–23.

16. Förstl H, Burns A, Levy R et al. Neuropathological correlates of behavioural disturbance in confirmed Alzheimer's disease. *Br J Psychiatry* (1993) **163:** 364–8.

17. Eastwood R, Reisberg B. Mood and behaviour. In Gauthier S (ed) *Clinical Diagnosis and Management of Alzheimer's Disease* (London: Martin Dunitz, 1996): 175–90.

18. Sandman O. Influence of the patient's environment on the progression of Alzheimer's disease. *Neurobiol Aging* (1995) **16:** 871–2.

19. Rabins PV. Behavioral disturbances of dementia: practical and conceptual issues. *Int Psychogeriatrics* (1996) **8(Suppl 3):** 281–3.

20. Reisberg B, Auer R, Monteiro I et al. Behavioral disturbances of dementia: an overview of phenomenology and methodologic concerns. *Int Psychogeriatrics* (1996) **8(Suppl 2):** 169–82.

21. Reisberg B, Borenstein J, Salob SP et al. Behavioral symptoms in Alzheimer's disease: phenomenology and treatment. *J Clin Psychiatry* (1987) **48(Suppl 5):** 9–15.

22. Tariot PN, Mack JL, Patterson MB et al. The Behaviour Rating Scale for Dementia of the Consortium to Establish a Registry for Alzheimer's Disease. *Am J Psychiatry* (1995) **152:** 1349–57.

23. Rosen WG, Mohs RC, Davis KL. A new rating scale for Alzheimer's disease. *Am J Psychiatry* (1984) **141:** 1356–64.

24. Lewin HS, High WM, Goethe KE et al. The Neurobehavioral Rating Scale: assessment of the behavioral sequelae of head injury by the clinician. *J Neurol Neurosurg Psychiatry* (1987) **50:** 183–93.

25. Cummings JL, Mega M, Gray K et al. The Neuropsychiatric Inventory: comprehensive assessment of psychopathology in dementia. *Neurology* (1994) **44:** 2308–14.

26. Cohen-Mansfield J, Billig N. Agitated behaviours in the elderly. I. A conceptual review. *J Am Geriatr Soc* (1986) **34:** 711–21.

27. Rosen J, Burgio L, Kollar M et al. The Pittsburgh Agitation Scale – a user-friendly instrument for rating agitation in dementia patients. *Am J Geriatr Psychiatry* (1994) **2:** 52–9.

28. Burns A, Jacoby R, Levy R. Psychiatric phenomena in Alzheimer's disease. 2. Disorders of perception. *Br J Psychiatry* (1990) **157:** 76–81.

29 Devanand D, Sano M, Tang M et al. Depressed mood and the incidence of Alzheimer's disease in the elderly living in the community.

Arch Gen Psychiatry (1996) **53:** 175–82.

30. Zubenko G, Moossy J, Kopp U. Neurochemical correlates of major depression in primary dementia. *Arch Neurol* (1990) **47:** 209–14.

31. Fernandez F, Levy JK, Lachar BL et al. The management of depression and anxiety in the elderly. *J Clin Psychiatry* (1995) **56(Suppl 2):** 20–9.

32. American Psychiatric Association. Practice guideline for the treatment of patients with Alzheimer's disease and other dementias of late life. *Am J Psychiatry* (1997) **154(Suppl):** 1–39.

33. Alzheimer A. About a peculiar case of cerebral cortex (1907). *Alz Dis Assoc Disorders* (1987) **1:** 7–9.

34. Drevets WC, Ubin EH. Psychotic symptoms and the longitudinal course of senile dementia of Alzheimer's type. *Biol Psychiatry* (1988) **25:** 39–48.

35. Leuchter AF, Spar JE. The late onset psychoses. *J Nerv Ment Dis* (1985) **173:** 488–94.

36. Lopez OL, Becker JT, Brenner RP et al. Alzheimer's disease with delusions and hallucinations: neuropsychological and electroencephalographic correlates. *Neurology* (1991) **41:** 906–12.

37. Folstein M, Folstein S, McHugh P. Mini-Mental State: a practical method for grading the cognitive state of patients for the clinician. *J Psychiat Res* (1975) **12:** 189–98.

38. Cummings JL. Organic delusions. *Br J Psychiatry* (1985) **146:** 184–97.

39. Schneider LS, Sobin PB. Non-neuroleptic medications in the management of agitation in Alzheimer's disease and other dementia: a selective review. *Int J Geriat Psychiatry* (1991) **6:** 691–708.

40. McKhann G, Drachman D, Folstein M et al. Clinical diagnosis of Alzheimer's disease: report of the NINCDS-ADRDA work group under the auspices of Department of Health and Human Services Task Force on Alzheimer's disease. *Neurology* (1984) **34:** 939–44.

41. Apter A, van Praag HM, Plutchik R et al. Interrelationships among anxiety, aggression, impulsivity, and mood: a serotonergically linked cluster? *Psychiatry Res* (1990) **32:** 191–9.

42. Teri L, Larson EB, Reifler BV. Behavioral disturbance in dementia of the Alzheimer's type. *J Am Geriatr Soc* (1988) **36:** 1–6.

43. Reifler BV. Depression, anxiety, and sleep disturbances. *Int Psychogeriatrics* (1996) **8(Suppl 3):** 415–18.

44. Markovitz P. Treatment of anxiety in the elderly. *J Clin Psychiatry* (1993) **54(Suppl 5):** 64–8.

45. Myers JK, Wissmann MM, Tischsler GI et al. Six month prevalence of psychiatric disorders in three communities 1980–1982. *Arch Gen Psychiatry* (1984) **41:** 959–67.

46. Lindesay J. Phobic disorders in the elderly. *Br J Psychiatry* (1991) **159:** 531–41.

47. Flint AJ. Epidemiology and comorbidity of anxiety disorders in the elderly. *Am J Psychiatry* (1994) **151:** 640–9.

48. Copeland JRM, Gurland BJ, Dewey ME et al. Range of mental illness among the elderly in the community: prevalence in Liverpool using the GMS-AGECAT package. *Br J Psychiatry* (1987) **150:** 815–23.

49. Bergmann K. The neuroses of old age. In Kay DWK, Walk A (eds) *Recent Developments in Psychogeriatrics: A Symposium. British Journal of Psychiatry Special Publication no. 6* (Ashford: Headley Brothers, 1971).

50. Copeland JRM, Gurland BJ, Dewey ME et al. Is there more dementia, depression and neurosis in New York? A comparative study of the elderly in New York and London using the computer diagnosis AGECAT. *Br J Psychiatry* (1987) **151:** 466–73.

51. Uhlenhuth EH, Balter MB, Mellinger GD et al. Symptom checklist syndromes in the general population: correlations with psychotherapeutic drug use. *Arch Gen Psychiatry* (1983) **40:** 1167–73.

52. Lawlor BA, Sunderland T. Use of benzodiazepines in the elderly. In Roy-Byrne PP, Cowley DS (eds) *Benzodiazepines in Clinical Practice: Risks and Benefits* (Washington, DC: American Psychiatric Press, 1991): 215–27.

53. Swales P, Soljin J, Sheikh J. Cognitive-behavioral therapy in older panic disorder patients. *Am J Geriatr Psychiatry* (1996) **4:** 46–60.

54. Jeste D, Calgiuri M, Paulsen J et al. Risk of tardive dyskinesia in older patients: a prospective longitudinal study of 266 patients. *Arch Gen Psychiatry* (1995) **52:** 756–65.

55. Harris MJ, Jeste DV. Late-onset schizophrenia: an overview. *Schizophr Bull* (1988) **14:** 39–55.

56. Pearlson GD, Kreger L, Rabins PV et al. A chart review study of late-onset and early-onset schizophrenia. *Am J Psychiatry* (1989) **146:** 1568–73.

57. Gannon MA, Wrigley M. Late paraphrenia. *Br J Hosp Med* (1995) **53:** 128–30.

58. Jeste DV, Eastham JH, Lacro JP et al. Management of late-life psychosis. *J Clin Psychiatry* (1996) **57(Suppl 3):** 39–45.

11
The violent patient in the community

Siegfried Kasper

Introduction

Violent patients generate many emotions among practitioners since they represent a rare situation where the practitioner fears for his or her safety or for the safety of the family or colleagues in the hospital. It is not often acknowledged that there may be a psychiatric disease behind this syndrome, and so practitioners often attempt not to treat violent patients. However, avoidance is not ideal: the clinician can meet such patients in any treatment setting – private offices and medical units as well as psychiatric treatment facilities. The assessment and management of violent patients have been thoroughly reviewed (e.g. by Tardiff[1]). The aims of this chapter are to give the clinician brief guidance about the aetiology of human violence, to suggest how the violent patient can be managed in the community and to point to further research that could be undertaken into violence among psychiatric patients and on how this could be dealt with.

Aetiology of human violence

Several factors contribute to violent behaviour, and these can be grouped into biological causes (or diseases) and psychological and socioeconomic influences as well as the physical environment itself (see Table 11.1). Violence can be the result of one of these factors alone but can also be a complex interaction of them all, as it is often the case. It may well be that biological or predisposing factors (such as neurophysiological dysfunction or certain psychiatric disorders) can tip the balance when a patient is in specific psychological surroundings that hold an additional, physical specification (for example, heat). These factors can contribute to impulsivity, irritability or irrational behaviour.

Among the neurophysiological factors, temporal lobe epilepsy (which is now termed partial complex seizure) plays an important role. Although violence is rare among epileptic patients during seizure, it can cause

Table 11.1   Factors that contribute to violent behaviour.

1) *Biological factors (diseases)*
   - Partial complex seizures
   - Alcohol and drug abuse
   - Psychosis and certain other forms of psychopathology
   - Subtle neurophysiological dysfunction secondary to head trauma, etc.
   - Chromosomal abnormalities
   - Decreased serotonin and impulsivity
   - Increased norepinephrine and dopamine
2) *Psychological factors*
   - Physical abuse as a child
   - Witnessing of domestic violence
   - Portrayal of violence in mass media
3) *Socioeconomic factors*
   - Subcultures
   - Racial inequality
   - Economic inequality
   - Absolute poverty
   - Marital and familial disruption
4) *Physical environment*
   - Crowding
   - Heat

substantial problems. In reported cases of patients with partial complex seizures, it has been found that aggressive behaviour is usually stereotyped, unsustained and not purposeful in nature.[2] Not only the disease itself but also other factors have been found to be associated with violence *per se* in patients with partial complex seizures (e.g. low socioeconomic status as well as problems in the individual's earlier development).

Evidence from neurotransmitter studies suggests that, in aggressive behaviour, there are increased levels of norepinephrine and dopamine[3] as well as lower activity in the serotonergic system as measured by cerebrospinal fluid levels of 5-hydroxyindoleacetic acid (5-HIAA).[4] The low serotonergic activity in this group of patients has been confirmed by investigations using the serotonergic probe fenfluramine – a presynaptic releaser of serotonin.[5] Studies conducted in this field revealed a blunted response of prolactin to fenfluramine in patients with personality disorders that included impulsive and aggressive behaviour. Since lower serotonergic activity is also found in self-destructive behaviour, it could well be that this represents a trait rather than a state-marker of violence.

Studies evaluating computed tomography (CT) and magnet resonance imaging (MRI) have revealed temporal-frontal abnormalities in violent patients. Further, other organic deficits that are the result of either a birth deficit or brain injury[6] have been associated with aggression.

Several attempts have been undertaken to characterize the specific genetic defects that are linked to violent behaviour. A number of surveys have indicated that men with the genetic abnormality XYY are disproportionately represented in prisons. However, a study conducted in Copenhagen[7] found no indication that sex chromosome abnormalities (XYY or XXY) have a specific role in violent behaviour. There seems, therefore, to be no indication that a specific chromosomal abnormality is associated with violent behaviour. However, inheritance studies support a genetic relationship for economic/property crimes but not for violence.

The role of psychiatric disorders in violent behaviour has long been the subject of research. In an early report, Boeker and Häfner[8] concluded that psychiatric patients do not have a higher incidence of criminality. However, Rabkin[9] concluded that there is an increase in violent crimes among psychiatric patients over time, which could be associated with the policy of discharging a number of patients with chronic psychiatric disorders into the community and not caring for them appropriately thereafter. This point has much relevance given the fact that, in some countries, there is a policy of reducing the number of hospital beds for such patients without replacing them with adequate outpatient treatment facilities. From the specific psychopathological point of view, it is of note that patients with psychotic disorders who are disturbed by their delusions are more likely to be seriously violent. Diagnosis and the course of the illness are therefore important factors in predicting the incidence of violence in hospitals.[10] The most important role of violent behaviour in the spectrum of psychiatric disorders is probably in the diagnosis of personality disorder.[11] Furthermore, alcohol and drug abuse (e.g. amphetamines, cocaine and hallucinogens) has been found to be associated with violent behaviour.[12]

Among the socioeconomic factors there seems to be a cycle that includes poverty and the need for the basic necessities of life, as well as disruptions to marriages, unemployment and difficulty in maintaining interpersonal ties (family structures and social control). Besides illness and psychological and socioeconomical determinants, there are also physical/environmental factors that play a substantial role in violence. Several studies have found a correlation between the ambient temperature of the environment and violent crime and riots.[13] There is a relation between heat and aggression in that aggression increases in higher ambient temperatures. In line with this finding are reports that rape and riots mainly occur in summertime. However, extremely hot temperatures seem to decrease aggression, leading to flight rather than fight.

Clinical situations

The frequency and patterns of violent behaviour vary from treatment centre to treatment centre and within different subspecialities (such as inpatient or outpatient unit and emergency room). The clinician's most important concern in this situation is, therefore, safety. If the clinician does not feel safe, this will interfere with his or her evaluation and may result in injury or even death. Physicians are, therefore, specifically not encouraged to play the role of the hero.

The American Psychiatric Association's Task Force on Clinician Safety[14] studied the frequency and the patterns of attacks on psychiatrists, psychiatric residents, nurses and psychologists, as well as social workers. It emerged that nurses are the most frequent victims of violence by psychiatric patients (80%). Some 40% of psychiatrists reported that they have experienced one or more attacks by patients during their professional lifetimes. Psychiatric residents are exposed to the same rate of violence by patients, but within the short time of their training. It also emerged that younger, inexperienced clinicians were at increased risk of being attacked by patients.

The first decision which the clinician must make concerns the best setting in which to interview the patient. There is a wide range of options. If the patient is not known to the clinician and exhibits violent behaviour, it is preferable to interview the patient with the staff present. The next step is to keep the office door open but to position the staff outside; a further step would be to close the office door. However, the clinician should ensure that he or she sits between the patient and the door in case an emergency escape is necessary.

Evaluation of violent patients

Table 11.2 summarizes interventions that can be used in emergency situations. Throughout this process, the clinician should present a calm appearance, demonstrating in his or her demeanour that he or she is in control of the situation, including the counter-transferent style that he or she has 'a safe feeling'. He or she should start by commenting, in a very neutral, concrete manner, on the most obvious aspect of the situation – for example, 'you look very angry' or 'something makes you very nervous'. However, emotional or pejorative comments (such as 'it is very stupid to act like this', etc.) should be avoided. Further, direct eye contact with the patient should be avoided and, most importantly, there should be plenty of space between the patient and the clinician.

If the patient permits it, a physical examination should be undertaken, including blood samples, electrocardiogram or X-rays. However, this is probably after emergency medication has been given.

Table 11.2   Guidelines for intervention in an emergency situation.

- Present a calm appearance – establish a 'safe feeling'
- Put space between yourself and the patient
- Do not adopt an authoritarian style, rather, indicate you are in control of the situation
- Show respect for the patient
- Avoid intense direct eye contact
- Speak softly in a nonprovocative and nonjudgemental manner
- Facilitate the patient's talking
- Listen to the patient
- Avoid early interpretations
- Do not make promises you cannot keep

When the emergency is under control, the clinician can take more time to evaluate the patient more carefully. This evaluation should include a detailed assessment of the violent behaviour (such as its date of onset, its frequency and target), any recurrent patterns and any situations where the aggressive behaviour tends to escalate (see Table 11.3). An assessment of illness should include both previous psychiatric illnesses (organic disorder, psychosis) and previous and present intake of psychoactive substances. The history of other impulsive behaviour (including suicidal behaviour) needs to be documented. The diagnostic procedures used in routine assessment, as well as additional tests based on clinical suspicion, are summarized in Table 11.4.

Table 11.3   Vital information for the assessment of violent behaviour.

Assessment of violent behaviour
- Date of onset of violent behaviour
- Frequency and target(s) of violent behaviour
- Are there recurring patterns and escalation?
- Severity of injuries to others
- Symptoms associated with violent episodes

Assessment of illnesses
- History of previous psychiatric illness
- History of neurological diseases, e.g. head injury, birth complications, serious childhood diseases and other developmental problems
- Past and current medical illnesses
- History of other impulsive behaviour, e.g. suicidal behaviour, destruction of property, reckless driving, sexual acting out, fire starting and criminal offences

Table 11.4   Diagnostic procedures for violent patients.

Routine assessment
- Complete blood count
- Blood chemistry (electrolytes, blood urea nitrogen, glucose, creatinine, calcium, phosphate and liver function tests)
- Thyroid (T_3, T_4, thyroid-stimulating hormone)
- Screening for syphilis
- Vitamins (B_{12}, folate, thiamine)
- Urinalysis
- Electrocardiogram
- Chest X-ray
- Drug and alcohol screen of blood and urine
- Electroencephalogram
- Rating scales for assessment of aggression and violence (e.g. the Overt Aggression Scale, see Figure 11.1)

Optional
- HIV antibodies
- Glucose tolerance test (hypoglycaemia)
- Ceruloplasmin, copper levels in urine and serum (Wilson's disease)
- Urine porphobilinogen (porphyria)
- Heavy metal screening (poisoning)
- Antinuclear antibodies (systemic lupus erythematosus)
- Lumbar puncture if intracranial pressure not elevated (infection, multiple sclerosis, haemorrhage)
- Magnetic resonance imaging and/or computed tomography (head trauma, tumour, etc.)
- Psychological tests (intelligence tests)

Yudofsky et al. have constructed a checklist to document violent/aggressive behaviour that can be used to rate verbal and physical aggression as well as its degree of seriousness, any injury and its duration and timing, and types of intervention[15] (Figure 11.1).

Restraint and seclusion

Restraint and seclusion are a rare but necessary response in specific emergency situations that necessitate effective and safe techniques. Depending on the country, specific legal steps must be undertaken to

Name of patient _____   Name of rater_____

Sex of patient _____   Date _____

Aggressive behavior (check all that apply)

Verbal aggression
☐ Makes loud noises, shouts angrily
☐ Yells mild personal insults (e.g., 'You're stupid')
☐ Curses viciously, uses foul language in anger, makes moderate threats to others or self
☐ Makes clear threats of violence toward others or self (e.g., 'I'm going to kill you') or requests help to control self

Physical aggression against objects
☐ Slams door, scatters clothing, makes a mess
☐ Throws objects down, kicks furniture without breaking it, marks the wall
☐ Breaks objects, smashes windows
☐ Sets fires, throws objects dangerously

Physical aggression against self
☐ Picks or scratches skin, hits self, pulls hair (with no or minor head injury only)
☐ Bangs heads, hits fist into objects, throws self onto floor or into objects (hurts self without serious injury)
☐ Small cuts or bruises, minor burns
☐ Mutilates self, makes deep cuts, bites that bleed, internal injury, fracture, loss of consciousness, loss of teeth

Physical aggression against other people
☐ Makes threatening gestures, swings at people, grabs at clothes
☐ Strikes, kicks, pushes, pulls hair (without injury to them)
☐ Attacks others, causing mild or moderate physical injury (bruises, sprain, welts)
☐ Attacks others, causing severe physical injury (broken bones, deep lacerations, internal injury)

Time incident began: _____   Duration: _____

Intervention: _____

Figure 11.1
The Overt Aggression Scale.[15]

protect the patient's rights and also the medical staff in any actions which they undertake. The indications for restraint and seclusion are primarily to prevent imminent harm to the patient or other persons when other means of control are ineffective or inappropriate. They are also designed to prevent significant damage being done to the physical environment, which, in turn, could again harm the patient or others. Restraint or seclusion can additionally be applied when seriously requested by the patient.

Restraint or seclusion should not be applied if the patient's medical status is unstable or unknown and/or further medical issues pertain – such as suspicious delirium, drug overdose or an inability to provide constant monitoring. Needless to say, restraint or seclusion should not be used as punishment or simply for the comfort or convenience of the staff or other patients.

An unstable medical status (such as infection or cardiac or metabolic illness) should be handled with close monitoring rather than restraint. However, restraint may be valuable in specific situations such as delirium or dementia. Since neuroleptics like phenothiacines can cause hyperthermia and since hyperthermic problems are also associated with restraint, it is advisable to monitor for hyperthermia very carefully.

When using restraint, constant observation by a staff member on a one-to-one basis should be seriously considered. The justification for this constant observation needs to be documented in the patient's record, and staff observations should be recorded on a regular basis (e.g. every 15–30 minutes). This will ascertain that there is no circulatory obstruction or other medical problem that could lead to a serious complication. Another possible adverse effect of restraint is aspiration, which can also be guarded by constant monitoring.

The need for restraint should be evaluated and documented at least every day, and the patient's mental or physical status should be assessed by the physician frequently. A concurrent medical problem will need more frequent visits.

If restraint is necessary, it is advisable to institute a standardized procedure in which someone from the medical staff can take the lead. After the decision to restrain the patient has been taken, no further discussions should be conducted with the patient. As soon as the patient is restrained, medication may be given if necessary.

The release from restraint is very often a very gradual process but can also be terminated instantly if the patient's symptoms are under control (see Table 11.5).

Emergency medication

When handling an emergency situation, there is no need for a thorough-going knowledge of the whole variety of psychopharmacology. However,

Table 11.5   When restraint or seclusion should *not* be applied.

- Only for the comfort or convenience of the staff or other patients
- As a punishment
- Unstable or unknown medical status
- Inability to provide constant monitoring for aspiration
- Self-mutilation (for seclusion)
- Drug overdose (for seclusion)
- Delirium (for seclusion)

knowing about a few medications and their dosages is essential in helping to control a situation rapidly. Before medication is used, a diagnosis (or at least a working diagnosis) needs to be established since organic brain dysfunction, for instance, needs either lower dosages or specific medication (as antiepileptics in an epileptic state, for example).

For patients with a manifest psychotic symptomatology, neuroleptic medication is the first line of treatment. Haloperidol can be given either orally, intramuscularly or intravenously. Very often, high-potency neuroleptics are combined with low-potency ones (such as levomepromazine, which is given in a dosage of up to 200 mg). Since low-potency neuroleptics have an alpha-1-adrenolytic receptor profile, the side-effect of postural hypotension needs to be observed. This may cause problems in elderly patients as it can worsen their cerebrovascular status. A successful strategy for psychotic disorders is to combine high-potency neuroleptics with benzodiazepines (such as lorazepam given in a dosage of up to 10 mg daily). Neuroleptics are also the treatment of choice for manic patients, and the same dosage as used in the treatment of acute schizophrenia is very often needed. Patients with organic brain syndromes very often require substantially lower dosages than patients with schizophrenic psychosis or mania.

To avoid fighting with the patient every day, a depot formulation should be considered as the basis for neuroleptic treatment (such as haloperidol decanoate, fluphenazine or the 3-day depot formulation zuclopenthixol). Extrapyramidal side-effects and orthostatic hypotension are the main complications that occur with this treatment regimen, and these need to be carefully observed (see Table 11.6).

Long-term treatment of patients with aggressive and violent behaviour

Since violence and aggression differ among patients and also between different diseases, there is no unique treatment strategy for them. Using

Table 11.6   Emergency medication for aggressive or violent behaviour.

1) **Neuroleptics**
   (a) *High potency*
   - Low-dose haloperidol 5 mg im every 4–8 hours (maximum daily dose 15–30 mg)
   - High-dose haloperidol 10 mg im every 4–8 hours (maximum daily dose 45–100 mg)

   (b) *Low potency*
   Levomepromazine (50–200 mg); watch out for postural hypotension

2) **Benzodiazepines** (with or without neuroleptics)
   - Lorazepam 2–4 mg by mouth (i.e. sublingual release formulation), with dose repeated 4–6 hours later if agitation and aggression continue (maximum daily dose 10 mg)
   - Lorazepam 2–4 mg (1–2 mL) iv slowly at the rate of 2 mg (1 mL) per minute repeated at 10-minute intervals if needed (maximum daily dose 10 mg)

Notes:
Doses should be adjusted based on the patient's age, weight, debilitation and other clinical considerations.
im = intramuscularly; iv = intravenously.

the established diagnosis, several psychopharmacological treatment approaches can be recommended.

If a diagnosis of schizophrenia is established, a depot formulation of either haloperidol or fluphenazine should be given in the dosage used for the treatment of schizophrenia. Clozapine has also been found to be effective for treatment of violent behaviour in schizophrenia and schizoaffective psychosis.[16] Side-effects such as extrapyramidal symptoms (akinesia, dystonia and further parkinsonian symptoms) need to be monitored carefully because they may constitute one of the reasons patients discontinue medication, therefore exposing themselves to the risk of another aggressive episode.

In addition to neuroleptics, carbamazepine has been recommended for the treatment of violent behaviour and might therefore be used either as an adjunctive or as the sole pharmacological treatment.[17] However, controlled trials are still awaited. Lithium has also been recommended for the management of aggression within different psychiatric diseases.[18] The plasma concentrations that need to be established are in the upper range for the treatment of bipolar disorder (from 0.7 to 1.0 mEq l). Benzodiazepines (such as clonazepam) might be helpful for the long-term man-

Table 11.7   Long-term treatment for patients exhibiting violent behaviour.

1) *Haloperidol*[a]
   (a) Haloperidol 0.5–2 mg by mouth for moderate symptoms and 3–5 mg by mouth for severe symptoms every 8–12 hours until psychosis is controlled. Dose rarely needs to exceed 15 mg/day. Maintenance dose rarely exceeds 8 mg/day. In chronic schizophrenia, higher doses may be needed until psychosis is controlled; maintenance dose rarely exceeds 20 mg/day
   (b) Haloperidol decanoate 25–100 mg im every 3–5 weeks. Initial dose is 10–15 times the oral dose but should not exceed 100 mg (2 mL)

2) *Fluphenazine*[a]
   Fluphenazine decanoate or enanthate 12.5–100 mg im every 1–3 weeks. Initial dose is 12.5 mg and dose is then increased by 12 mg every 2–3 weeks until maintenance level is achieved, but dose should not exceed 100 mg every 2–3 weeks

3) *Benzodiazepines*[a]
   Clonazepam 1–10 mg/day

4) *Lithium, carbamazepine*
   In dosages (e.g. carbamazepine: 300–800 mg/day) and in plasma levels (for lithium, upper range: 0.7–1.0 mmol l)

Notes:
Doses should be adjusted based on the patient's age, weight, physical status and other clinical considerations.
[a] Other medications of the same class may be used in doses relative to the ones recommended here.
im = intramuscularly.

agement of violent behaviour. Clonazepam with a dosage between 1 and 10 mg daily may be implemented for treatment of aggression and violence, mainly in schizoaffective disorder.

Since aggressive and impulsive behaviour is believed to be associated with low levels of serotonergic activity, several lines of research have indicated that enhancement of the serotonergic tone (with, for example, selective serotonin reuptake inhibitors) is helpful. Fluoxetine, for instance, has been shown to be beneficial in borderline personality disorders in a higher dosage range than that used for depression (60 mg)[19] (Table 11.7).

In parallel with pharmacotherapy, psychosocial management (including behavioural therapy) needs to be implemented to ensure that the patient can cope successfully not only with the treatment but also with everyday life.[20]

References

1. Tardiff K. *Assessment and Management of Violent Patients* (2nd edn) (Washington, DC, and London: American Psychiatric Press, 1996).

2. Leicester J. Temper tantrums, epilepsy and episodic dyscontrol. *Br J Psychiatry* (1982) **141:** 262–6.

3. Eichelman B, Elliott GR, Barchas J. Biomedical, pharmacological and genetic aspects of aggression. In Hamburg DA, Trudeau MB (eds) *Behavioral Aspects of Aggression* (New York: A R Liss, 1981): 278–91.

4. Brown GL, Ebert MH, Goyer PF et al. Aggression, suicide, and serotonin: relationship to CSF amine metabolites. *Am J Psychiatry* (1982) **136:** 741–6.

5. Coccaro EF, Harvey PD, Kupsaw-Lawrence E et al. Development of neuropharmacologically based behavioral assessments of impulsive aggressive behavior. *J Neuropsychiatry Clin Neurosci* (1991) **3:** 544–51.

6. Tonkonogy JM. Violence and temporal lobe lesion: head CT and MRI data. *J Neuropsychiatry Clin Neurosci* (1991) **3:** 189–96.

7. Schiavi RC, Theilgaard A, Owen DR et al. Sex chromosome abnormalities, hormones and aggressivity. *Arch Gen Psychiatry* (1984) **41:** 93–9.

8. Boeker W, Häfner H. *Eine psychiatrisch-epidemiologische Untersuchung in der Bundesrepublik Deutschland* (Berlin, Heidelberg and New York: Springer, 1973).

9. Rabkin JG. Criminal behavior of discharged mental patients: a critical review of the research. *Psychol Bull* (1979) **86:** 1–27.

10. Krakowski M, Volavka J, Brizer D. Psychopathology and violence: a review of the literature. *Compr Psychiatry* (1986) **27:** 131–48.

11. Tardiff K, Koenigsberg HW. Assaultive behavior among psychiatric outpatients. *Am J Psychiatry* (1985) **27:** 960–3.

12. Nurco DN, Ball JC, Shaffer JW et al. The criminality of narcotic addicts. *J Nerv Ment Dis* (1985) **173:** 94–102.

13. Bell PA, Baron RA. Ambient temperature and human violence. In Brain PF, Benton D (eds) *Multidisciplinary Approaches in Aggression Research* (Amsterdam: Elsevier/North Holland, 1981): 263–80.

14. American Psychiatric Association, Task Force on Clinician Safety. *Clinician Safety (Task Force Report no. 33)* (Washington, DC: American Psychiatric Association, 1993).

15. Yudofsky SC, Silver JM, Jackson W et al. The Overt Aggression Scale for the objective rating of verbal and physical aggression. *Am J Psychiatry* (1986) **143:** 35–9.

16. Ratey JJ, Leveroni C, Kilmer D et al. The effects of clozapine on severely aggressive psychiatric inpatients in a state hospital. *J Clin Psychiatry* (1993) **54:** 219–23.

17. Evans RW, Gualtieri CT. Carbamazepine: a neuropsychological and psychiatric profile. *Clin Neuropharmacol* (1985) **8:** 221–41.

18. Sheard MH. Lithium in the treatment of aggression. *J Nerv Ment Dis* (1975) **160:** 108–18.

19. Coccaro EF, Astill JL, Herbert JL et al. Fluoxetine treatment of impulsive aggression in DSM-III-R personality disorder patients. *J*

Clin Psychopharmacol (1990) **10:** 373–5 (letter).

20. Lion TR, Tardiff K. The long-term treatment of the violent patient. In Hales RE, Frances AJ (eds) *Psy-chiatry Update, American Psychiatric Association Annual Review* (Washington, DC: American Psychiatric Press, 1987) **6:** 537–48.

12
The hyperactive child

Peter Hill

Introduction

Hyperactivity in children is not uncommon but is elusively difficult to assess and treat comprehensively. Comorbid developmental, educational and social problems are extremely common. The differential diagnosis of a primary hyperactivity disorder needs to be considered, rather than identifying the condition by 'colour matching' to a list of diagnostic features. Only then can a comprehensive management strategy be considered. This will need to address more than hyperactivity symptoms if the long-term prognosis is to be improved.

Assessment

Hyperactivity is more than overactivity and indicates restlessness coupled with inconsistent attention and excitable, impulsive, disinhibited behaviour. Hyperactive children have a strong distaste for delay and are impatient. Their inattentiveness is most marked when challenged by a requirement to think. Hyperactivity is therefore a pattern of behaviour. If it is primary and unexplained by another clinical disorder, then it may be understood as a disorder in its own right. Quite possibly such a disorder has its roots in an inherited deficiency of mental executive function but this is controversial and the clinical, behavioural manifestations remain the primary issue. For a hyperactivity disorder to be present, this pattern of inattentive, restless, excitable, impulsive, impatient behaviour must be primary, excessive and pervasive (manifest in different kinds of situation) and must impair the child's ordinary functioning or development. Currently, the nosological emphasis is placed on inattentiveness and restlessness as the most salient features.

Establishing the diagnosis is only part of the assessment process but is, of course, critical. The two major diagnostic schemes have categories for a primary hyperactivity disorder but they are not quite the same. In ICD-10, the criteria are best spelt out in the research edition.[1] The items listed are almost exactly the same as in DSM-IV[2] but the combination rules are different. In DSM-IV attention deficit hyperactivity disorder (ADHD), the diagnosis may be made if either hyperactive-impulsive *or* inattentive elements are present. In ICD-10 hyperkinetic disorder, items from *both* the hyperactivity *and* the inattentiveness scales (*as well as* the impulsiveness scale in the research but not the clinical edition) are present. In both schemes, pervasiveness and impaired functioning are required.

In other words, ADHD is a broader diagnostic concept than hyperkinetic disorder. It is effectively a syndrome whereas hyperkinetic disorder is more like a unitary disorder. Not surprisingly it is more prevalent – 4% of the school-age population have ADHD rather than about 0.5–1% for hyperkinetic disorder.[3] It is possible to have hyperactivity as a feature of a disorder such as autism. But ADHD and hyperkinetic disorder are disorders of exclusion, indicating a primary condition, and the diagnostic rules preclude their association with comorbid autism or psychotic disorder.

The first phase of assessment obviously revolves around whether a pattern of hyperactive behaviour exists and whether it fulfils diagnostic criteria. Mere presence of behaviours listed in classificatory schemes is not enough; they must be beyond the normal range for mental age. Additionally, the combination of behaviours has to be pervasive and impairing.

If this can be established, the differential diagnosis of a child who shows the pattern of hyperactivity includes several primary disorders, which can have prominent hyperactivity as a feature. In other words there is a true differential diagnosis to be made from general learning disability, pervasive developmental disorders, hyperthyroidism, mania, agitated depression and general anxiety. Usually this is straightforward since features of the primary condition will be evident at the time of assessment. A primary condition often missed is developmental language impairment with verbal comprehension difficulty. This is sometimes associated with marked inattentiveness to other people's verbal communications and also with understandable academic difficulties which give rise to bored restlessness in a classroom. The same is true for hearing impairment; turning the head to present the preferred ear in monaural deafness can mimic inattentiveness.

A few disorders can produce a picture superficially similar to primary hyperactivity but the clue as to their existence is located in the personal history of the child. The quality of inattentive restlessness is, in fact, different from that found in a primary hyperactivity disorder, but the mindless application of diagnostic elements from a list without a proper developmental history can mislead the inexperienced. Particular instances include disinhibited attachment disorder, and closed head injury. Usually a history and clinical examination will provide enough information upon which to base the distinction.

The task of assessment also includes identifying conditions which are comorbid with a primary hyperactivity disorder, not producing or mimicking inattentive restlessness in the case in question but associated with it. These include some of the disorders mentioned above which can have hyperactivity as a secondary feature (general learning disability, communication disorders, affective and anxiety disorders) but can also coexist with a primary hyperactivity disorder. The distinction between differential and comorbidity is a matter of judgement: can the hyperactivity symptoms be wholly explained by another primary condition?

Antisocial behaviours and attitudes are commonly associated with hyperactivity disorders and may be sufficiently pronounced to fulfil criteria for oppositional-defiant or conduct disorder. The nature of the link is much discussed and essentially unresolved, though there is evidence that hyperactivity is disruptive to family and social conditions that would ordinarily promote prosocial development.[4] In addition, specific developmental disorders (academic skills difficulties such as dyslexia, motor planning disorders, language disorders) and Tourette's syndrome are markedly increased over population baseline levels in children with a primary hyperactivity disorder.[5] There are also other clinical issues that require assessment although they may not be conditions in their own right: low self-esteem, illicit substance abuse, relationships with others (peers, teachers and parents), educational underachievement and the resourcefulness of the parents and the child's school.

As part of an initial assessment, a baseline measure of behaviour should be obtained by, for instance, Conners' questionnaires for parents and teachers.[6] It is also wise to take a problem list of issues from both parents and child as well as inquiring about a family history of childhood hyperactivity in other family members. If there are apparent speech difficulties then a language assessment by a speech and language therapist is needed. Similarly, any academic problems indicate that a psychological assessment should be carried out by a clinical psychologist. Each of these assessments takes several hours to arrange, carry out, score, report and feedback, so it is not likely that many services will carry them out routinely.

If the child is seen simultaneously with the parents there are opportunities for observation, not just of the child's restlessness, inattention to questions or instructions, or interruptions, but of parental behaviour and attitudes too. Many hyperactive children are more abnormal in a group situation than in a one-to-one interview. Indeed, it is not uncommon for them to be initially compliant and reasonably self-contained in an interview with a sympathetic mental health professional. The most productive observations will be made when the child is challenged cognitively during psychometric testing or, if time allows, in the classroom during a school visit.

Particularly with older children, an individual interview enables assessment of mental state and an appreciation of the child's point of view.

Only at a private interview will full details of antisocial behaviour and of parental and teachers' behaviour towards the child emerge. The opportunity should also be taken to conduct a brief neurological examination, though it is not likely that anything positive will emerge beyond a few soft signs or minor physical anomalies, the presence or absence of which will not alter management.

Treatment

Information and advice

The conventional treatment approach is multimodal. Although many children with severe combined ADHD or hyperkinetic disorder will need medication, the general view of the point of medication is that it allows a so-called window of opportunity. In other words, medication produces a period of near-normality to supervene during which positive influences on development (good parenting, good sibling and peer relationships, good teaching) can be perceived attentively by the child and not be disrupted by his or her disruptive behaviour or inattentiveness. The core components of an adequate treatment are thus several – psychoeducational, supportive measures, more specific behavioural interventions (provided by parents and teachers) and medication. Some children will also benefit from dietary manipulation and a few from cognitive therapy. Comorbid conditions and problems will need addressing in their own right.

The first steps in treatment are psychoeducational. It is still the case that many people believe that hyperactivity disorders are caused by inadequate parenting[7] even though the evidence is that they are initially caused by genetic and biological mechanisms with psychosocial factors maintaining or escalating initial manifestations.[8] A handout or recommended book, followed by a discussion of particular points which child or parents wish to raise, are invaluable. In similar vein, contact with a self-help group or nearby families who also have a hyperactive child provides access to experience, literature and a range of suggestions most of which are helpful even though prejudices and biases inevitably operate, particularly on the Internet.

The child's school will almost always welcome similar information and professional advice. In some areas, an educational psychologist will prove to be the best placed professional. It has to be said though that, only too often, educational psychology is a scarce resource as far as classroom interventions are concerned and the organization of a particular school may be inimical to optimal management. Hyperactive children require structure, frequent interventions and, quite commonly, supplementary or corrective education to compensate for underachievement or comorbid learning difficulties.

In other words, most hyperactive children will have special educational needs that should be recognized and documented. Clinicians may be asked to contribute to this and may find that the most significant contribution they can make is to emphasize the child's deficiencies. Not many teachers recognize that hyperactive children cannot wait for praise or an incentive; they require immediate and frequent reinforcement and instruction. This will put a substantial strain on a class teacher and is an argument for a classroom aide. It also means that the child should be positioned near the teacher who may thus find his or her movement round the class constrained. It is also often necessary to point out that the child's difficulties extend to peer relationships as well as academic difficulties and classroom behaviour so that social education needs to extend to the playground.

Behavioural and cognitive management

Management of behaviour at home and school can be hard. Affected children live their lives to a soundtrack of criticism from adults and other children. Their self-esteem suffers and parents find themselves driven into a habit of nagging. Basic parenting skills of clear instructions, planning, use of pointed praise, limit setting, justifiable rules and the use of parental authority through example and praise rather than intimidation and excessive physical punishment need discussion with both parents. Special efforts to build self-confidence, to extend settled behaviour and the completion of tasks, and to encourage negotiation rather than confrontation will be required in many instances. Aggressive, oppositional behaviours are common in association with hyperactivity disorders.[9] They arise or are maintained by several mechanisms – irritable mood caused by the critical or hostile comments of others, copying the management styles of harassed parents, impulsive responses, a failure to have learnt negotiation tactics, fragile self-esteem causing a reluctance to give way to others, impatience and so forth.

The management of hyperactive behaviours, aggression, noncompliance with authority, self-esteem problems and social skills deficits requires different strategies for separate issues. This is particularly true for classroom management, where the topic is well studied.[10] Time-out, for instance, is hard to employ effectively for hyperactive behaviours (disruptive overactivity, impulsiveness and impatience, inattention, disorganization and poor task completion) simply because of their high frequency in any time period. On the other hand, it is effective as an intervention to reduce aggressive behaviours. It may be rational to consider a response cost system (loss of points from a total established at the outset of a time period) for hyperactive behaviours and time-out for less frequent aggressive responses. The system should be understandable to the child and kept reasonably simple to ensure consistency and fairness. Coupling responses cost with an incentive scheme (in which the child earns points and praise for compliance) can lead to the child feeling outraged as hard-won points are lost in a fine for a minor misdemeanour. In other words, a behaviour or a shortcoming is identified as a priority and worked on while other behaviours are left to be dealt with in their own right later on.

Where and when such approaches are implemented is an issue. School-based interventions along the above lines are effective but, not surprisingly, are more effective within a special classroom than within a general classroom.[11] Combining school and home interventions is better than either alone.[12] Comparable work with other conditions suggests that, in home-based behavioural interventions, parents will work best if they feel their priorities are being dealt with first.[13]

Behavioural interventions are carried out in the home by parents, not the clinic. Effectively the parents change their behaviour first and the work is with them. This is time consuming since their observations and records need appraisal and the rationale or feasibility of schemes has to be explored with them. Although it is possible for a psychiatrist or paediatrician to manage behavioural interventions, not all will have the experience or time to coach the parents in their implementation. It is usually preferable for a clinical psychologist or a nurse with special expertise to be the key clinician in running a behavioural intervention.

Work on cognitive interventions has shown that selected patients may benefit in the short term, mainly with intelligent children who understand their own difficulties.[14] Teaching covert self-instruction to delay and consider responses or evaluate one's own social problem-solving and task completion can be done and can be successful in a supervised situation. Some schools with a special interest in hyperactive children teach such strategies and encourage children to use them in class, for instance. Otherwise the problem in real life is that children fail to use what they have learnt and early enthusiasm has waned.[15] Intelligent teenagers can often grasp the principles but usually need coexisting medication to promote their own introspection and it is very unusual for a patient to benefit from a cognitive intervention alone.

Dietary interventions

A proportion of hyperactive children will improve when particular foods are removed from their diet. The size of such improvement is modest – by no means as large as that obtained by medication – but certainly significant. The main problem is that there is much incorrect advice and a common assumption that diets are easy to implement.

There have been a number of assertions about diet which have been shown to be groundless or wrong. Blanket exclusion diets ('cutting out the E numbers', eliminating all red foods, the Feingold diet, removing sugar or gluten) are useless in routine clinical practice.[16] The occasional child will respond to such manoeuvres,[17] which is probably what perpetuates the myth of their general utility.

Almost certainly the reason for this is the demonstration in controlled trials that a severe ('oligo-antigenic' or 'few-foods') diet restricted to a single meat, one vegetable and one fruit over a 3-week period will produce an improvement in a number of hyperactive children.[18] Foods can then be incrementally reintroduced, one-by-one. If there is a relapse, that food can be identified as pathogenic and permanently removed from the child's diet. A tailor-made exclusion diet is then established for that child.

In practice, most parents of hyperactive children with dietary sensitivities have already identified which foods cause trouble.[19] The contribution of the clinician is often to help them to systematize their observations and avoid excluding innocent foods. The mechanism for food intolerance is not established and the earlier claim that it is an allergy is not justified. Awkwardly, a number of independent allergy clinics have yet to show scientific restraint in this area, and promote skin testing for dietary allergic responses even though this is valueless.

Different clinics have different views about the usefulness of dietary interventions. It probably depends on the enthusiasm of the clinician. Diets can be expensive and place restrictions on the child's social life. They come to preoccupy families who develop conceptual tunnel vision so that a worsening of the child's behaviour is inevitably blamed on the child cheating on his or her diet. If the child has not broken his or her diet then there will be bad feeling and the likelihood that the real reason for relapse goes unidentified. In a few cases an excessively restricted diet can lead to malnutrition or be a vehicle for child abuse. Nevertheless, the possibility of diet restriction contributing to management, perhaps especially in young children, needs to be borne in mind, especially for children whose parents are opposed to medication. The supervision of a paediatric dietician is important for children placed on restriction diets for any length of time.

Medication

Psychopharmacology is the mainstay of treatment for severe hyperactivity. It should probably not be the only treatment intervention since medication provides only a temporary relief from hyperactivity symptoms and is not curative. It therefore creates, during this time, an opportunity for education, competent parenting and other psychological influences on personal development to act as they would in ordinary children. For the duration of its action, medication allows near-normality to supervene so that the child can enjoy more normal peer relationships, attend to what is being taught by teachers or parents and learn for him or herself that tasks can be completed. It prevents the child creating for him or herself a social environment that is critical or hostile.

The most powerful drugs are the stimulants, of which only methylphenidate and dexamphetamine are available in the UK and only in standard (not slow-release) tablet form). Methylphenidate has become the most popular, mainly because it lacks the street reputation of an amphetamine. It is often argued that methylphenidate is also a little more powerful than dexamphetamine, a little less likely to reduce growth velocity, but that dexamphetamine is less ictogenic. The evidence on which these claims are made is rather old and thin. Indeed, a recent meta-analytic appraisal for the MTA trial suggested that dexamphetamine might be marginally more effective.[9] Nevertheless, methylphenidate will be the drug of first choice for nearly all clinicians because of general professional familiarity. Two-thirds of children with ADHD will respond[20] and it is probable that a higher proportion of the more severe and selective condition of hyperkinetic disorder will do likewise.

There is no need to postulate a condition-specific paradoxical effect for stimulants. They have the same effect in at least some children without hyperactivity.[21] A response to stimulants does not confirm the diagnosis of a hyperactivity disorder. In general terms they appear to promote dopaminergic activity, directly and through noradrenergic systems.[22] This, in turn, is thought to promote higher cortical functions, particularly in the right cerebral hemisphere, through cortico-striatal tracts. Although it seems likely that orbito-frontal activity might also be enhanced, performance on laboratory tasks of executive function has not been shown to improve.[23] The ultimate effect is a general increase in all aspects of attention, impulse control and activity moderation, and a decrease in aggressive behaviours.[22] The size of such improvements is impressive but not sufficient to return the child to normality in these areas. There are also gains in the quality of mother–child interaction,[24] in peer group popularity[25] and in academic achievement.

The standard preparation of methylphenidate is absorbed promptly and a clinical effect is evident within about 40 minutes, lasting about 3 hours. Tolerance is not a problem[26] so that once a daily dose is established it can be maintained, if necessary, for years. The most usual way to decide what the daily dose should be is to proceed with a stepwise increase in doses rather than apply a mg/kg approach,[27] titrating amount and time of dose against clinical gain. Blood levels are of no value. The adverse effects, which supervene at higher doses, are insomnia, auditory hallucinations and an overfocused, perseverative 'zombie' state in which the child sits quietly but does very little.[28] Parents have no difficulty identifying this but it can sometimes go unnoticed (or even welcomed) in a large classroom. Its presence may be unsuspected if rating scales only are used to monitor treatment.

With this in mind, the usual regimen is to start with 5 mg after breakfast and after lunch, adding a mid-afternoon dose if indicated, inquiring as to benefit and increasing the dose after a few days (see Table 12.1). The impact of an increase in dose is evident within a couple of days provided that like environment is compared with like. There is a general consensus that the conventional maximum daily dose is about 50 mg (35 mg for children weighing less than 25 kg).[19] A few children will require more, though this is probably better managed in consultation with an expert centre. Stimulants have their greatest effect on attention control and activity moderation in structured settings in which the child is being posed cognitive challenges and has to think, plan and organize.[29] The gains at school are greater than the gains at home and these are greater than those in free play with peers. Monitoring the impact of treatment therefore needs to include information from both home and school, most conveniently by the use of the questionnaires developed by Conners.[6] It is good practice to include a measure of academic achievement too, though earlier concerns that stimulant doses sufficiently high to control disruptive behaviour would have deleterious effects on learning may have been unfounded.[23]

Because of insomnia, most children will not tolerate a stimulant dose after about 4 p.m., but some will. A few are troubled by a withdrawal rebound effect in the late afternoon, in which case a 5 mg dose of methylphenidate at that time can ease matters.

In the initial stages of treatment it is not uncommon for children to complain of stomach-ache and for parents to notice a loss of appetite. It is standard practice to monitor height and weight at least every 6 months and modify treatment accordingly, though growth retardation is not common and follow-up studies have not shown any stunting of adolescent height in most children.[24] Nevertheless, most authorities would be cautious about prescribing stimulants to children with pre-existing growth retardation. The relevance of drug holidays is not established because of contradictory results from studies.[24] In practice, growth retardation is only an occasional concern.

Because the effects of stimulants are greater at school and because of the short duration of their action, it is often a good idea to start medication at a weekend or during a school holiday so that parents can see the benefit.

Table 12.1   Protocol for methylphenidate administration (mg).

After breakfast	After lunch	Mid-afternoon
5	5	(5)
10	10	(5)
15	15	(5–10)
20	20	(10)

Attitudes to psychoactive medication vary and can be a major impediment to treatment. Parents and teachers may be concerned that what is happening is sedation or that the 'root cause' is not being tackled. In most instances the root cause is assumed by them to be poor parenting or the child's inferred emotional insecurity. Some headteachers are alarmed by the fact that stimulants are controlled drugs and have a street value leading to the possibility of playground trading or robbery. Most adults will want to know the risks of dependency (addiction to stimulants has not been found to be a problem in follow-up studies[30]). Children dislike having to take tablets, particularly in school, even though they usually declare that they notice no change in themselves when taking them or that they feel 'calmer'. Effort spent in providing parents, teachers and children with unbiased information is a good investment. There is counter-propaganda available on the Internet and through Scientology pamphlets which any parent, relative, teacher or child needs to know how to evaluate.

Contraindications to stimulant medication are few and generally relative. It would be foolhardy to use stimulants to treat attentional problems associated with schizophrenia because of the risk of hallucinosis as an adverse effect. Most clinicians find that stimulants are less effective or have a higher rate of adverse effects when used for hyperactivity in preschool children or hyperactivity in association with pervasive developmental disorders, severe mental retardation (in ICD terms), acquired brain injury and high levels of anxiety.[31] In particular, dysphoria seems to be more prevalent in such instances. It is generally thought to be wiser to use dexamphetamine than methylphenidate in children with poorly controlled epilepsy since it raises the convulsive threshold,[32] though either can be used in children with a controlled seizure disorder. The same probably applies to tic disorders. The literature is contradictory as to whether exacerbation of tics occurs,[33] but in practice either stimulant can be used with simple tics on a cautious basis. It is still conventional to be cautious about the use of stimulants in hyperactivity associated with Tourette's syndrome though it is thought at least possible that earlier reports of Tourette's syndrome being caused by stimulants may be documenting the coincidence of a comorbid disorder.

Age is assumed by many to be a relative contraindication but the logic behind this is not clear. Most clinicians would be wary of prescribing stimulants for children below the age of 5 years, at least in part because the diagnosis of a primary hyperactivity disorder is difficult in this age group.

Because stimulants will cause tachycardia and elevate systolic blood pressure, extreme caution as to their use in the presence of congenital heart disease, coarctation, Marfan's syndrome or secondary hypertension is only sensible.

Idiosyncratic adverse reactions to stimulants are rare. White cell count suppression has been known though it is not clear that regular blood counts will predict this and most centres do not do these.

There are possible adverse interactions with other drugs, the most serious instances being MAOIs (monoamine oxidase inhibitors). In practice the most likely drugs to be prescribed in combination with a stimulant are clonidine and, just possibly but with great caution, a tricyclic antidepressant. Since either of these can produce cardiac dysrhythmias and stimulants increase heart rate and blood pressure, it is wise to carry out a baseline and subsequent intermittent ECGs, consulting with a paediatric cardiologist if changes appear. Existing drug misuse in an adolescent or in other members of the household would represent an obvious contraindication for most clinicians.

Good practice with antihyperactivity medication is to test for continuing effect by periodic withdrawal, placebo controlled if there is ambiguity. The value of placebo is questionable as patients can often detect which is the active agent, by taste or subjective effect.[34] A workable schedule is to discontinue after 12 months of active drug treatment and, if there is relapse, to continue for another year. Relapse on withdrawal at this point is an indication for continuing treatment, usually until the mid-teens when further discontinuation can be attempted. In practice, there are sufficient interruptions to treatment (tablets forgotten, repeat prescriptions delayed, etc.) for withdrawal to be tested without the need for specific arrangements.

It is generally believed that if one stimulant is ineffective, the other may work,[19,35] though the hard evidence for this is scant. The usual problem with hyperkinetic disorder is not so much ineffectiveness but problems with the duration of effect of each dose, intolerance of adverse effects such as insomnia, abdominal pain or a school that is unwilling to handle a controlled drug. In such circumstances, addition of other agents or substitution of an alternative type of medication is often considered.

Stimulants in combination with other agents

The common problem of evening hyperactivity, either uncontrolled or accentuated by rebound, may not be satisfactorily dealt with by a further dose of stimulant because of subsequent insomnia. A moderately popular but poorly evaluated remedy is to provide an evening dose of clonidine (25–250 µg). In its own right, clonidine has been shown to moderate overactivity[36] but has little effect on inattention. Its unwanted effect of drowsiness makes it useful in this context, though this is a problem when clonidine is used alone. Awkwardly, clonidine can sometimes produce unsettled sleep and it is sensible to start with a low dose and increase weekly by 25 µg intervals checking blood pressure. Abrupt discontinuation is dangerous and cardiac dysrhythmias can occur on a steady dose.[37]

Another combination, also scientifically unevaluated but popular with some, is to combine methylphenidate with risperidone in low doses (3 mg a day or less). Advocates of this regimen point to anecdotal evidence for a marked effect on aggressive and oppositional behaviour (which can indeed be impressive) and rather less in the way of insomnia. Risperidone in the short term is not entirely innocuous, however, and the long-term risks for children are still unknown. The beneficial effect can wear off so that doses have to be increased and some children put on excessive weight.

Many families with a hyperactive child on a stimulant who will not sleep experiment with a variety of hypnotics such as antihistamines or with melatonin but with varying success, and no unequivocally effective combination has emerged.

Alternatives to stimulants

Tricyclic antidepressants have been the best studied group of agents, which can be shown to have a beneficial effect on hyperactive behaviours.[31] Imipramine (25–75 mg/day) is quite widely used. Its action is prolonged and a single daily dose can often be used. Unfortunately, it is less powerful than the stimulants, acts mainly on behaviour rather than cognition and the antimuscarinic effects are not always well tolerated. Desipramine has been well studied[31] but its cardiotoxicity is a problem and ECG monitoring is advisable, departures from a baseline value, particularly for PR and QT intervals, requiring discussion with a paediatric cardiologist. Given the extensive use of imipramine for enuretic children over the years it seems a counsel of perfection to carry out regular ECGs on a child taking imipramine.

Other antidepressants have been less studied, mainly in open trials, and reports of the effectiveness of various MAOIs (including moclobemide)[31] and bupropion[38] have appeared, and venlafaxine has been effective in open trials with ADHD in adults.[39,40] Anecdotal reports (and an open trial)[41] of the effectiveness of SSRIs (specific serotonin reuptake inhibitors) have probably been balanced by reports of ineffectiveness and disinhibition.

Clonidine has been used, particularly for ADHD, predominantly hyperactive type and in preschool children, and there is a respectable literature to support this.[36] Risperidone used alone probably has no effect on core symptoms. Traditional phenothiazines are not usually of use, though some young children with ADHD (hyperactive type) will respond to low-dose haloperidol (500 µg to 3 mg/day).[42] It pays to ask oneself whether behavioural control is being achieved at the expense of sedation (are *all* activities being suppressed?).

Duration of pharmacological treatment

As stated above, medication is a means to an end: to facilitate the beneficial impact of teaching, training and ordinary psychological influences on personality development. Routine discontinuation will test whether it is still required or whether normal control over attention, impulsiveness and activity has been developed. Most children will no longer need stimulants after their mid-teens but a minority will.[31]

Follow-up studies of hyperactive children have been bedevilled by biased sample selection initially or by large drop-out rates. The best study from which to draw data[43] suggests that some 8% of hyperactive children will continue to have problems with self-organization, impulsiveness and restlessness in their mid-twenties. The impact of methylphenidate on symptoms in this age group seems variable but beneficial to some,[44] particularly when observers' ratings rather than simply subjective ratings are included. Experience of general adult psychiatrists with this group of patients is limited and there are inconsistencies in the literature, yet it seems likely that a small proportion of hyperactive children will benefit from continued treatment, psychological or psychopharmacological, in early adult life. It is possible that taking the subjective experience of having a hyperactivity disorder into account (as is possible with adult patients) may lead to greater popularity of antidepressant medication (especially SSRIs) since, in many series, that is what adult patients prefer. With that in mind, it would be rational to question children closely about their subjective symptoms as well as the complaints of their parents and teachers.

Conclusion

Symptomatic treatment, although effective, may not do much to alter ultimate prognosis, partly because the problem appears to be a vulnerability factor for serious social pathology which may be a more substantial problem in the longer term. Many such children prove eventually to be remarkably expensive to the state, requiring expenditure from not just health, but education, social security and the criminal justice systems. Getting their management right is a priority if this is to be minimized. It may also be the case that concentrating on improvement in behaviour misses an important aspect of the condition, namely, its subjective symptomatology about which, little is currently known.

References

1. World Health Organization. *ICD-10 Diagnostic Criteria for Research* (Geneva: World Health Organization, 1993).

2. American Psychiatric Association. *Diagnostic and Statistical Manual of Mental Disorders (DSM-IV)* (4th edn) (Washington, DC: American Psychiatric Association, 1994).

3. Buitelaar JK, van Engeland H. Epidemiological approaches. In Sandberg S (ed) *Hyperactivity Disorders of Childhood* (Cambridge: Cambridge University Press, 1996): 26–68.

4. Sandberg S, Garralda ME. Psychosocial contributions. In Sandberg S (ed) *Hyperactivity Disorders of Childhood* (Cambridge: Cambridge University Press, 1996): 280–328.

5. Barkley RA. Guidelines for defining hyperactivity in children. In Lahey BB, Kazdin AE (eds) *Advances in Clinical Child Psychology. Vol. 5* (New York: Plenum, 1982): 153–80.

6. Conners CK. *Conners' Rating Scales-Revised* (North Tonawanda, NY: Multi-Health Systems Inc. and Windsor: NFER, 1997).

7. Klasen H. Conceptualizing hyperactivity: a qualitative study of parents' explanatory models. University of London, MSc thesis, 1996.

8. Hinshaw SP. *Attention Deficits and Hyperactivity in Children* (Thousand Oaks, CA: Sage, 1994).

9. Taylor E, Sandberg S, Thorley G, Giles S. *The Epidemiology of Childhood Hyperactivity. Maudsley Monograph no. 33* (Oxford: Oxford University Press, 1991).

10. Pfiffner LJ, Barkley RA. Educational placement and classroom management. In Barkley RA (ed) *Attention-Deficit Hyperactivity Disorder: A Handbook for Diagnosis and Treatment* (New York: Guilford Press, 1990): 498–539.

11. Barkley R, Copeland AP, Sivage C. A self-control classroom for hyperactive children. *J Autism and Devel Disorders* (1980) **10:** 75–89.

12. Gittelman-Klein R, Abikoff H, Pollack E et al. A controlled trial of behavior modification and methylphenidate in hyperactive children. In Whelan CK, Henker C (eds) *Hyperactive Children: The Social Ecology of Identification and Treatment* (New York: Academic Press, 1980): 221–43.

13. Howlin P, Rutter M. *Treatment of Autistic Children* (Chichester: Wiley, 1987).

14. Bugental DB, Whalen CK, Henker B. Causal attributions of hyperactive children and motivational assumptions of two behavior-change approaches: evidence for an interactionist position. *Child Devel* (1977) **48:** 874–84.

15. Abikoff H. Cognitive training in ADHD children: less to it than meets the eye. *J Learning Disabil* (1991) **24:** 205–9.

16. Mattes JA, Gittelman R. Effects of artificial food colorings in children with hyperactive symptoms. *Arch Gen Psychiatry* (1981) **38:** 714–18.

17. Weiss B, Williams JH, Margen S et al. Behavioral responses to artificial food colors. *Science* (1980) **207:** 1487–9.

18. Carter CM, Urbanowitz M, Hemsley R et al. Effects of a few-food diet in attention-deficit disorder. *Arch Dis Childhood* (1993) **69:** 564–8.

19. Greenhill LL, Abikoff HB, Arnold LE et al. Medication treatment strategies in the MTA study: relevance to clinicians and research. *J Am Acad Child and Adolescent*

Psychiatry (1996) **34:** 1304–13.

20. Elia J, Borcherding BG, Rapoport JL, Keysor CS. Methylphenidate and dextroamphetamine treatments of hyperactivity: are there true non-responders? *Psychiatry Res* (1991) **36:** 141–55.

21. Rapoport JL, Buchsbaum MS, Zahn TP et al. Dextroamphetamine. Cognitive and behavioral effects in normal prepubertal boys. *Science* (1978) **199:** 560–3.

22. Wilens T, Biederman J. The stimulants. *Psychiat Clin N Am* (1992) **15:** 191–222.

23. Oosterlain J. Short and long term effects of methylphenidate on cognitive functioning in ADHD children. Paper presented at the 8th Eunethydis meeting, Lisbon, 1997.

24. Barkley RA, Karlsson J, Strzelecki E, Murphy JV. The effects of age and dosage of Ritalin on the mother–child interactions of hyperactive children. *J Consult Clin Psychol* (1984) **52:** 750–8.

25. Whalen CK, Henker B, Buhrmeister D et al. Does stimulant medication improve the peer status of hyperactive children? *J Consult Clin Psychol* (1989) **57:** 545–9.

26. Safer D, Allen RP. Absence of tolerance to the behavioral effects of methylphenidate in hyperactive and inattentive children. *J Pediatr* (1989) **115:** 1003–8.

27. Rapport MD, Denney C. Titrating methylphenidate in children with attention deficit/hyperactivity disorder: is body mass predictive of clinical response? *J Am Acad Child and Adolescent Psychiatry* (1997) **36:** 523–30.

28. Tannock R, Schachar R. Methylphenidate and cognitive perseveration in hyperactive children. *J Child Psychol Psychiatry* (1992) **33:** 1217–28.

29. Whalen CK, Collins BE, Henker B et al. Behavior observations of hyperactive children and methylphenidate (Ritalin) effects in systematically structured classroom environments: now you see them, now you don't. *J Pediatr Psychol* (1978) **3:** 177–87.

30. Biederman J, Wilens T, Mick E, Milberger S et al. Psychoactive substance use disorder in adults with attention deficit hyperactivity disorder. *Am J Psychiatry* (1995) **152:** 1652–8.

31. Spencer T, Biederman J, Wilens T et al. Pharmacotherapy of attention deficit hyperactivity disorder across the life cycle. *J Am Acad Child and Adolescent Psychiatry* (1996) **35:** 409–32.

32. Taylor E. Physical treatments. In Rutter M, Taylor E, Hersov LA (eds) *Child and Adolescent Psychiatry: Modern Approaches* (Oxford: Blackwell Scientific, 1994). 880–99.

33. Gadow K, Sverd J, Sprafkin J et al. Efficacy of methylphenidate for ADHD in children with tic disorder. *Arch Gen Psychiatry* (1995) **52:** 444–55.

34. Gualtieri CT, Ondrusek MG, Finely C. Attention deficit disorders in adults. *Clin Neuropharmacol* (1985) **8:** 343–56.

35. Taylor E, Hemsley R. Treatment of hyperkinetic disorders in childhood. *Br Med J* (1995) **310:** 1617–18.

36. Hunt RD, Minderaa BB, Cohen DJ. Clonidine benefits children with attention deficit disorder and hyperactivity: report of a double blind placebo-crossover therapeutic trial. *J Am Acad Child Psychiatry* (1985) **24:** 617–29.

37. Cantwell DP, Swanson J, Connor DF. Case study: adverse response to clonidine. *J Am Acad Child and Adolescent Psychiatry* (1997) **36:** 539–44.

38. Conners CK, Casat CD, Gualtieri CT et al. Bupropion hydrochloride

in attention deficit disorder with hyperactivity. *J Am Acad Child and Adolescent Psychiatry* (1996) **34:** 1314–21.

39. Findling RL, Schwartz MA, Flannery DJ, Manos MJ. Venlafaxine in adults with attention-deficit/hyperactivity disorder: an open clinical trial. *J Clin Psychiatry* (1995) **57:** 184–9.

40. Hedges D, Reimherr FW, Rogers A et al. An open trial of venlafaxine in adult patients with attention deficit hyperactivity disorder. *Psychopharmacol Bull* (1995) **31:** 779–83.

41. Barrickman L, Noyes R, Kuperman S et al. Treatment of ADHD with fluxoetine: a preliminary trial. *J Am Acad Child and Adolescent Psychiatry* (1991) **30:** 762–7.

42. Barker P, Fraser IA. A controlled trial of haloperidol in children. *Br J Psychiatry* (1968) **114:** 855–7.

43. Mannuzza S, Klein RG, Bessler A et al. Adult outcome of hyperactive boys. *Arch Gen Psychiatry* (1993) **50:** 565–76.

44. Spencer T, Wilens T, Biederman J et al. A double blind, crossover comparison of methylphenidate and placebo in adults with childhood-onset attention-deficit hyperactivity disorder. *Arch Gen Psychiatry* (1995) **52:** 434–43.

13
Ways of improving compliance

Martina Hummer and W Wolfgang Fleischhacker

Introduction

Despite the 37 130 articles on compliance that have been published so far (Medline Search since 1966), this topic is rarely discussed and is, hence, poorly understood in daily clinical life. Considering this enormous number of publications, it is astonishing that the compliance rate in schizophrenic patients is only about 41%[1] and is 20–57%[2] in patients with bipolar affective disorder. This may be an indication that it is easier to discuss this problem than to provide remedies for it. When dealing with compliance one has to realize, first of all, that this word is not used uniformly. On one hand, the term can mean complying with pharmacological treatment while, on the other, it can mean adherence to the overall treatment plan (including social-therapeutic and psychotherapeutic measures as well as the willingness to start treatment and keeping to scheduled appointments). Further, compliance is not an 'all or nothing' phenomenon. For these reasons, compliance is influenced by many factors and its definition varies widely.

Scientifically, compliance is commonly expressed as the ratio between an observed treatment behaviour and given treatment standards.[3] This definition includes patient-related factors as well as other kinds of variables, such as for instance drug-induced adverse effects and the doctor–patient relationship. In the scientific literature, compliance is most often considered in the context of drug treatment. Only about one-third of patients are reported to be fully compliant.[4–6] Another third are partially compliant, meaning they will either reduce the dose of the drug prescribed or fail to take drugs from time to time. The remaining patients do not follow prescription instructions at all. Not only failing to take the medication but also taking more than the prescribed daily dose or not taking it in the proper dosing pattern can be defined as noncompliance. Clinicians who have attempted to judge which of their patients will eventually comply with treatment have been shown to fail miserably.[7] Therefore, it is important to know the characteristics of the patients who are more prone to noncompliance.

Factors influencing compliance

Although the factors that influence compliance (see Table 13.1) often overlap or influence each other, it is possible to differentiate between factors that are related to the patient, the environment, the physician and the treatment. Although this differentiation may in some ways be artificial, it could help clinicians in their daily clinical work in assessing the various reasons why a particular patient has become noncompliant.

Patient-related factors

First, the nature of the patient's illness has a strong impact on the patient's insight about, and acceptance of, the treatment. Hence, non-compliance may be a more extensive and complex issue in psychiatric disorders than in general medicine.[8] Patients who feel persecuted or poisoned will be reluctant to take drugs. Grandiose or manic patients are, for the most part, not interested in their own treatment. Manic patients often miss the exhilaration or excess energy experienced during their previous episodes.[9] Additionally, both patients with negative symptoms and depressive patients (who are suffering from motivational deficits) have been shown to be poor compliers. In any kind of disorder, the patient's subjective attitudes towards taking drugs – which will always be tainted by the patient's illness – need to be taken into account.[10,11]

If the time of relapse following drug discontinuation has been such that the patient in good remission may not relapse for several months after stopping medication, this could lead to a false sense of security after a short interruption of treatment.[12] It will, moreover, reinforce the patient's reluctance to continue drug-taking.

Table 13.1   Factors that influence compliance.

- *Patient related*
  Psychopathology, cognitive impairment, age, comorbidity

- *Environment related*
  Social support, financial support, attitude towards treatment, supervision of treatment, social rank of illness

- *Physician related*
  Lack of guidelines, belief in treatment, doctor–patient relationship, aftercare management, provision of information

- *Treatment related*
  Side-effects, route of administration, pattern of dosing, length of treatment, costs of treatment, polypharmacy

Another reason for noncompliance could be that the psychopharmaco-logical treatment has not been as effective as the patient had expected it to be. If patients are in full remission, they may stop taking medication because they experience no further symptoms; they may think they no longer require medication.

An illness's social rank may also be of fundamental importance for compliance. If the illness's social ranking is low, the patient may try to avoid everything connected with the illness, including its treatment. Apart from the illness itself, comorbid alcohol or other substance abuse is a strong predictor of noncompliance.[13–15]

A patient's age is also of importance for compliance. It has been shown that older patients have more problems with compliance.[16] One reason for this may be the memory deficits that are often prevalent in this group of patients. In addition, multiple morbidity in such patients often requires complex prescription plans which such patients have difficulty following. On the other hand, young patients have also been found to be poor compliers.[17,18] One reason for this could be that young adults asso-ciate any kind of treatment or keeping scheduled appointments as typical features of the generation they are trying to be different from. Taking medication and hence not being allowed to drink alcohol or spend the whole night out without sleeping make such young patients feel different from their friends. It is important for young people to feel they belong to a group who have the same characteristics as themselves – more so than for any other age group. Contradictory results, however, have been found when investigating the influence of gender or ethnicity on compliance.

Environment-related factors

The patient's environment can be a major factor influencing compli-ance.[19,20] Negative attitudes towards psychiatric treatment in the patient's social surroundings have an adverse effect on the patient's compliance. This is reflected in the fact that inpatients are better compliers than patients living in the community. In addition, poor social support (particu-larly when the patient lives alone[21]) is associated with poor compliance. Alternatively, stressful social interactions may negate the positive influ-ence on compliance that may be exerted when the patient lives with others.[22] For example, an overemotional family[23] may counteract any pos-itive effects that may be had from living with related significant others, or the family may be unable to assist or supervise in the patient's medica-tion. In addition, the sensationalist reports that appear in the media about the alleged adverse effects medications can have may impact on patients and hence their compliance to a much greater extent than is often realized. Lack of money to pay for the treatment or to pay for travel-ling to the pharmacy or outpatient department must also be considered when establishing reasons for noncompliance.[24]

Physician-related factors

First, the compliance problems physicians may create when they do not follow certain therapy guidelines must be mentioned. A European and an American study have both shown considerable discrepancies between treatment guidelines and common clinical practice.[25,26] Apart from the difficulty patients experience in following treatment guidelines, it must also be noted that psychiatric guidelines are still far from perfect. Treatment decisions may, therefore, be accompanied by a certain degree of uncertainty. As a result of different treatment recommendations, the patient feels uncertain and may ask several specialists for their advice so that the patient can form his or her own opinion. The strength of a doctor's belief in his or her prescribed medication has also been found to be associated with compliance.[21]

The doctor–patient relationship is particularly significant in compliance.[27–29] Such a relationship is a prerequisite for a working therapeutic alliance, and reliable information is its cornerstone. The patient must be provided with facts about the various treatment possibilities, including a detailed explanation of their effectiveness and any anticipated side-effects. The notion that information about side-effects will lead to noncompliance is a common misconception.[30]

It may also be a consequence of better compliance that patients who are involved in clinical trials often achieve better results than patients receiving routine treatment. This could, to a certain extent, be a consequence of the additional effort and the rigidity of structure that are a feature of clinical studies. Patients receive scheduled appointments that the doctor will keep and that will not be rescheduled even if the doctor's workload would indicate otherwise. The structured nature of therapy signals to the patient the importance of the therapeutic measures that are being taken. Nelson et al. found that the single best predictor of medication compliance among discharged schizophrenic patients was the patient's perception of the physician's interest in the patient as a human being.[31]

Marder et al. demonstrated that in-patients suffering from schizophrenia and who consented to neuroleptic treatment were more satisfied with the ward staff and their own physicians. They felt that their physicians understood them, had their best interests at heart and had explained the reasons for taking the medication and their potential side-effects.

Although the results of studies conflict to some extent, it seems that the way the patient is informed about his or her medication seems to be of relevance. Additional, circumscribed interventions aimed at providing information about schizophrenia and its treatment have been of variable effect in increasing compliance. Neither 30–50 minute information sessions[33] nor educational sessions provided once a week for 3 weeks could be demonstrated to have had an influence on compliance, although an increase in knowledge about the illness was documented.[34] Alternatively, a randomized controlled trial that investigated the effectiveness of compliance therapy through a brief, pragmatic intervention that targeted treatment adherence in psychotic disorders found significant improvements in the compliance therapy group.[35] Seventy-four patients received 4–6 sessions of either compliance therapy or nonspecific counselling. The patients' insight, attitudes to treatment and observer-rated compliance were better in the specific therapy group over the follow-up period of 18 months. Eckman et al. designed a medication management module that improved compliance from 67% before training to 82% after training.[36] The module included information about medication, administering medication and evaluating its benefits, identifying side-effects and negotiating medication with healthcare providers. The patients were trained for 3 hours per week over 15–20 weeks.

The health model with which patients are provided is also a major determinant of general noncompliance. According to this model, noncompliance is a function of the patient's perception of his or her susceptibility to illness, the severity of the illness, the efficacy of treatment and the costs (practical and emotional) of treatment.[37–39]

Treatment-related factors

It must be taken into consideration that almost every psychiatric therapy (with the exception of the anxiolytic effect of benzodiazepines) has a delayed onset of effects. Psychopharmacological drugs may even worsen the patient's initial status. This is generally the result of early side-effects, which often precede clinical benefits.[40] The negative effect of these drugs can be counteracted by informing patients about this potential problem, and by providing them with additional support in the difficult initial stages of treatment.

Van Putten was the first to show that side-effects that occur during the first hours of the therapy can lead to a substantial impairment of compliance.[40] Not only the objective but also the subjective symptoms of side-effects are of major importance. Objective side-effects (which are clearly evident to the doctor) lead to prompt therapeutic intervention in many cases and, therefore, to a relief of symptoms. The diagnosis of subjective side-effects requires a more thorough examination and extensive discussion with the patient. These adverse effects are difficult to evaluate as they cannot be measured and, for this reason, the doctor must trust the patient's report concerning their severity and relevance. Consequently, a discussion of the treatment's benefits and risks must be held with the patients themselves and, ideally, with their significant others. This discussion may be a decisive factor in the successful outcome of therapy.

In clinical practice, the clinician's subjective value system is the basis of most decision-making. However, for successful long-term therapy it is important to consider the patient's subjective value system even if this is difficult for the doctor to comprehend. Extensive discussion will determine if the patient is prepared to accept the existing side-effects or if a change of treatment should be considered. The side-effects that are regularly encountered as having a negative impact on compliance are extrapyramidal motor side-effects, weight gain and changes in sexual libido.

The route of treatment administration has an influence on compliance and thus on treatment outcome. While a review of 26 studies[41] showed compliance advantages in administering depot neuroleptics compared with oral neuroleptics, a change to depot neuroleptics in noncompliant patients did not seem to be effective. Van Putten et al. investigated schizophrenia outpatients and found that 83% of habitual noncompliant schizophrenic outpatients who had been switched to depot neuroleptics did not return regularly for injections.[42] Comparable results were found by Falloon et al.[43] These authors showed that patients who were irregular in their tablet taking also missed at least one injection in 12 months. These results are supported by Buchanan, who found no differences in compliance rates over 2 years postdischarge for patients treated with either depot or oral neuroleptics.[44] Although no certain compliance advantage can be found for depot neuroleptics, depot neuroleptics have the advantage that noncompliance can be detected immediately with the possibility of early intervention. The pharmaceutical industry has recently been drawing physicians' attention to the benefits of prescribing liquid formulations, especially to older patients. While it is easier to swallow liquids, it takes more effort on the patient's part to count drops or measure syrup quantities several times during the day or to use liquids when travelling.

Apart from the type of medication application, simplified therapy schemes are necessary for improved compliance. Provided the medication's half-life permits once-a-day dosing or two doses at most, this is to be preferred to more frequent administrations.[45] Complicated treatment schemes clearly lead to impairment of compliance. If the patient has to administer many different medications (which may happen when side-effects are treated with other medications) this may make intake as prescribed by the clinician more unlikely. When dealing with multimorbid patients, individual specialists should consult one another to simplify pharmacological treatment as much as is feasible.

Measuring compliance

The meaningful measurement of compliance is fraught with difficulties. If intravenous or intramuscular injections are not used, compliance can only be tested by indirect methods. The easiest way is to count the patient's remaining tablets at each visit, and to tally this number with the amount of tablets prescribed. A more sophisticated method is the medication event monitoring system (MEMS) – a microprocessor-based means of monitoring compliance continuously (a microelectronic circuit records the date and time of each opening and closing of the medication's container).[46]

Another method is to measure plasma concentrations. However, such measurements cannot always detect whether the patient has been non-compliant days or weeks before the tests, or has only taken the medication immediately before being tested. Results of blood tests can also be influenced by inter- and intraindividual metabolic variations. Urinary drug markers (such as riboflavin or salvia screens) can be used, but these have not proved useful outside research settings. Clinical outcome – which is often used as measure of adherence to treatment – is also not valid as an indicator.

Patient self-reports and information gleaned from significant others are relevant indicators of compliance in daily clinical work. A drawback of this method is that its accuracy depends primarily on the doctor–patient relationship and the trust that exists between them. However, regular discussion about therapy can lead to an improvement in this relationship and hence to an improvement in compliance.

Prerequisites for improving compliance

Intervention at various levels can have a positive influence on compliance.[6,29,47,48] Apart from routine compliance assessment, the factors that

Table 13.2   Prerequisites for improving compliance.

- Make sure the treatment follows evidence-based guidelines
- Choose agents and dosages that allow maximum efficacy and minimal side-effects
- Regularly assess the factors that influence compliance
- Assess and treat side-effects
- Discuss risk/benefit considerations with the patient and his or her significant others frequently
- Provide health models for different psychiatric disorders
- Provide information booklets about the illness and treatment that are written in nontechnical language patients and relatives can understand
- Plan outpatient aftercare at the time of inpatient treatment
- Try to resolve the patient's request to discontinue treatment for financial reasons
- Provide organizers who can reduce the patient's confusion over which medication to take and when, or to help decide if a patient has already taken his or her medication

influence adherence to treatment in each individual patient have to be analysed. The general interventions given in Table 13.2 are the absolute essentials. These include evidence-based treatment, a regular check of treatment efficacy and side-effects and a risk–benefit discussion with patients and their significant others. Information should not only be given verbally but also in written form. Aftercare must be planned at the time of inpatient treatment. Guidelines should be provided not only for the physician but also for the patient and his or her family. If the family and patient are informed about the guidelines, they will then know what they can expect and demand of the physician – which will keep the doctor on his or her toes! A sound relationship between patients, significant others and clinicians, based on the balanced provision of information on all sides, will hence serve as the basis for a good, working, therapeutic alliance.

References

1. Fenton WS, Blyler CR, Heinssen RK. Determinants of medication compliance in schizophrenia: empirical and clinical findings. *Schizophr Res* (1997) **23:** 637–51.

2. Elixhauser A, Eisen SA, Romeis JC et al. The effects of monitoring and feedback on compliance. *Medical Care* (1990) **28:** 883–93.

3. Fleischhacker WW, Meise U, Günther V et al. Compliance with antipsychotic drug treatment: influence of side-effects. *Acta Psychiatr Scand* (1994) **382(Suppl):** 11–15.

4. Blackwell B. Treatment adherence. *Br J Psychiatry* (1976) **129:** 513–31.

5. Lima J, Nazarian L, Charney E et al. Compliance with short term antimicrobial therapy. Some techniques that help. *Pediatrics* (1976) **57:** 383–6.

6. Wright EC. Non-compliance – or how many aunts has Matilda? *Lancet* (1993) **342:** 909–13.

7. Sleator EK. Measurement of compliance. *Psychopharmacol Bull* (1985) **21:** 1089–93.

8. Kane JM. Compliance issues in outpatient treatment. *J Clin Psychopharmacol* (1985) **5(Suppl):** 22S–27S.

9. Schou M. The combat of non-compliance during prophylactic lithium treatment. *Acta Psychiatr Scand* (1997) **95:** 361–3.

10. McEvoy JP, Apperson LJ, Appelbaum PS et al. Insight in schizophrenia. Its relationship to acute psychopathology. *J Nerv Ment Dis* (1989) **177:** 43–7.

11. Pan PC, Tantam D. Clinical characteristics, health beliefs and compliance with maintenance treatment: a comparison between regular and irregular attenders at a depot clinic. *Acta Psychiatr Scand* (1989) **79:** 564–70.

12. Kane JM. Prevention and treatment of neuroleptic non-compliance. *Psychiat Ann* (1996) **16:** 576–9.

13. Drake RE, Osher FC, Wallach MA. Alcohol use and abuse in schizophrenia. *J Nerv Ment Dis* (1989) **177:** 408–14.

14. Kashner TM, Rader LE, Rodell DE et al. Family characteristics, substance abuse and hospitalization

patterns of patients with schizophrenia. *Hosp Comm Psychiat* (1991) **42:** 195–7.

15. Owen RR, Rischer EP, Booth BM et al. Medication non-compliance and substance abuse among patients with schizophrenia. *Psychiat Serv* (1996) **47:** 853–8.

16. Schwartz D, Wang W, Zeitz L et al. Medication errors made by elderly, chronically ill patients. *Am J Public Health* (1962) **52:** 2018–29.

17. Danion JM, Neunruther C, Krieger-Finance F et al. Compliance with long-term lithium treatment in major affective disorders. *Pharmacopsychiatry* (1987) **20:** 230–1.

18. Swett J, Noones J. Factors associated with premature termination from outpatient treatment. *Hosp Comm Psychiat* (1989) **40:** 947–51.

19. Blackwell B. Drug therapy. *N Engl J Med* (1973) **2:** 249–52.

20. Hoge SK, Appelbaum PS, Lawlor T et al. A prospective, multicenter study of patients' refusal of antipsychotic medication. *Arch Gen Psychiatry* (1990) **47:** 949–56.

21. Irwin DS, Weitzell WD, Morgan DW. Phenothiazine intake and staff attitudes. *Am J Psychiatry* (1971) **127:** 1631–5.

22. Reilly EL, Wilson WP, McClinton HK. Clinical characteristics and medication history of schizophrenics readmitted to the hospital. *Int J Neuropsychiat* (1967) **39:** 85–90.

23. Tamminga CA, Schulz SC. *Schizophrenia Research. Advances in Neuropsychiatry and Psychopharmacology. Vol. 1* (New York: Raven Press, 1991).

24. Sullivan G, Wells KB, Morgenstern H et al. Identifying modifiable risk factors for rehospitalization: a case-control study of seriously mentally ill persons in Mississippi. *Am J Psychiatry* (1995) **152:** 1749–56.

25. Meise U, Kurz M, Fleischhacker WW. Antipsychotic maintenance treatment of schizophrenia patients: is there a consensus? *Schizophr Bull* (1994) **20:** 215–25.

26. Lehmann AF, Steinwachs DM. Patterns of usual care for schizophrenia: initial results from the schizophrenia patient outcomes research team (PORT) client survey. *Schizophr Bull* (1998) **24:** 11–20.

27. Meise U, Günther V, Gritsch S. Die Bedeutung der Arzt-Patienten-Beziehung für die Patientencompliance. *Wien Klin Wochenschr* (1992) **104:** 267–71.

28. Ley P, Spelman MS. Communication in an outpatient setting. *Br J Soc Clin Psycholog* (1965) **4:** 114–16.

29. Linden M. Therapeutische Ansätze zur Verbesserung von Compliance. *Nervenarzt* (1979) **50:** 109–14.

30. Albus M, Burkes S, Scherer J. Welche Faktoren beeinflussen die Medikamenten-Compliance? *Psychiat Praxis* (1995) **22:** 228–30.

31. Nelson AA, Gold BH, Huchinson RA et al. Drug default among schizophrenic patients. *Am J Hosp Pharmacy* (1975) **32:** 1237–42.

32. Marder SR, Mebane A, Chien CP et al. A comparison of patients who refuse and consent to neuroleptic treatment. *Am J Psychiatry* (1983) **140:** 470–2.

33. Boczkowski JA, Zeichner A, DeSanto N. Neuroleptic compliance among chronic schizophrenic outpatients: an intervention outcome report. *J Consult Clin Psychiatry* (1985) **53:** 666–71.

34. Macpherson R, Jerrom B, Hughes A. A controlled study of education about drug treatment in schizophrenia. *Br J Psychiatry* (1996) **168:** 709–17.

35. Kemp R, Kirov G, Everitt B et al.

Randomised controlled trial of compliance therapy. *Br J Psychiatry* (1998) **172:** 413–19.

36. Eckman TA, Lieberman RP, Phipps CC et al. Teaching medication management skills to schizophrenic patients. *J Clin Psychopharmacol* (1990) **10:** 33–8.

37. Becker M, Maiman CA. Sociobehavioral determinants of compliance with health and medical care recommendations. *Medical Care* (1975) **13:** 10–24.

38. Kasi SA, Cobb S. Health behavior, illness behavior and sick role behavior. *J Health Illness Behav Arch Environment Health* (1966) **12:** 246–66.

39. Rosenstock IM. Why people use health services. *Millbank Mem Fund Q* (1966) **44:** 94–127.

40. Van Putten T, May PRA, Marder SR. Akathisia with haloperidol and thiothixene. *Arch Gen Psychiatry* (1984) **41:** 1036–9.

41. Young JL, Zonana HV, Shepler L. Medication non-compliance in schizophrenia: codification and update. *Bull Am Acad Psychiat Law* (1986) **14:** 105–22.

42. Van Putten T, Crumpton E, Yale C. Drug refusal in schizophrenia and the wish to be crazy. *Arch Gen Psychiatry* (1976) **33:** 1433–46.

43. Falloon IRH, Watt DC, Shepherd M. A comparative controlled trial of pimozide and fluphenazine decanoate in the continuation therapy of schizophrenia. *Psycholog Med* (1978) **8:** 59–70.

44. Buchanan A. A two-year prospective study of treatment compliance in patients with schizophrenia. *Psycholog Med* (1992) **22:** 787–97.

45. Eisen SA, Miller DK, Woodward RS et al. The effect of prescribed daily dose frequency on patient medication compliance. *Arch Intern Med* (1990) **150:** 1881–4.

46. Kruse W, Weber E. Dynamics of drug regimen compliance – its assessment by microprocessor-based monitoring. *Eur J Pharmacol* (1990) **38:** 561–5.

47. Diamond RJ. Enhancing medication use in schizophrenic patients. *J Clin Psychiatry* (1983) **44:** 7–14.

48. Falloon RH. Developing and maintaining adherence to long-term drug taking regimens. *Schizophr Bull* (1984) **10:** 412–17.

Index

Abnormal Involuntary Movement Scale (AIMS) 26
acamprosate in alcoholism 165–7, 173
acyclovir in chronic fatigue syndrome (CFS) 146
ADAS non-cog (Alzheimer's Disease Assessment Scale, noncognitive part) 187
addiction, biological basis 155
affective disorders 48
aggressive behaviour
  checklist 205
  in dementia 191
  long-term treatment 207–9
agitation in dementia 192
agoraphobia 77–9, 85–6, 88, 90
alcoholism 155, 163
  comorbid psychiatric disorder 170–2
  new agents 165–70
  pharmacotherapy 165–73
  prevalence 156
  relapse prevention 165, 172, 173
alpha-methyldopa in tardive dyskinesia (TD) 27
alprazolam
  in anxiety in dementia 190
  in panic disorder 82–4
Alzheimer's disease (AD) 185–90
  behavioural domain symptoms 187
  see also dementia
American Psychiatric Association 6
  Task Force on Clinician Safety 202
aminoglutethimide in obsessive–compulsive disorder (OCD) 102
amitriptyline
  in bipolar disorder 45
  in manic-depressive illness 49
amphetamines 164
anorexia nervosa 109–33
  aetiology 113–16
    family factors 115–16
    genetic component 114–15
    psychological factors 116
    social factors 115
  biological factors 113–15
  blood chemistry 119
  cardiovascular problems 118

comorbidity 111
  with physical problems 119
  dental changes 117
  diagnosis 110–11
  diagnostic criteria 112
  effects on central nervous system (CNS) 117–18
  endocrine system 118
  epidemiology 111
  fertility and reproductive function 118
  gastrointestinal tract 118–19
  haematology 119
  history 109–10
  medical complications 116–19
  musculoskeletal problems 116–17
  prevalence 112
  prognosis 123
  skin and hair changes 116
  treatment 120–3
    current models 121–2
    essential facets 121
    inpatient treatment 122
    medication 122
    outpatient psychotherapy or counselling 121–2
    service acceptability 122
    transtheoretical approach 120
anticonvulsants
  in bipolar disorder 49
  in refractory schizophrenia 13
antidepressants 183
  combining 66–7
  in unipolar depression 60
anxiety disorder in dementia 190, 193–4
apomorphine in tardive dyskinesia (TD) 27
attention deficit hyperactivity disorder (ADHD) 214, 216, 220
  in hyperactive child 224

baclofen in panic disorder 85
BEHAVE-AD scale 187
behavioural disturbances
  in dementia 185–90
  in old age 181–98
  in panic disorder 77
behavioural psychotherapy in obsessive–compulsive disorder (OCD) 103–5

benzodiazepines
    in anxiety disorder in dementia 190,
        194
    in bipolar disorder 48, 208
    in emergency medication 207
    in manic-depressive illness 50
    in panic disorder 79, 81, 82, 84, 88–91
    in refractory schizophrenia 13
    in sleep disturbance in dementia 192
    in violent behaviour 208, 209
Berlin Ageing Study 183
bipolar disorder
    algorithmic approach to
        pharmacological treatment 43–6
    amitriptyline in 45
    anticonvulsants in 49
    benzodiazepines in 48, 208
    calcium channel antagonists (CCAs) in
        49
    calcium channel blocking agents in 49
    carbamazepine in 43, 45, 47
    clonazepam in 48
    diagnostic classification 46
    gabapentin in 49
    lamotrigine in 49
    lithium in 41–3, 45, 47, 49
    noncompliance 45
    patterns affecting initial drug selection
        41–3
    pharmacological treatment 41–9
    prophylactic pharmacotherapy 37, 42
    thyroxine in 45
    valproate in 43, 47
borderline personality disorder (BPD)
        99–100
botulinum toxin (BTX-a) in tardive
        dyskinesia (TD) 26
Brief Psychiatric Rating Scale (BPRS) 4
brofaromine in panic disorder 81
bromocriptine
    in alcoholism 170
    in tardive dyskinesia (TD) 27
BRSD (Behaviour Rating Scale for
        Dementia) 187
bulimia nervosa 113
buprenorphine in substance abuse 162
bupropion in hyperactive child 224
buspirone
    in alcoholism 165
    in anxiety disorder in dementia 194
    in obsessive–compulsive disorder
        (OCD) 102
    in panic disorder 84–5
    in unipolar depression 68

calcium channel antagonists (CCAs) in
        bipolar disorder 49
calcium channel blocking agents
    in bipolar disorder 49
    in tardive dyskinesia (TD) 26

carbamazepine
    in alcoholism 173
    in bipolar disorder 43, 45, 47
    in manic-depressive illness 37, 38, 50
    in panic disorder 85
    in refractory schizophrenia 13
    in unipolar depression 68
    in violent behaviour 209
catecholamine 7
CERAD (Consortium to Establish a
        Registry for Alzheimer's Disease)
        programme 187
cerebrospinal fluid (CSF) 7
children
    hyperactivity, see hyperactive child
    obsessive–compulsive disorder (OCD)
        98
chlorpromazine in refractory schizophrenia
        4, 6, 15
cholinomimetic drugs in tardive dyskinesia
        (TD) 28
chronic fatigue syndrome (CFS) 135–53
    acyclovir in 146
    aetiology 137
    and psychiatric disorder 138
    behavioural factors 141–2
    clinical description 136–7
    cognitive dysfunction in 138–9
    diagnosis 135
    epidemiology 135–6
    evening primrose oil in 146
    factors contributing to development and
        maintenance 140
    illness attributions and cognitions 141
    immune system in 138
    immunoglobulins in 146
    insurance assessment 147–8
    magnesium in 146
    multifactorial model 139
    muscle dysfunction in 137
    neuroimaging in 139
    neuropsychiatry 138–9
    operational criteria 136
    outpatient treatment 142
    perpetuating factors 141
    predictors of outcome 147
    predisposing and precipitating factors
        139–41
    prevalence 135–6
    prognosis 137
    referral to psychiatric service 147
    rehabilitation programme 142–6
    role of spouse/parent 148
    traditional treatment approaches 146
    viral infection in 137
    see also cognitive behaviour therapy
        (CBT)
citalopram
    in alcoholism with comorbid psychiatric
        disorder 170

in depression in old age 184
in manic-depressive illness 49
in panic disorder 81
Clinical Global Impression (CGI) 4, 50
clomipramine
   in obsessive–compulsive disorder
      (OCD) 102, 103
   in panic disorder 81, 83–4
clonazepam
   in aggressive behaviour 209
   in bipolar disorder 48
   in obsessive–compulsive disorder
      (OCD) 102
   in violent behaviour 208–9
clozapine
   as mood stabilizer 48
   in dementia with Lewy bodies (DLB) 191
   in late-life psychosis 195
   in refractory schizophrenia 6–10, 12,
      15, 16
   in tardive dyskinesia (TD) 28
CMAI (Cohen–Mansfield Agitation
      Inventory) 187
cocaine use disorders 161, 163–4
   treatment 163–4
cognitive behaviour therapy (CBT) 142–6
   active scheduling 144–5
   assessment 143
   engagement of patient 143
   evidence for efficacy of 146–7
   in panic disorder 85–9
   modifying negative and unhelpful
      thinking 145
   psychosocial problems 146
   rationale for treatment 143–4
   sleep routine 145
   structure of treatment 144
cognitive dysfunction in chronic fatigue
      syndrome (CFS) 138–9
compliance/noncompliance 229–38
   doctor–patient relationship 232
   environment-related factors 231
   factors influencing 230
   measuring compliance 234–5
   patient-related factors 230
   physician-related factors 232–3
   prerequisites for improving compliance
      235–6
   route of treatment administration 234
   side-effects 233
   treatment-related factors 233–4
compulsions, see obsessive–compulsive
      disorder (OCD)
computed tomography (CT) 7, 201
corticotropin releasing factor (CRF) 118
Cross-National Collaborative Panic Study
      80
cyproterone acetate in
      obsessive–compulsive disorder
      (OCD) 102

delusions in dementia 190–1
dementia
   aggression in 191
   agitation in 192
   anxiety disorder in 190, 193–4
   behavioural disturbances in 185–90
   delusion in 190–1
   depression in 188
   differential diagnosis 189
   electroencephalogram (EEG) in 191
   hallucinations in 190–1
   sexual disinhibition in 193
   sleep disturbances in 192 3
   symptoms 187
   wandering in 192
dementia with Lewy bodies (DLB),
      clozapine in 191
depression
   differential diagnosis 189
   in dementia 188
   in old age 181–4
      pharmacological treatment 183–4
desipramine
   in cocaine use disorders 164
   in stimulant abuse 164
detoxification 155
dexamphetamine in hyperactive child 220
diaphragmatic breathing 86–7
diazepam in panic disorder 88
dinor-LAAM 161
dopamine-D2 receptors 6
dopamine receptor antagonist in tardive
      dyskinesia (TD) 24, 27
dopaminergic drugs in alcoholism 165,
      169–70
drug abuse, see substance abuse
Drug Abuse Reporting Program 156
Drug Abuse Treatment Outcome Study
      157

elderly persons, see old age
electroconvulsive therapy (ECT)
   in manic-depressive illness 50
   in refractory schizophrenia 13
   in treatment-resistant depression 68
   in unipolar depression 57, 67
electroencephalogram (EEG) in dementia
      191
entactogenic
      methylenedioxyamphetamines/buta
      mines 164
Epidemiological Catchment Area Study
      (ECA) 181
evening primrose oil in chronic fatigue
      syndrome (CFS) 146
extrapyramidal side-effects (EPS) 6, 24,
      31

5–HT metabolites 170
5–hydroxyindoleacetic acid (5–HIAA) 200

fluoxetine
   in aggressive behaviour 209
   in alcoholism with comorbid psychiatric
      disorder 170
   in cocaine use disorders 164
   in depression in old age 184
   in manic-depressive illness 49
   in unipolar depression 66
flupenthixol
   in alcoholism 170
   in cocaine use disorders 164
fluphenazine
   in emergency medication 207
   in violent behaviour 209
fluvoxamine
   in depression in old age 184
   in manic-depressive illness 49
   in panic disorder 81, 83
follicle stimulating hormone (FSH) 118
free radicals 25-6

gabapentin in bipolar disorder 49
genetic defects and violent behaviour 201

hallucinations 163
   in dementia 190-1
hallucinogenic methoxyphenethylamines
   164
hallucinogens 155, 156
haloperidol
   in dementia 191
   in emergency medication 207
   in manic-depressive illness 50
   in refractory schizophrenia 4, 15
   in tardive dyskinesia (TD) 29
   in violent behaviour 209
heroin
   abstinence-orientated treatment 156
   consumption 158
   in opioid-dependent patients 162
homovanillic acid 7
hyperactive child 213-28
   alternatives to stimulants 224
   antisocial behaviours and attitudes 215
   assessment 213-16
   behavioural management 217-18
   cognitive management 217-18
   contraindications to stimulant
      medication 222
   diagnosis 213-14
   dietary interventions 218-19
   duration of pharmacological treatment
      225
   individual interview 215-16
   information and advice 216-17
   medication 219-25
   psychopharmacology 219-23
   stimulants in combination with other
      agents 223-4
   treatment 216-18

hypothalamic–pituitary–adrenal (HPA)
   system 113, 118
hypothalamic–pituitary–gonadal axis
   118
hypothalamic–pituitary–thyroid (HPT) axis
   40, 47

imipramine
   in alcoholism with comorbid psychiatric
      disorder 172
   in panic disorder 79, 82-4
   in stimulant abuse 164
   in unipolar depression 64
immune system in chronic fatigue
   syndrome (CFS) 138
immunoglobulins in chronic fatigue
   syndrome (CFS) 146
inositol in panic disorder 85
isocarboxazid in unipolar depression 61

Kluver-Bucy syndrome 186

LAAM 161
laevo-alpha-acetylmethadol (LAAM) 161
lamotrigine in bipolar disorder 49
late-life paraphrenia 195
late-life psychosis 194-5
late-life schizophrenia 195
levodopa in tardive dyskinesia (TD) 27
levomepromazine in emergency
   medication 207
lithium
   in aggressive behaviour 208
   in bipolar disorder 41-3, 45, 47, 49
   in manic-depressive illness 37, 38, 49,
      50
   in obsessive–compulsive disorder
      (OCD) 102
   in refractory schizophrenia 12-13
   in unipolar depression 61, 61-4
   in violent behaviour 209
   interference with thyroid axis 40
   modalities and consequences of
      discontinuation 50-1
lorazepam
   in bipolar disorder 48
   in emergency medication 207
   in manic-depressive illness 50
   in violent behaviour 208
luteinizing hormone (LH) 118

magnesium in chronic fatigue syndrome
   (CFS) 146
magnetic resonance imaging (MRI) 7,
   117, 139, 201
manic-depressive illness 37-56
   amitriptyline in 49
   benzodiazepines in 50
   carbamazepine in 37, 38, 50
   citalopram in 49

electroconvulsive therapy (ECT) in 50
epidemiology and course 37–8
fluoxetine in 49
fluvoxamine in 49
frequency and characteristics of rapid
cycling 38–41
haloperidol in 50
lithium in 37, 38, 49, 50
lorazepam in 50
optimization of prophylaxis 45
paroxetine in 49
pathophysiology 38
sertraline in 49
treatment of depressive breakthrough
episodes 49–50
treatment of manic breakthrough
episodes 50
valproate in 37, 38, 50
see also bipolar disorder
MAOIs
in depression in old age 183–4
in hyperactive child 223, 224
in panic disorder 84, 91
in treatment-resistant depression 61
in unipolar depression 61, 66, 67
maprotiline in panic disorder 81
medication event monitoring system
(MEMS) 234–5
melperone in sleep disturbance in
dementia 192
methadone maintenance 157–61
drugs contraindicated 159
drugs which may increase plasma
levels 160
drugs which may lower plasma levels
159
drugs whose pharmacokinetics may be
altered by 160
3-methoxy-4-hydroxyphenylglycol (MHPG)
186
methylphenidate in hyperactive child 220,
224
mianserin in depression in old age 183–4
microsomal ethanol oxidising system
(MEOS) 161
Mini-Mental State Examination (MMSE) 190
mirtazapine in depression in old age 184
moclobemide
in anxiety in dementia 190
in depression in dementia 188
in depression in old age 184
in hyperactive child 224
monoamine oxidase inhibitors, see MAOIs
mood stabilizers 46–9, 67–8, 173
adjunctive and new drugs 47
alternatives 47
choice of second drug 47

morphine sulphate in substance abuse
162

muscle dysfunction in chronic fatigue
syndrome (CFS) 137
myalgic encephalomyelitis (ME) 135

nalmefene in alcoholism 165, 167–9
naltrexone
in alcoholism 165, 167–9, 173
in opioid-dependent patients 162–3
NBRS (Neurobehavioral Rating Scale) 187
nefazodone in panic disorder 85
neuroimaging in chronic fatigue syndrome
(CFS) 139
neuroleptics
in bipolar disorder 48
in elderly patients 191
in emergency medication 207
in violent behaviour 208
neurosurgery in obsessive–compulsive
disorder (OCD) 105
nifedipine in tardive dyskinesia (TD) 26
NMDA (N-methyl-D-aspartate) antagonists
165–7
noncompliance, see
compliance/noncompliance
NPI (Neuropsychiatric Inventory) 187
N-substituted amphetamines 164

obsessive–compulsive disorder (OCD)
97–108
aminoglutethimide in 102
behavioural psychotherapy in 103–5
buspirone in 102
clomipramine in 102, 103
clonazepam in 102
comorbid diagnoses 99
comorbid psychopathology 100
complicating diagnoses 99–100
cyproterone acetate in 102
diagnostic difficulties 97–9
hospitalization 104
in children 98
in pregnancy 101
lithium in 102
neurosurgery in 105
pathogenesis 100–1
phenelzine in 103
pindolol in 102
SSRIs in 100–3
tramadol in 102
treatment-refractory 101–5
venlafaxine in 103
olanzapine
in late-life psychosis 195
in refractory schizophrenia 6, 10–11
in tardive dyskinesia (TD) 24, 29
old age
behavioural disturbances in 181–98
suicides in 183
ondansetron in panic disorder 85
opiate antagonists in alcoholism 165

opioid agonists 157–62
opioid antagonists 162–3
  in alcoholism 167–9
opioid dependence 155–7
  pharmacological treatment 157
  possible pharmacological agents 157
opioid detoxification 158
oxazepam in sleep disturbance in
  dementia 192
oxypertine in tardive dyskinesia (TD) 27

panic disorder 77–96
  alprazolam in 82–4
  alternative drug treatments 84–5
  baclofen in 85
  behavioural strategies 86–7
  benzodiazepines (BZDs) in 79, 81, 82,
    84, 88–91
  brofaromine in 81
  buspirone in 84–5
  carbamazepine in 85
  citalopram in 81
  clinical problems 77
  clomipramine in 81, 83–4
  cognitive-behavioural therapy (CBT) in
    85–9
  comparison of drugs with psychological
    treatments 88
  diagnostic criteria 78
  diazepam in 88
  differential diagnosis 79
  drug treatment 80
  duration of treatment 83–4
  efficacy of combined treatments 89
  fluvoxamine in 81, 83
  imipramine in 79, 82–4
  inositol in 85
  long-term pharmacotherapy 83–4
  main features 77–9
  management of difficult patients 89–91
  MAOIs in 84, 91
  maprotiline in 81
  nefazodone in 85
  ondansetron in 85
  paroxetine in 81, 83–4
  pharmacotherapy 79–81
  phenelzine in 84
  prevalence 77, 78
  propranolol in 85
  psychosocial treatments 88
  psychotherapy 85–6
  sertraline in 81, 83
  severity 79
  short-term management of drug therapy
    81–3
  SSRIs in 79–82, 84, 88, 89, 91
  TCAs in 79, 82–4, 91
  tranylcypromine in 84
  valproate in 85
  verapamil in 85

paranoid syndromes in the elderly 194–5
paroxetine
  in depression in old age 184
  in manic-depressive illness 49
  in panic disorder 81, 83–4
partial complex seizure 199
PAS (Pittsburgh Agitation Scale) 187
phenelzine
  in obsessive–compulsive disorder
    (OCD) 103
  in panic disorder 84
  in unipolar depression 66
pindolol
  in obsessive–compulsive disorder
    (OCD) 102
  in unipolar depression 61, 67
pipamperone in sleep disturbance in
  dementia 192
Positive and Negative Symptom Scale
  (PANSS) 12
pregnancy, obsessive–compulsive
  disorder (OCD) in 101
propranolol
  in panic disorder 85
  in tardive dyskinesia (TD) 27
psychiatric disorders 79
  in violent behaviour 201
psychosocial treatments in panic disorder
  88
psychostimulant abuse 156
psychosurgery in treatment-resistant
  depression 68

quetiapine in late-life psychosis 195

rapid cycling disease (RCD) 38–41
  female gender 39
  risk factors 38–41
  thyroid dysfunction in 40
  tricyclic antidepressants (TCAs) in 38–9
refractory schizophrenia 3–22
  anticonvulsants in 13
  atypical neuroleptics 8–11, 13, 15
  benzodiazepines in 13
  carbamazepine in 13
  chlorpromazine in 4, 6, 15
  clozapine in 6–10, 12, 15, 16
  definition 3–6
  electroconvulsive treatment (ECT) in 13
  haloperidol in 4, 15
  lithium in 12–13
  noncompliance 7
  olanzapine in 6, 10–11
  pharmacological treatment 7–16
  resistance to neuroleptic treatment 15
  risperidone in 3, 6, 10, 12
  sertindole in 6
  treatment recommendations 13–16
  treatment resistance
    criteria 4–7

degrees 5
  factors associated with 7
  prevalence of 6–7
  treatment strategy 14
  typical neuroleptics 7–8, 16
  valproic acid in 13
  zotepine in 11, 12
relaxation technique 86–7
reserpine in tardive dyskinesia (TD) 26–7
risperidone
  in dementia 191
  in hyperactive child 224
  in late-life psychosis 195
  in refractory schizophrenia 3, 6, 10, 12
  in tardive dyskinesia (TD) 24, 28–9

schizophrenia
  late-life 195
  see also refractory schizophrenia
selective serotonin reuptake inhibitors, see
    SSRIs
selegiline in tardive dyskinesia (TD) 26
serotonergic drugs in alcoholism with
    comorbid psychiatric disorder 170,
    171
serotonin–dopamine antagonists (SDAs)
    30, 31
  in tardive dyskinesia (TD) 28–9
serotonin–dopamine receptor antagonists
    24
sertindole
  in late-life psychosis 195
  in refractory schizophrenia 6
sertraline
  in depression in old age 184
  in manic-depressive illness 49
  in panic disorder 81, 83
sex hormones in unipolar depression 68
sexual disinhibition in dementia 193
single photon emission computerized
    tomography (SPECT) 117, 139
sleep disturbances in dementia 192–3
SSRIs
  in aggressive behaviour 209
  in alcoholism 165
    with comorbid psychiatric disorder
      170
  in anxiety in dementia 190
  in cocaine use disorders 164
  in depression 49, 60
    in dementia 188
    in old age 183–4
  in hyperactive child 224
  in obsessive–compulsive disorder
    (OCD) 100–3
  in panic disorder 79–82, 84, 88, 89, 91
  in rapid cycling disease 39
  in stimulant abuse 164
  in unipolar depression 61, 64, 66
stimulant abuse 164

substance abuse 155–79
  buprenorphine in 162
  comorbid psychiatric disorder 155
  morphine sulphate in 162
  prevalence 156
suicides in old age 183
Sydenham's chorea 98

tardive dyskinesia (TD) 23–35, 48
  alpha-methyldopa in 27
  apomorphine in 27
  botulinum toxin (BTX-a) in 26
  bromocriptine in 27
  calcium channel blockers in 26
  cholinomimetic drugs in 28
  clozapine in 28
  diagnostic criteria 23
  disabling 29–30
  discontinuing antipsychotics 25
  dopamine agonists in 27
  dopamine receptor antagonist in 24
  educating patients and families 24–5
  haloperidol in 29
  levodopa in 27
  management strategy 24–5, 29–31
  nifedipine in 26
  olanzapine in 24, 29
  overview 23–4
  oxypertine in 27
  propranolol in 27
  relatively mild 30–1
  reserpine in 26–7
  risk factors 24
  risperidone in 24, 28–9
  selegiline in 26
  serotonin–dopamine antagonists in
    28–9
  tetrabenazine in 26–7
  treatment strategies of mild to severe
    24–5
  vitamin E in 25–6, 30, 31
TCAs
  in alcoholism with comorbid psychiatric
    disorder 171–2
  in cocaine use disorders 164
  in depression 49
    in old age 183–4
  in panic disorder 79, 82–4, 91
  in rapid cycling disease 38–9
  in unipolar depression 58, 60, 61, 64–7
temporal–frontal abnormalities 201
temporal lobe epilepsy 199
tetrabenazine in tardive dyskinesia (TD)
    26–7
thioridazine in dementia 191
thyroid axis, lithium interference with 40
thyroid dysfunction in RCD 40
thyroid hormone augmentation 47–8
  in unipolar depression 64–6
thyroid-stimulating hormone (TSH) in

unipolar depression 66
thyrotropin-releasing hormone in unipolar
    depression 66
thyroxine in bipolar disorder 45
tiapride in alcoholism 170
Tourette's disorder 99
Tourette's syndrome 101
tramadol in obsessive–compulsive
    disorder (OCD) 102
tranylcypromine
    in panic disorder 84
    in unipolar depression 61
Treatment Outcome Prospective Study
    156–7
trichotillomania 99
tricyclic antidepressants, see TCAs
tri-iodothyronine in treatment-resistant
    unipolar depression 65
tryptophan in unipolar depression 68

unexplained bright objects (UBOs) 139
unipolar depression
    antidepressants in 60
    augmentation strategies 67–8
    buspirone in 68
    carbamazepine in 68
    combined antidepressant drugs 66–7
    ECT in 67, 68
    efficacy of antidepressants used
        following treatment failure 60
    electroconvulsive therapy (ECT) in 57
    fluoxetine in 66
    imipramine in 64
    isocarboxazid in 61
    lithium in 61
    MAOIs in 61, 66, 67
    pindolol in 61, 67
    prognosis 57
    psychosurgery 68
    sex hormones in 68
    SSRIs in 61, 64, 66
    staging of depression based on past
        treatment responses 59
    TCAs in 58, 60, 61, 64–7
    thyroid hormone augmentation in 64–6
    tranylcypromine in 61
    treatment-resistant 57–75
        definitions 57–8
        lithium augmentation 61–4
        relapse and recurrence 59
        strategies 60–1

tri-iodothyronine in 65
tri-iodothyronine in 65
tryptophan in 68
valproate in 68

valproate
    in alcoholism 173
    in bipolar disorder 43, 47
    in manic-depressive illness 37, 38, 50
    in panic disorder 85
    in unipolar depression 68
valproic acid in refractory schizophrenia
    13
venlafaxine
    in depression in old age 184
    in obsessive compulsive disorder
        (OCD) 103
verapamil in panic disorder 85
violent behaviour 199–211
    aetiology 199–201
    and genetic defects 201
    assessment 203
    clinical situations 202
    diagnostic procedures 204
    emergency medication 206–7
    evaluation of patients 202–3
    factors contributing to 200
    guidelines for intervention in emergency
        situation 203
    long-term treatment 207–9
    psychiatric disorders in 201
    restraint and seclusion 204–6
    socioeconomic factors 201
viqualine in alcoholism with comorbid
    psychiatric disorder 170
viral infection in chronic fatigue syndrome
    (CFS) 137
vitamin E in tardive dyskinesia (TD) 25–6,
    30, 31

wandering in dementia 192

zimeldine in alcoholism with comorbid
    psychiatric disorder 170
zolpidem in sleep disturbance in dementia
    193
zopiclone in sleep disturbance in
    dementia 193
zotepine in refractory schizophrenia 11, 12
zuclopenthixol in emergency medication
    207